Prenatal Care

Editor

SHARON T. PHELAN

OBSTETRICS AND GYNECOLOGY CLINICS OF NORTH AMERICA

www.obgyn.theclinics.com

Consulting Editor
WILLIAM F. RAYBURN

September 2023 • Volume 50 • Number 3

ELSEVIER

1600 John F. Kennedy Boulevard • Suite 1800 • Philadelphia, Pennsylvania, 19103-2899

http://www.theclinics.com

OBSTETRICS AND GYNECOLOGY CLINICS OF NORTH AMERICA Volume 50 Number 3
September 2023 ISSN 0889-8545, ISBN-13: 978-0-443-12953-7

Editor: Kerry Holland
Developmental Editor: Hannah Almira Lopez

Obstetrics and Gynecology Clinics (ISSN 0889-8545) is published quarterly by Elsevier Inc., 360 Park Avenue South, New York, NY 10010-1710. Months of issue are March, June, September, and December. Periodicals postage paid at New York, NY, and additional mailing offices. Subscription price per year is $355.00 (US individuals), $757.00 (US institutions), $100.00 (US students), $428.00 (Canadian individuals), $956.00 (Canadian institutions), $100.00 (Canadian students), $487.00 (international individuals), $956.00 (international institutions), and $225.00 (international students). To receive student/resident rate, orders must be accompanied by name of affiliated institution, date of term, and the signature of program/residency coordinator on institution letterhead. Orders will be billed at individual rate until proof of status is received. Foreign air speed delivery is included in all *Clinics* subscription prices. All prices are subject to change without notice. POSTMASTER: Send address changes to *Obstetrics and Gynecology Clinics*, Elsevier Health Sciences Division, Subscription Customer Service, 3251 Riverport Lane, Maryland Heights, MO 63043. **Customer Service: Telephone: 1-800-654-2452 (U.S. and Canada); 314-447-8871 (outside U.S. and Canada). Fax: 314-447-8029. E-mail: journalscustomerservice-usa@elsevier.com (for print support); journalsonlinesupport-usa@elsevier. com (for online support).**

Reprints. For copies of 100 or more of articles in this publication, please contact the Commercial Reprints Department, Elsevier Inc., 360 Park Avenue South, New York, New York 10010-1710. Tel.: 212-633-3874; Fax: 212-633-3820; E-mail: reprints@elsevier.com.

Obstetrics and Gynecology Clinics of North America is also published in Spanish by McGraw-Hill Interamericana Editores S.A., P.O. Box 5-237, 06500, Mexico; in Portuguese by Reichmann and Affonso Editores, Rio de Janeiro, Brazil; and in Greek by Paschalidis Medical Publications, Athens, Greece.

Obstetrics and Gynecology Clinics of North America is covered in MEDLINE/PubMed (Index Medicus), Excerpta Medica, Current Concepts/Clinical Medicine, Science Citation Index, BIOSIS, CINAHL, and ISI/BIOMED.

Contributors

CONSULTING EDITOR

WILLIAM F. RAYBURN, MD, MBA
Affiliate Professor, Department of Obstetrics and Gynecology and College of Graduate Studies, Medical University of South Carolina, Charleston, South Carolina; Emeritus Distinguished Professor, Department of Obstetrics and Gynecology University of New Mexico School of Medicine Albuquerque, New Mexico

EDITOR

SHARON T. PHELAN, MD, FACOG
Professor Emeritus, Department of Obstetrics and Gynecology, University of New Mexico Health Science Center, Albuquerque, New Mexico, USA

AUTHORS

BRENNA BANWARTH-KUHN, BS
Medical student, University of New Mexico School of Medicine, Albuquerque, New Mexico, USA

MARGARITA BERWICK, MD
Department of Obstetrics and Gynecology, University of Florida College of Medicine, University of Florida, Gainesville, Florida, USA

JENNIFER N. CRAWFORD, PhD
Departments of Psychiatry and Behavioral Sciences, and Obstetrics and Gynecology, University of New Mexico, Albuquerque, New Mexico, USA

TAYLOR M. DUNN, MS, CGC
Department of Genetics, University of Alabama at Birmingham, Birmingham, Alabama, USA

TAMARA J. GARDNER, MSN, CNM, PMHNP-BC
Perinatal Associates of New Mexico, Albuquerque, New Mexico, USA

SARAH JEAN HANSON, MD
Division of Global and Community Health, Department of Obstetrics and Gynecology, Beth Israel Deaconess Medical Center, Instructor of Medicine, Harvard Medical School, Boston, Massachusetts, USA; Department of Obstetrics and Gynaecology, Princess Marina Hospital, Lecturer of Medicine, University of Botswana, Gaborone, Botswana

NINA E. HIGGINS, MD
Reproductive Psychiatry Fellowship Director, Departments of Psychiatry and Behavioral Sciences, and Obstetrics and Gynecology, University of New Mexico, Albuquerque, New Mexico, USA

LISA G. HOFLER, MD, MPH, MBA
Department of Obstetrics and Gynecology, University of New Mexico School of Medicine, Albuquerque, New Mexico, USA

RESHMA KHAN, MD
Shifa Free Clinic, Medical University of South Carolina, Charleston, South Carolina, USA

TEKOA KING, CNM, MPH
University of California, San Francisco, School of Nursing, San Francisco, California, USA

JAMIE W. KRASHIN, MD, MSCR
Assistant Professor, Department of Obstetrics and Gynecology, University of New Mexico Health Sciences Center, Albuquerque, New Mexico, USA

THERESA KURTZ, MD
Department of Obstetrics and Gynecology, University of Utah Health, Salt Lake City, Utah, USA

KATHERINE LEE, MD
Harbor–UCLA Medical Center, University of California Los Angeles, Torrance, California, USA

ADETOLA F. LOUIS-JACQUES, MD
Department of Obstetrics and Gynecology, University of Florida College of Medicine, University of Florida, Gainesville, Florida, USA

BRENNA McGUIRE, MD
Department of Obstetrics and Gynecology, University of New Mexico Hospital, UNM Obstetrics and Gynecology, Albuquerque, New Mexico, USA

MIRIAM McQUADE, MD
Complex Family Planning Fellow, University of New Mexico Health Sciences Center, Albuquerque, New Mexico, USA

DAWN PALASZEWSKI, MD
Associate Professor of Obstetrics and Gynecology, University of South Florida Morsani College of Medicine, Tampa, Florida, USA

ALEX F. PEAHL, MD, MSc
Department of Obstetrics and Gynecology, University of Michigan, Institute for Healthcare Policy and Innovation, Ann Arbor, Michigan, USA

SHARON T. PHELAN, MD, FACOG
Professor Emeritus, Department of Obstetrics and Gynecology, University of New Mexico Health Science Center, Albuquerque, New Mexico, USA

WILLIAM RAYBURN, MD, MBA
Affiliate Professor, Department of Obstetrics and Gynecology and College of Graduate Studies, Medical University of South Carolina, Charleston, South Carolina; Emeritus Distinguished Professor, Department of Obstetrics and Gynecology, University of New Mexico School of Medicine, Albuquerque, New Mexico

MARQUETTE J. ROSE, MD
Department of Psychiatry and Behavioral Sciences, University of New Mexico, Albuquerque, New Mexico, USA

MARIAM SAVABI, MD, MPH
General Obstetrician and Gynecologist, HealthCare Anti-Oppression Institute (Founder), Tacoma, Washington, USA

MARCELA C. SMID, MD, MS
Department of Obstetrics and Gynecology, University of Utah Health, Salt Lake City, Utah, USA

SINDHU SRINIVAS, MD, MSCE
Department of Obstetrics and Gynecology, University of Pennsylvania Perelman School of Medicine, Philadelphia, Pennsylvania, USA

AKILA SUBRAMANIAM, MD, MPH
Division of Maternal Fetal Medicine, Department of Obstetrics and Gynecology, University of Alabama at Birmingham, Birmingham, Alabama, USA

BEATRIZ TENORIO, MD, Capt, USAF, MC
Resident Physician, Department of Gynecologic Surgery and Obstetrics, Navy Medicine Readiness and Training Command Portsmouth, Portsmouth, Virginia, USA

LAUREN THAXTON, MD, MBA, MS
Department of Women's Health, Dell Medical School, University of Texas, Austin, Texas, USA

MARK TURRENTINE, MD
Department of Obstetrics and Gynecology, Baylor College of Medicine, Houston, Texas, USA

JULIE R. WHITTINGTON, MD, LCDR, MC, USN
Assistant Professor, Attending in Maternal-Fetal Medicine, Department of Gynecologic Surgery and Obstetrics, Navy Medicine Readiness and Training Command Portsmouth, Portsmouth, Virginia, USA

CHRISTOPHER M. ZAHN, MD
American College of Obstetricians and Gynecologists, Washington, DC, USA

Contents

> The one-size-fits-all model of prenatal care has remained largely un-
> changed since 1930. New models of prenatal care delivery can improve
> its efficacy, equity, and experience through tailoring prenatal care to
> meet pregnant people's medical and social needs. Key aspects of recently
> developed prenatal care models include visit schedules based on needed
> services, telemedicine, home measurement of routine pregnancy parame-
> ters, and interventions that address social and structural drivers of health.
> Several barriers that affect the individual, provider, health system, and pol-
> icy levels must be addressed to facilitate implementation of new prenatal
> care delivery models.

> Group prenatal care (GPC) is a novel model of health care delivery for preg-
> nant patients. In GPC, a small group of patients of similar gestational age
> meet at scheduled intervals for both medical care and facilitated educa-
> tional discussions. This care model encourages better communication
> and engages patients and providers in a supportive community. There is
> evidence that GPC leads to improved patient and provider satisfaction,
> health equity, and maternal and neonatal outcomes. Delivery of prenatal
> care in a group setting is a significant change from the traditional model
> and takes willingness, planning, and commitment for implementation
> and continued success.

> Conditions that often present with vaginal bleeding before 20 weeks are
> common and can cause morbidity and mortality. Clinically stable patients
> can choose their management options. Clinically unstable patients require
> urgent procedural management: uterine aspiration, dilation and evacua-
> tion, or surgical removal of an ectopic pregnancy. Septic abortion requires
> prompt procedural management, intravenous antibiotics, and intravenous
> fluids. Available data on prognosis with expectant management of pre-via-
> ble rupture of membranes in the United States are poor for mothers and
> fetuses.

The number of prenatal genetic screening options, including aneuploidy screening and carrier screening, has drastically increased with rapid advancements in DNA sequencing technologies. Noninvasive prenatal screening analyzing cell-free DNA has quickly been integrated into routine prenatal care as it is the most sensitive and specific screening method for pregnancies at increased and average risk of fetal aneuploidy. The aim of this article is to outline current recommendations for cell-free DNA screening and carrier screening, important aspects of pretest and posttest counseling for obstetric providers, and which patients should be referred to a genetic specialist.

Pregnancy care should include open discussions with patients about their ideal family size and pregnancy spacing. With these patient-voiced goals in mind, clinicians should review contraceptive tools to meet these goals, including special considerations after birth. For patients that desire contraception, it is important to prioritize the provision of their chosen method as soon as safely possible and desired after birth.

Modifications of prenatal care will be needed in expected weight gain, nutritional recommendations, screening tests, thromboprophylaxis, ultrasound, antenatal testing, and timing and mode of delivery.

Patients experience many new and concerning symptoms during pregnancy and it is the role of the obstetric clinician to provide appropriate guidance, recommendations, and treatment options. Often times, these symptoms are related to hormonal and physiologic changes that occur and will resolve in the postpartum period. However, clinicians must be able to recognize more concerning pathologic symptoms that require further evaluation and treatment. This review provides updates on the evaluation and management of some of the common symptoms during pregnancy.

Breastfeeding is the gold standard of infant nutrition and current guidelines suggest exclusive breastfeeding for 6 months, with continued breastfeeding through 24 months or beyond. Obstetric care professionals can encourage and educate their patients about breastfeeding through the prenatal period when many expectant parents make decisions about their infant feeding choices. Education and support should extend through the postpartum period and include parents who may have concerns surrounding medical comorbidities, breast augmentation, or substance use disorders.

these requires an effective screening process during prenatal care. The challenges include selection of an appropriate tool for use in pregnancy; incorporating the tool into the clinical flow to ensure screening of all pregnant patients; and developing an approach to address the issues, be it providing emotional support, management within the clinic, or referring to outside resources.

The challenges of providing prenatal care for undocumented immigrants require patience. Pregnant undocumented immigrant women should receive routine prenatal care tailored to their specific needs, with an emphasis on basic needs (eg, housing, safety, food, transportation to appointment). Financial, cultural, and language barriers can impede undocumented immigrants from receiving adequate or optimal prenatal care. Adverse maternal and fetal outcomes may be more common but have not been well-quantified and cannot be compared with outcomes if care had been provided in their country of origin. An example of a community-funded clinic is described in minimizing cost and optimizing outcomes.

OBSTETRICS AND GYNECOLOGY CLINICS

SERIES OF RELATED INTEREST

Clinics in Perinatology
www.perinatology.theclinics.com
Pediatric Clinics of North America
https://www.pediatrics.theclinics.com

THE CLINICS ARE AVAILABLE ONLINE!
Access your subscription at:
www.theclinics.com

Foreword

Prenatal Care: New Perspectives About an Often Used Health Service

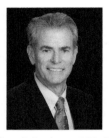

William F. Rayburn, MD, MBA
Consulting Editor

Formal prenatal care began nearly a century ago and has remained one of the most often used health services. Women in the United States who eventually deliver with no prenatal care are rare. However, 10% of African American and 7.7 % of Hispanic women have higher rates of inadequate or no prenatal care. This issue of *Obstetrics and Gynecology Clinics of North America* pertains to the essential need of obstetricians and their coclinicians to reexamine their practices of prenatal care. Originally published in 2008, the issue has been updated and reedited by Sharon T. Phelan, MD, a leading obstetrician who has dedicated her career to optimal, evidence-based delivery of prenatal care.

Throughout this issue, the reader is reminded that prenatal care is about risk assessment, health promotion and education, and therapeutic intervention. Ideally, a comprehensive prenatal service begins before pregnancy and extends into the postpartum and interpregnancy periods. Prenatal care involves a coordination of medical care, continuous risk assessment, and psychosocial support. Otherwise, declining care is associated with an increase in stillbirth, neonatal deaths, maternal deaths, preterm births, and special care nursery admissions. While commonly viewed as a series of office visits, prenatal care is opening access or improving efficiency with group care and use of telehealth with phone or video conferencing.

The goals are birth of a healthy infant and minimizing maternal risk. Optimal prenatal care can prevent or lead to timely recognition and treatment of maternal and fetal complications as described in this issue. Components of quality prenatal care include early and accurate gestational dating, identifying pregnancies at increased risk, anticipation of problems with intervention to prevent or minimize morbidity, health promotion, and prenatal counseling (ie, nutrition, contraception, breastfeeding). This is accomplished

Obstet Gynecol Clin N Am 50 (2023) xiii–xiv
https://doi.org/10.1016/j.ogc.2023.04.001
0889-8545/23/© 2023 Published by Elsevier Inc.

obgyn.theclinics.com

using shared decision making. Recognizing the impact of social determinants of health has gained much attention and is well-covered by two articles in this issue. A newer challenge, advocating for undocumented pregnant immigrants, is also described.

Prenatal care is comprehensive, including timing of initiation of care, number and spacing of visits, type and quality of care, clinician type/training, setting for providing care, ancillary services, and prenatal care systems. The effectiveness of many of these components alone or in combination has generally been evaluated in randomized trials. Data as to what constitutes the optimal number and frequency of prenatal visits, and the optimal content of those visits are limited. Pregnant patients should be counseled about signs and symptoms that should be reported because of potential serious maternal or fetal consequences (eg, vaginal bleeding, leakage of fluid per vagina, decreased fetal activity, preterm contractions, preeclampsia, substance use).

Ongoing assessments during prenatal care include blood pressures measurements, weight gain, fetal heart rate changes, signs and symptoms of potential problems, and events before a visit such as recent travel, illness, stressors, and exposure to infection. Risk assessments are often dependent on the gestational age from early to late in gestation and include screening for depression and anxiety; substance use; medical challenges of morbid obesity; neural tube defects and other congenital anomalies; genetic assessment for trisomy 21 and other aneuploidies and carrier status; short cervical length; diabetes, anemia, red blood cell antibody; fetal growth; fetal presentation; sexually transmitted infections; rectovaginal group B beta-hemolytic streptococcus colonization; and preparation for labor, birth, and postpartum.

I appreciate the efforts of Dr Phelan and her team of experienced obstetricians for their timely and thoughtful recommendations on many relevant topics. Multiple evidence-based options are provided, and expert-based pearls add depth to these discussions. Regardless of whether the patient's care is provided by the same clinician, it is important to clearly identify and follow up with the appropriate team-based care during this rewarding period in caring for the expectant mother and her unborn baby.

William F. Rayburn, MD, MBA
Department of Obstetrics and Gynecology
Medical University of South Carolina
1721 Atlantic Avenue
Sullivan's Island, SC 29482, USA

E-mail address:
wrayburnmd@gmail.com

Preface

Advances and Changes in the Components of Prenatal Care

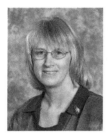

Sharon T. Phelan, MD, FACOG
Editor

Over the past couple of decades, there is more appreciation of the limitations and challenges of the "traditional" components of prenatal care. New testing activities, both laboratory and imaging, were tacked on to the original prenatal care schedule that was developed before 1950. Few researchers attempted a critical review of the logistics and content of prenatal care.

Over the past few years, several developments and events have seriously challenged this traditional approach to prenatal care. The inclusion of recently developed genetic testing requires a more in-depth understanding and counseling regarding interpretation of results for both provider and patient. The second major development was the need to alter the number and content of prenatal visits. Despite that for a number of years many women found the traditional 14+ prenatal visits cumbersome and problematic due to employment, childcare, and transportation, a reduction in visits was not research or promoted. With the COVID-19 pandemic, practices had to quickly seek ways to safely decrease the number of visits and make them more efficient. The result was a critical review of the timing and content of prenatal visits. This approach was supplemented as needed by virtual visit with phone or video conferencing.

Research is determining that fewer well-timed visits provide comparable outcomes, are accepted by patients, and improve efficiency overall relative to prenatal care. Finally, the focus on maternal mortality by the Centers for Disease Control and Prevention has identified numerous contributing causes to the country's increasingly continually high rates of pregnancy-related deaths (with 20% occurring prior to delivery) despite the increased use of technology and frequent prenatal care and screening.

The impact of social determinants, including behavioral activities, economics, race, geographic location, access to care, employment, and education (both providers, patients, and patient's families), on pregnancy outcomes is better understood now. There

Obstet Gynecol Clin N Am 50 (2023) xv–xvi
https://doi.org/10.1016/j.ogc.2023.03.001
0889-8545/23/© 2023 Elsevier Inc. All rights reserved.

is acknowledgment that obstetric providers need to expand the scope of their care to not only incorporate the new technology but also acknowledge these social determinants of health. The articles that follow address these new developments to help the reader understand the need for changes in our concept of traditional prenatal care "standards."

Sharon T. Phelan, MD, FACOG
Department of Obstetrics and Gynecology
University of New Mexico Health Science Center
Albuquerque, NM 87106, USA

601 Park Lake Circle
Helena, AL 35080, USA

E-mail address:
stphelan@salud.unm.edu

Routine Prenatal Care

Alex F. Peahl, MD, MSc[a,b,*], Mark Turrentine, MD[c],
Sindhu Srinivas, MD, MSCE[d], Tekoa King, CNM, MPH[e], Christopher M. Zahn, MD[f]

KEYWORDS

- Prenatal care • Telemedicine • Social determinants of health
- Social drivers of health • Blood pressure monitoring • Prenatal visits • Antenatal care

KEY POINTS

- The traditional, one-size-fits-all, medical model of prenatal care fails to address the comprehensive needs and preferences of pregnant people.
- New tailored models of prenatal care include alternative visit schedules, telemedicine, home monitoring, and incorporation of screening and management of social and structural drivers of health.
- Shared decision-making should guide the selection of prenatal care options when there is clinical equipoise.
- Implementation of new prenatal care models requires overcoming barriers at the individual, provider, health system, and policy levels.

INTRODUCTION

Prenatal care is one of the most common preventive services provided in the United States. Prenatal care is designed to improve the health of almost 4 million pregnant people and their infants annually.[1] During the past century, there have been revolutionary innovations in prenatal care technology, including the discovery of Rho(D) immune globulin, fetal ultrasound, home pregnancy tests, and noninvasive prenatal genetic testing.[2] Simultaneously, there has been growing recognition of the significant impact of social and structural drivers (also known as social and structural determinants) of health access to pregnancy care and health outcomes.[3] Yet, there have been relatively few changes in how prenatal care is delivered. The traditional medical model—clinically

[a] Department of Obstetrics and Gynecology, University of Michigan, 1500 East Medical Center Dr., Ann Arbor, MI 48109, USA; [b] University of Michigan Institute for Healthcare Policy and Innovation, 2800 Plymouth Road, Ann Arbor, MI 48109, USA; [c] Department of Obstetrics and Gynecology, Baylor College of Medicine, 6651 Main Street, Suite F1020, Houston, TX 77030, USA; [d] Department of Obstetrics and Gynecology, University of Pennsylvania Perelman School of Medicine, 3400 Civic Center Boulevard, Philadelphia, PA 19104, USA; [e] University of California, San Francisco School of Nursing, 2 Koret Way, San Francisco, CA 94143, USA; [f] American College of Obstetricians and Gynecologists, 409 12th Street Southwest, Washington, DC 20024, USA
* Corresponding author.
E-mail address: alexfrie@med.umich.edu

Obstet Gynecol Clin N Am 50 (2023) 439–455
https://doi.org/10.1016/j.ogc.2023.03.002

focused, in-person visits every 4 weeks until 28 weeks' gestation, every 2 weeks until 36 weeks' gestation, and weekly until childbirth—has remained unchanged since it was first published in 1930.[4]

The traditional prenatal care model has significant limitations. First, it is a one-size-fits-all schedule that does not provide specific care recommendations for pregnant people with medical or social risk factors.[5] This failure to individualize care results in too much care for medically low-risk pregnant people and the wrong kind of care for pregnant people with social risk factors. Second, the model has failed to grow with emerging technology—telemedicine is widely used across specialties and can provide more flexible, accessible care without requiring missed work, transportation, or childcare.[6] Finally, the traditional model of prenatal care was designed to detect complications of pregnancy, specifically preeclampsia.[2,7] This medical model of care fails to address the social and structural drivers of health that adversely affect perinatal outcomes.

The COVID-19 pandemic catalyzed the most rapid adoption of changes in prenatal care delivery in almost a century.[8,9] Social distancing and resource conservation led to the successful implementation of reduced visit schedules and telemedicine, opening the door to new recommendations for prenatal care delivery that have continued beyond the acute public health crisis.[8,10–15] In this article, we review recent innovations in prenatal care delivery including key definitions, evidence, and recommendations from the Plan for Appropriate Tailored Healthcare (PATH) in pregnancy panel (**Fig. 1**) to inform a new era of prenatal care designed to comprehensively address individuals' medical and social needs.

DEFINITIONS

Prenatal care spans the entire pregnancy—from identification of pregnancy to the postpartum period—and seeks to achieve 3 key goals: (1) Medical care: screening for and management of chronic conditions and pregnancy complications; (2) Anticipatory guidance: preparation for pregnancy, birth, the postpartum period, and parenting; and (3) Psychosocial support: management of the mental health and nonmedical factors that affect pregnant people's ability to access care and achieve healthy outcomes. Below, we define key considerations in prenatal care delivery as developed for the PATH panel.

PRENATAL CARE SERVICES VERSUS PRENATAL CARE DELIVERY

In considering different approaches to the provision of prenatal care, it is important to first recognize the difference between "prenatal care services" and "prenatal care

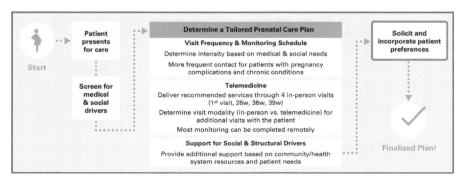

Fig. 1. Overview of the plan for appropriate tailored healthcare in pregnancy panel recommendations.

delivery." Prenatal care *services* include evidence-based services (eg, laboratory tests, vaccinations, and ultrasonography), as recommended and summarized in the American College of Obstetricians and Gynecologists (ACOG) Antepartum Record[16] (**Fig. 2**). Prenatal care *delivery* focuses on how prenatal services are administered. Delivery includes the frequency of prenatal care visits and encounters, as well as their modality or how visits are administered (eg, individual in-person encounters, group care, virtual visits). Delivery also includes the frequency and modality of assessing routine pregnancy parameters, such as blood pressure (BP) and weight. Although evidence-based assessments and interventions have been identified to some degree, they have been "squeezed into" the historical framework of prenatal care delivery, as opposed to being used to inform appropriate timing, frequency, and modality of visits. The COVID-19 experience forced a rapid change in prenatal care delivery, with many practices successfully adopting new visit schedules and telemedicine, several examples of which have been published.[8,10–15,17]

Prenatal Visit Frequency

Description

The traditional prenatal care visit schedule paradigm consists of 12 to 14 visits: an office visit every 4 weeks until 28 weeks of gestation, every 2 weeks until 36 weeks of gestation, and weekly thereafter.[18] This standardized timetable is still used, despite guidance suggesting that the frequency of obstetric visits should be individualized.[18] Alternative prenatal visit schedules for patients without comorbidities or complications in pregnancy include a total of 8 to 9 visits and include (1) visit schedules based on services, that is, timing visits around needed services throughout the pregnancy (see **Fig. 2**) and (2) less-intense visit schedules, that is, visits every 6 weeks until 28 weeks, monthly until 36 weeks, and every 2 weeks until birth.

	8w	12w	16w	20w	24w	28w	32w	36w	40w
History & Exam	• Full History & Physical							• Birth preparation	
Laboratory Testing	• Prenatal labs • Aneuploidy screen		• Aneuploidy screen		• Diabetes screen • Complete blood count • Rh antibody screen[b] • Repeat STI testing[b]			• Group B strep screen	
Imaging	• Dating ultrasound • Nuchal translucency			• Anatomy ultrasound				• Assess for fetal presentation	
Injections[a]						• Tetanus, Diphtheria, Pertussis • RhIG[b]			
Anticipatory Guidance	• Weight gain • Expected course of prenatal care • Nutrition • Toxoplasmosis • Use of medications • Sexual activity • Exercise • Dental care/referral • Avoidance of saunas/hot tubs • Seat belt use • Childbirth classes/hospital facilities • Breastfeeding			• Signs and symptoms of preterm labor • Selecting a newborn care clinician • Reproductive life planning and contraception • Postpartum care planning		• Fetal movement monitoring • Signs and symptoms of preeclampsia • Labor signs • Cervical ripening/labor induction counseling • Post-term counseling • Infant feeding • Newborn education • Family Medical Leave or disability forms • Postpartum depression • Birth preferences			
Screening for Social/Structural Drivers	• Depression/Anxiety • Substance use disorder • Intimate partner violence • Social and structural drivers of health			• Depression/Anxiety • Substance use disorder • Intimate partner violence		• Depression/Anxiety • Substance use disorder • Intimate partner violence			

Fig. 2. Prenatal services and timing as recommended by the American College of Obstetricians and Gynecologists.[a]Seasonal vaccines given as appropriate.[b]As appropriate. (*Adapted from* the ACOG Antenatal Record. American College of Obstetricians and Gynecologists. Obstetric Patient Record Forms. Available at https://www.acog.org/clinical-information/obstetric-patient-record-forms; with permission)

Evidence

Since 2015, 3 systematic reviews have evaluated the frequency and timing of prenatal care visit schedules relative to various maternal and neonatal outcomes.[17,19,20] The most recent, which included the recognized literature from the 2 previous reviews, identified 10 studies (among 13 publications) from 5 randomized controlled trials and 5 nonrandomized studies with 14,735 pregnant people.[20] All studies compared reduced prenatal care schedules (6–10 visits) with a traditional visit schedule (12–15 visits). Included studies were limited to high-income countries. The majority of included studies enrolled "low-risk" pregnant people. Data on the effects of visit frequency in pregnant people with medical and social risk factors are limited.[17] **Table 1** lists the strength of evidence for each primary outcome identified in the 3 recent systematic reviews. Comparisons of a reduced versus traditional prenatal care schedule demonstrated similar rates of all maternal and neonatal outcomes between the 2 schedule approaches. It is difficult to determine if the lack of differences in results across studies reflects the effect of different visit schedules or whether there is just insufficient evidence or sample sizes to evaluate such potential differences.

Measurement of Routine Pregnancy Parameters: Frequency

Description

Parameters routinely measured during pregnancy, including BP, fetal heart tones (FHTs), weight, and fundal height, are assessed to monitor for adverse pregnancy outcomes. Current guidance suggests that obstetric care providers should evaluate these

Table 1
Evidence profile for reduced versus traditional prenatal visit schedules

Outcome	Systematic Review Strength of Evidence		
	Dowswell et al,[19] 2015	Barrera et al,[17] 2021	AHRQ 2022[20]
Maternal quality of life	Not addressed	Insufficient	Insufficient
Maternal anxiety	Not addressed	Insufficient	Low
Maternal depression	Not addressed	Insufficient	Insufficient
Satisfaction with antenatal care	Insufficient	Insufficient	Insufficient
Lost work time	Not addressed	Not addressed	Insufficient
Completion of ACOG-recommended services	Not addressed	Not addressed	Insufficient
Unplanned visits	Insufficient	Insufficient	Insufficient
Delayed diagnoses	Not addressed	Not addressed	Insufficient
Gestational age at birth	Not addressed	Not addressed	Moderate
Preterm birth	Moderate	Low	Low
Small for gestational age	Moderate	Moderate	Moderate
Low birthweight	Low	Low	Low
Apgar score	Not addressed	Not addressed	Moderate
NICU admissions	Moderate	Not addressed	Moderate
Breastfeeding	Not addressed	Not addressed	Insufficient

Abbreviations: ACOG, American College of Obstetricians and Gynecologists; NICU, neonatal intensive care unit.

parameters at "appropriate gestational ages."[18] These parameters are typically assessed in essentially every prenatal visit; however, the optimal frequency and timing of these assessments are not known.

Evidence

Evidence for optimal monitoring of these pregnancy parameters is limited. Systematic reviews that assess the effects of reduced prenatal clinic visits can be considered a surrogate for a lower frequency of maternal and fetal assessments.[17,19,20] These studies found reduced frequency of measurements was not associated with any differences in maternal or fetal outcomes. Similar rates were noted for the diagnosis of hypertensive disorders of pregnancy, small for gestational age infants, intrauterine fetal growth restriction, and stillbirth.[20] Although this may suggest that a reduced frequency of maternal and fetal assessment in low-risk populations provides adequate surveillance, studies were underpowered to detect these adverse outcomes. Specifically, experts have questioned the value of measuring fundal height in the assessment of fetal growth, particularly when compared with the diagnostic accuracy of ultrasound and inaccuracy of fundal height in individuals with a high body mass index.[21,22] Others, however, have advocated for continued monitoring of fundal height given a lack of alternative, cost-effective screening tools.[17] Additionally, observational data suggests higher detection rates of fetal growth restriction when fundal height is more routinely measured in pregnancy.[23]

Prenatal Visits: Modality (Telemedicine)

Description

Telemedicine in obstetric care can include multiple care delivery modalities including virtual visits (one-on-one appointments between maternity care professionals and pregnant people) and remote monitoring. Several potential advantages of telemedicine in obstetrics include decreasing the burden of travel, reducing missed work or need for additional childcare, and improving access to services—particularly for people living in health care deserts.[13,15] In spite of its promise, until the COVID-19 pandemic, the use of telemedicine in obstetrics was fairly limited, with most use related to text messaging and remote monitoring in high-risk pregnancies.[13,15]

The rapid expansion of telemedicine that occurred during the COVID-19 pandemic provided opportunities for developing a better understanding of the potential advantages and greater use of telemedicine in prenatal care. For example, much of the routine prenatal education, counseling, and anticipatory guidance can be performed virtually.

Evidence

Recently, 3 systematic reviews compared prenatal care schedules for groups of people who had a hybrid schedule, including both telemedicine and in-person visits, with those who only had in-person visits to evaluate how the schedules affected various maternal and neonatal outcomes.[14,17,20] The 3 reviews identified studies using various modalities of telemedicine hybrid prenatal schedules (either audio only or audio-video) compared with the traditional all in-person visit approach.[14,17,20] Most of the identified studies compared the perception of care by the pregnant person or care provider between the 2 models. Of the 4 studies that reported maternal or fetal outcomes (1 randomized controlled trial and 3 observational trials), no discernable differences in outcomes were detected.[24–27] However, outcomes were sparsely reported across studies, and none of these studies was powered to detect differences in rare adverse events. Additionally, access to care and disparities were not directly addressed;

further research is unquestionably needed to assess the potential impact of telemedicine use on access to prenatal care and pregnancy outcomes in more diverse populations.

Measurement of Routine Pregnancy Parameters: Modality (Telemedicine)

Description

With recent expansions in technology, assessment of routine parameters including BP, FHTs, weight, and fundal height can now be self-performed outside of the clinical setting. Home measurement could remove barriers to care access and improve the pregnant person's autonomy, knowledge, and engagement in care. Further, remote monitoring, including serial assessment of routine parameters such as BP, may provide better surveillance for the development of pregnancy complications.[28] In particular, home monitoring of BP has been proven to be accurate as well as feasible.[29,30] Remote monitoring systems for parameters can be connected to the electronic medical record (EMR) via applications, streamlining data reporting, tracking, documentation, and follow-up.[31–33]

There are several important considerations when implementing remote monitoring, many of which overlap with telemedicine implementation: (1) access to appropriate (eg, cuff size) equipment that is validated for use in pregnancy; (2) patient education and training on device use (eg, arm placement, position, timing of measurements), expected and abnormal values, and when to report results to their care team; (3) staff training in recognition of abnormal values and appropriate response; (4) health system ability to document and track data so that abnormal values are reviewed and acted on; and (5) implementation of safeguards when monitoring systems are integrated into the EMR to ensure pregnant individuals have sufficient Internet connectivity.[34] Failure to address each of these considerations could result in further exacerbation of existing health system inequities. For example, although individuals may obtain devices through several avenues such as a health savings account or durable medical equipment benefit, insurance coverage widely varies, which may limit access and result in inequities in telemedicine utilization.[35,36]

Evidence

Limited studies have shown that remote monitoring of maternal BP, weight, and FHTs with home devices can be used successfully in a reduced prenatal visit schedule.[24,37] Although the primary outcome of these studies was satisfaction with prenatal care, these trials do demonstrate feasibility. Existing data on the incorporation of remote BP and FHT monitoring with a reduced visit schedule are from research conducted in tertiary academic centers with limited population demographic diversity; further research is needed to assess access to devices and applicable support in using the devices in a more diverse population.[12,24,37]

The accuracy and potential benefits of home monitoring for BP and glucose have been reported for other clinical scenarios, although concerns exist related to accuracy and validation of instruments used in home assessments.[38–43] Clinical outcomes data on the use of home, or remote, monitoring of the routine parameters assessed in pregnancy are very limited—particularly for FHT and fundal height assessments, although preliminary data related to feasibility of weight, BP, and fetal heart rate monitoring are promising.[24,31,33,44–47] Additional investigation is needed to further determine the role of home or remote monitoring of routine pregnancy parameters, and the proper balance to accurately detect complications without generating false positives.

Incorporating Social and Structural Drivers of Health into Prenatal Care Delivery

Description

Social drivers of health are the nonmedical conditions into which people are born, grow, live, work, and play. Social drivers include material conditions, psychologic conditions, social support conditions, and demographic characteristics (**Fig. 3**).[48–50] Further upstream, structural drivers of health are the social, economic, and political conditions that affect social determinants.[51,52] Together, social and structural drivers of health are the most powerful contributors to population health—more so than clinical care or health behaviors.[53,54]

The National Academy of Medicine framework for addressing social drivers of health includes 5 key areas: (1) Awareness: identifying social risks through systematic screening with a standardized tool; (2) Adjustment: modifying clinical care activities to accommodate identified social needs; (3) Assistance: linking people to resources and referrals; (4) Alignment: developing partnerships with community-based organizations

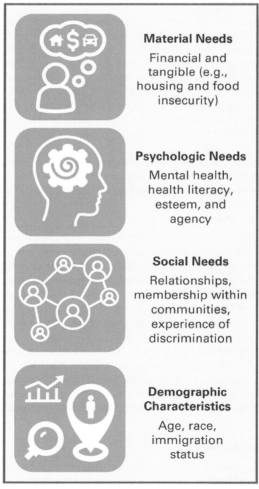

Material Needs

Financial and tangible (e.g., housing and food insecurity)

Psychologic Needs

Mental health, health literacy, esteem, and agency

Social Needs

Relationships, membership within communities, experience of discrimination

Demographic Characteristics

Age, race, immigration status

Fig. 3. Social and structural drivers of health suggested by the PATH panel.

to facilitate care; and (5) Advocacy: working at the policy level to address social needs.[55] Although areas 1 to 3 may occur largely at the individual-provider level, areas 4 and 5 require a more systems-based approach to effecting change. Evidence for effectiveness of screening for and managing social drivers of health in pregnancy is limited.[56]

Evidence

Multiple decades of work have documented the relationship between social drivers such as race (as a proxy for systemic racism and structural inequities), public insurance (as a proxy for poverty), and education on maternal outcomes. Yet multiple systematic reviews have highlighted gaps in data about other social drivers that may have significant effects on maternal and fetal outcomes independently, or as part of the causal pathway.[3,56] Further, as many social needs assessments are conducted through nonclinical programs, data on the prevalence of unmet social needs are lacking. Although there have been efforts to better document social needs in claims data, uptake has been limited, with an estimated less than 1% of people having a documented "Z code" for social needs.[3,57]

Even when a person's social needs are identified, how to best address them is not clear. Studies of social needs interventions in primary care demonstrate that less than half of people with unmet social needs accept assistance, and even fewer actually receive help.[58,59] This gap suggests that to be effective, social needs programs must address stigma, alleviate doubt that the health system can actually help, and be autonomy-supportive. The promise of innovative maternity care delivery programs such as home visiting, group prenatal care, and peer mentoring programs lies in their ability to simultaneously address medical and social drivers but evidence for many of these interventions is lacking, or if positive, it is based on studies with a small number of participants.[60–62]

In summary, although the strong relationship between social drivers of health and poor pregnancy outcomes is clear, the current prevalence of many specific needs, as well as the best ways to identify and address them, are unclear.

"Average-Risk" Versus "High-Risk"

Many factors determine an individual's level of risk, including their comorbidities, the experience of the obstetric professional, and available resources.[5] There is no widely accepted definition of a "high-risk" pregnancy. One practical definition of "average-risk" refers to individuals not requiring care from a maternal–fetal medicine subspecialist. This definition intentionally includes individuals with "common" conditions in pregnancy such as gestational diabetes, chronic hypertension, depression, and anxiety, recognizing there is geographic variation in which pregnant people are cared for by maternal–fetal medicine specialists.

"Average-risk" or "high-risk" is a blunt measure of pregnant people's needs—with careful history and evaluation, few pregnant people are truly "uncomplicated." A more individualized assessment of medical, social, and structural drivers of health, as well as available resources, is necessary to identify which pregnant people are at risk for which outcomes, and to inform the most appropriate individualized interventions.

Pregnant People's Perspectives

It is also important to consider pregnant people's perspectives and preferences in the use of telemedicine and home or remote monitoring; indeed, their perspective is paramount to consider in the shared decision-making approach to alternative prenatal care delivery. Reduced visit schedules, incorporating virtual visits and remote monitoring, have been associated with increased care satisfaction and less pregnancy-related stress.[12,14,24,31] Additionally, pregnant people may prefer having fewer in-person visits while still retaining contact with their health-care teams between visits by phone or EMR portal.[12,63] It has also been reported that a reduced visit schedule implemented during the COVID-19 pandemic actually *improved* access to prenatal care.[12] Comfort with remote monitoring tools is also an important consideration; preliminary data suggest that pregnant people are comfortable with remote monitoring, including assessment of FHTs.[63]

LIMITATIONS IN EXISTING EVIDENCE

At present, there are significant gaps in evidence to guide policy change on prenatal care delivery, including visit frequency, modality, and incorporation of social and structural drivers of health. Systematic reviews that address prenatal care delivery have noted inconsistencies in which outcomes are routinely collected and reported.[17,19,20] There is a need for consistent reporting of maternal and fetal outcomes in future clinical trials that incorporate different frequency of visits and use of telemedicine.

Core outcome sets (COS) are key tools for ensuring consistent, homogenous reporting of outcomes across studies. Use of COS can improve clinical practice via standardization of outcomes across studies, thereby making it easier to compare outcomes. Furthermore, the use of COS can reduce the risk of outcome-reporting preference.[64] Currently, no COS look at the frequency of prenatal visit schedules. A recent systematic review prioritized 15 outcomes that were deemed both important and likely to be affected by changes to routine antenatal visit schedules.[20] Results of an ongoing trial for the development of a stakeholder-informed COS on the Frequency Of pRenatal CA viSiTs (FORCAST) is an important step in determining the most critical outcomes to consider.[65]

GUIDELINES
PATH Overview

In October 2020, following the sweeping changes in prenatal care delivery that were catalyzed by the COVID-19 public health crisis, ACOG partnered with the University of Michigan to develop revised guidance on prenatal care delivery. Panel leaders were selected from leading maternity care organizations to rapidly develop rigorous guidance. Leaders selected the RAND/UCLA Appropriateness Method, a modified eDelphi approach that combines existing evidence and expert opinion.[66] Six systematic reviews were completed to support the panel. Reviews covered 3 topics: prenatal visit frequency and timing, routine pregnancy assessments, and use of telemedicine across 2 populations: pregnant people with and without medical conditions.[17] The full panel included 19 stakeholders from maternity care, public health, advocacy, and equity organizations. Two public representatives were also included in the panel. Given the urgency of developing new recommendations, the panel planned to solicit broader stakeholder input following initial recommendations, to inform final consensus guidelines in the following years.[48]

The final product of panel deliberations was the PATH in pregnancy: a nuanced, comprehensive prenatal care plan designed to address pregnant people's medical, social, and structural drivers of health, as well as their preferences (see **Fig. 1**). PATH includes 5 key aspects of care delivery, which were considered across specific chronic conditions (hypertension, diabetes), pregnancy complications (gestational hypertension, gestational diabetes), social and structural drivers (eg, housing insecurity, pregnancy-related anxiety) to serve as a template for other conditions. Each recommendation is reviewed below.

Screen for medical and social drivers of health from the beginning of pregnancy

The PATH panel recommended that all pregnant people receive comprehensive screening for medical and social drivers to identify risk factors, optimize management of preexisting conditions, and inform care planning. This screening can be conducted by any trained member of the maternity care team, in-person or virtually as determined by clinic operations, and should ideally occur between 6 and 10 weeks' gestation. If a pregnant person presents for care after this time, screening should still be completed, and the care team should ensure the person feels supported and welcomed.

For specific risk factors to be screened, the panel affirmed the medical risk factors previously identified by ACOG.[18] They developed a list of social and structural drivers of health for inclusion through iterative review, which included material needs, psychological needs, social needs, and demographic characteristics (see **Fig. 3**). The panel did not select a specific screening tool for addressing social and structural drivers of health.

Match prenatal visit frequency and monitoring of routine parameters to risk factors

The panel provided recommendations on key aspects of prenatal visit frequency and monitoring, including the timing of the first prenatal visit and ultrasound, the frequency of routine prenatal visits, and the appropriateness of monitoring routine parameters in pregnancy. The panel identified 7 to 10 weeks' gestation as the ideal timing of the first prenatal ultrasound for pregnant people with and without chronic medical conditions. They identified the ideal window for the first prenatal visit as 6 to 10 weeks' gestation for pregnant people with chronic medical conditions and 7 to 10 weeks' gestation for those without chronic medical conditions. They again emphasized that pregnant people should be welcomed whenever they present for care, even if it occurs after the ideal window.

The panel affirmed a prenatal visit schedule based on recommended services for pregnant people without chronic conditions. This visit schedule included visits every 6 weeks in the first and second trimester, every 4 weeks in the early third trimester, and every 2 weeks in the late third trimester. For pregnant people with chronic medical conditions or pregnancy complications, the panel endorsed a traditional visit schedule with visits every 4 weeks in the first and second trimester, every 2 weeks in the early third trimester, and weekly until delivery. For all conditions, the frequency of routine pregnancy assessments including measurement of BP, weight, FHTs, and fundal height matched visit frequency, aside from people with chronic hypertension, where the recommendation for monitoring BP in the second trimester was more frequent than the recommended visit frequency (**Fig. 4**).

Offer telemedicine, including home monitoring of routine parameters, for prenatal visits that do not require in-person services

The panel identified which prenatal appointments could be delivered through telemedicine based on which recommended services required in-person delivery. After clustering evidence-based in-person services including physical examinations, laboratory tests, ultrasounds, and vaccinations into the most efficient time points, they concluded that a minimum of 4 key in-person visits were needed for all pregnant people: the initial prenatal visit, and visits at 28 weeks' gestation, 36 weeks' gestation, and 39 weeks' gestation. Ultrasounds, which may be delivered by the routine maternity care professional or other providers (eg, radiology, maternal–fetal medicine

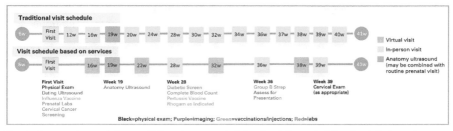

Fig. 4. Comparison of the traditional prenatal visit schedule and visit schedule based on services, with corresponding prenatal services by gestational age.

specialists), were not considered in the determination of the key in-person visits. The panel also recognized that pregnant people with additional risk factors may require additional in-person services (eg, nonstress tests, ultrasounds) and emphasized that these considerations should be used to determine visit modality.

For all other prenatal visits where in-person services were not required, the panel supported shared decision-making between pregnant people and providers to determine visit modality. The panel did not make a firm recommendation on what home devices are required for virtual visits but suggested, at minimum, a BP monitor be available. The panel agreed that most routine pregnancy assessments could be completed by pregnant people at home. Home collection of BP and weight were considered appropriate in all trimesters. Collection of FHTs was considered appropriate after the first trimester. Home collection of fundal height was seen as appropriate in the early third trimester, and possibly in the second and late third trimesters. Panelists emphasized the importance of universal access to high-quality home devices, specifically BP monitors, and adequate training on how to use them (see **Fig. 4**).

Ensure social needs are met with appropriate health system and community resources
The panel recognized the significant effect of social and structural drivers of health on care access and pregnancy outcomes. They highlighted the importance of managing social and structural drivers in routine pregnancy care, and the unique position of the maternity care professional to identify unmet social needs. In addition to screening for social needs in pregnancy, the panel recommended connection to community and health system resources where possible. They highlighted that maternity care professionals may not have the time or training to manage social needs themselves but team-based models of care and a strong referral basis could ensure pregnant people's needs were addressed.

When social needs could be met with existing resources, they concluded most pregnant people could with few exceptions receive new care models, including reduced visit schedules and telemedicine. They recommended caution when considering reduced visit schedules for people with low health literacy, pregnancy-associated anxiety, and intimate partner violence because these individuals may benefit from increased contact with the health-care system. In-person prenatal visits may be the only opportunity for people experiencing intimate partner violence to be away from their abuser. Panel recommendations were less clear when a person's social needs could not be met by existing resources. Although additional prenatal visits would be unlikely to address the underlying social needs, more visits might afford opportunities to adapt care and screen for medical consequences. The panel called for increased infrastructure to address unmet social needs.

In areas of clinical equipoise, incorporate each person's preference for determining care plans

The panel emphasized the importance of incorporating people's voices into prenatal care plans. Specifically, they suggested that in areas of clinical equipoise, such as telemedicine, shared decision-making between pregnant people and providers should guide final prenatal care plans. This was seen as an important part of ensuring equity in prenatal care delivery, particularly for people who face the greatest barriers to care.

DISCUSSION

PATH is not the first attempt to change prenatal care delivery to be more effective and efficient. A 1989 panel commissioned by the National Institutes of Health similarly attempted to make sweeping changes to prenatal care delivery for average-risk pregnant people, yet until the COVID-19 pandemic, prenatal care delivery remained largely the same as it had since 1930.[67] What then is needed to maintain the seismic shift in prenatal care delivery seen during the COVID-19 pandemic and ensure recommendations do not sit idly?

Reduced visit schedules have become the standard of care in many settings—in peer nations, as well as some health systems in the United States. The success of these models depends on supportive payment plans that recognize that the same care is being delivered—just organized more efficiently for people. Additionally, health system infrastructure must be aligned to provide high-quality education, social support, and access to providers for urgent questions and concerns in schedules with longer intervals between visits. Preparation for new models in particular is critical for ensuring pregnant people feel supported and are prepared to detect warning signs.

Continued policy support in all states, for the provision of telemedicine is also sorely needed to maintain the flexible care delivery made possible during the public health crisis. Maintenance of payment parity for telemedicine visits, coverage of high-quality home devices, and access to broadband Internet are just a few of the steps needed to make telemedicine accessible and equitable for all. On the practice and provider levels, telemedicine has become increasingly common. Maintaining the availability and quality of this convenient and accessible option requires investment in training, education, and support.

Integrating social and structural drivers of health into routine prenatal care requires investment in partnerships between community-based organizations and prenatal care clinics. Infrastructure building on the community and practice levels may require new staffing models and workforce considerations to ensure a smooth transition from screening to management. Providers must be ready to respond to people's unmet needs with understanding and empathy, even if they are not the ones providing direct resources. Team-based care used in primary care settings may be promising avenues for accomplishing these goals, incorporating diverse professionals such as social workers, nutritionists, and community health workers. Models of care such as group prenatal care that provide extensive education and peer support may also help health-care systems better address social and structural determinants of health.[62] Payment models that support these wraparound services will be critical for ensuring people's needs are met comprehensively.

Finally, the success of any prenatal care model depends on the contributions of those using it—pregnant people and the complex network who cares for them. It is critical that these end-users be intimately involved in the development and implementation of new initiatives to ensure recommendations are acceptable and desirable for those using them.

For this reason, we will be conducting a national listening tour of key stakeholders including pregnant people and advocacy groups, maternity care providers, public health representatives, policymakers, and payers. The goal of the listening tour is to understand the real-world implementation of new prenatal care recommendations in practice, including barriers and facilitators to uptake, needed implementation tools, effects on equity, and potential unintended consequences.[68] Findings from the listening tour will be added to existing evidence and expert opinion to generate new final consensus recommendations for prenatal care delivery.

SUMMARY

Prenatal care delivery is due for redesign, from an outdated one-size-fits-all model of individual in-person visits to an individualized, person-centered approach to care. Innovations that were implemented during the COVID-19 pandemic have paved the way for change, and early evidence on alternative care delivery methods including targeted visit schedules and telemedicine is nascent but promising. Social and structural drivers of health are critical drivers of maternity care access and equity, and must be integrated into current care delivery models to optimize pregnancy outcomes and experience. An ongoing national listening tour will bring diverse perspectives from pregnant people, providers, health systems, and policymakers into new formal prenatal care delivery guidance: through building a model *for* users, *with* users we hope to improve the efficacy, equity, and experience of prenatal care for all pregnant people.

CLINICS CARE POINTS

- The traditional model of prenatal care fails to comprehensively address pregnant people's medical *and* social needs.
- Social and structural drivers of health are significant contributors to maternity care access and health outcomes, and must be screened for and addressed through routine prenatal care.
- More flexible models of tailored prenatal care, including alternative visit schedules, telemedicine, home monitoring, and incorporation of social and structural drivers of health, are needed to improve prenatal care efficacy, equity, and experience.
- Forthcoming prenatal care guidelines will incorporate feedback from multiple stakeholders to ensure recommendations meet the needs of all users, particularly those from historically marginalized groups.

DISCLOSURE

Dr A.F. Peahl is a paid consultant for Maven Clinic. The remaining authors report no conflicts of interest.

REFERENCES

1. Osterman M, Hamilton B, Martin JA, et al. Births: final data for 2020. Natl Vital Stat Rep 2021;70(17):1–50.
2. Peahl AF, Howell JD. The evolution of prenatal care delivery guidelines in the United States. Am J Obstet Gynecol 2021;224(4):339–47.

3. Wang E, Glazer KB, Howell EA, et al. Social Determinants of Pregnancy-Related Mortality and Morbidity in the United States: A Systematic Review. Obstet Gynecol 2020;135(4):896–915.

4. United States Department of Labor Children's Bureau. Prenatal Care. Available at: https://www.mchlibrary.org/history/chbu/2265-1930.PDF. Accessed 8 October, 2021.

5. Peahl AF, Gourevitch RA, Luo EM, et al. Right-sizing prenatal care to meet patients' needs and improve maternity care value. Obstet Gynecol 2020;135(5): 1027–37.

6. Whittington JR, Ramseyer AM, Taylor CB. Telemedicine in Low-Risk Obstetrics. Obstet Gynecol Clin North Am 2020;47(2):241–7.

7. Alexander GR, Kotelchuck M. Assessing the role and effectiveness of prenatal care: history, challenges, and directions for future research. Public Health Rep 2001;116(4):306–16.

8. Peahl AF, Smith RD, Moniz MH. Prenatal care redesign: creating flexible maternity care models through virtual care. Am J Obstet Gynecol 2020;223(3):389 e1–e389 e10.

9. Limaye MA, Lantigua-Martinez M, Trostle ME, et al. Differential uptake of telehealth for prenatal care in a large New York City Academic Obstetrical Practice during the COVID-19 Pandemic. Am J Perinatol 2021;38(3):304–6.

10. Aziz A, Zork N, Aubey JJ, et al. Telehealth for high-risk pregnancies in the setting of the COVID-19 pandemic. Am J Perinatol 2020;37(8):800–8.

11. Fryer K, Delgado A, Foti T, et al. Implementation of Obstetric Telehealth During COVID-19 and Beyond. Matern Child Health J 2020;24(9):1104–10.

12. Peahl AF, Powell A, Berlin H, et al. Patient and provider perspectives of a new prenatal care model introduced in response to the coronavirus disease 2019 pandemic. Am J Obstet Gynecol 2021;224(4):384 e1–e384 e11.

13. Lowery C, DeNicola N, American College of Obstetricians and Gynecologists' Presidential Task Force on Telehealth. ACOG Committee Opinion 798: Implementing Telehealth in Practice. Obstet Gynecol 2020;135(2):e73–9.

14. Cantor AG, Jungbauer RM, Totten AM, et al. Telehealth strategies for the delivery of maternal health care : a rapid review. Ann Intern Med 2022;175(9):1285–97.

15. DeNicola N, Grossman D, Marko K, et al. Telehealth interventions to improve obstetric and gynecologic health outcomes: a systematic review. Obstet Gynecol 2020;135(2):371–82.

16. American College of Obstetricians and Gynecologists. Obstetric Patient Record Forms. Available at: https://www.acog.org/clinical-information/obstetric-patient-record-forms. Accessed 14 September, 2022.

17. Barrera CM, Powell AR, Biermann CR, et al. A review of prenatal care delivery to inform the michigan plan for appropriate tailored health care in pregnancy panel. Obstet Gynecol 2021;138(4):603–15.

18. Kilpatrick SJ, Papile L, and Macones GA. Guidelines for perinatal care, 8th ed., 2017, American Academy of Pediatrics/The American College of Obstetricians and Gynecologists. Available at: https://publications.aap.org/aapbooks/book/522/Guidelines-for-Perinatal-Care?autologincheck=redirected.

19. Dowswell T, Carroli G, Duley L, et al. Alternative versus standard packages of antenatal care for low-risk pregnancy. Cochrane Database Syst Rev 2015;(7): CD000934. https://doi.org/10.1002/14651858.CD000934.pub3.

20. Balk EM, Konnyu KJ, Cao W, et al. Schedule of Visits and Televisits for Routine Antenatal Care: A Systematic Review. Comparative Effectiveness Review No. 257 (Prepared by the Brown Evidence-based Practice Center under Contract

No. 75Q80120D00001). AHRQ Publication No 22-EHC031. 2022;https://doi.org/10.23970/AHRQEPCCER257.

21. Pay AS, Wiik J, Backe B, et al. Symphysis-fundus height measurement to predict small-for-gestational-age status at birth: a systematic review. BMC Pregnancy Childbirth 2015;15:22.

22. Goetzinger KR, Tuuli MG, Odibo AO, et al. Screening for fetal growth disorders by clinical exam in the era of obesity. J Perinatol 2013;33(5):352–7.

23. Zafman KB, Cudjoe E, Srinivas SK, et al. Adjustment of prenatal care during COVID was associated with an increased risk of undetected FGR. Am J Obstet Gynecol 2022;226(1 Suppl):S578–9.

24. Butler Tobah YS, LeBlanc A, Branda ME, et al. Randomized comparison of a reduced-visit prenatal care model enhanced with remote monitoring. Am J Obstet Gynecol 2019;221(6):638 e1–e638 e8.

25. Duryea EL, Adhikari EH, Ambia A, et al. Comparison between in-person and audio-only virtual prenatal visits and perinatal outcomes. JAMA Netw Open 2021;4(4):e215854.

26. Palmer KR, Tanner M, Davies-Tuck M, et al. Widespread implementation of a low-cost telehealth service in the delivery of antenatal care during the COVID-19 pandemic: an interrupted time-series analysis. Lancet 2021;398(10294):41–52.

27. Pflugeisen BM, McCarren C, Poore S, et al. Virtual visits: managing prenatal care with modern technology. MCN Am J Matern Child Nurs 2016;41(1):24–30.

28. Yeh PT, Rhee DK, Kennedy CE, et al. Self-monitoring of blood pressure among women with hypertensive disorders of pregnancy: a systematic review. BMC Pregnancy Childbirth 2022;22(1):454.

29. Pealing LM, Tucker KL, Mackillop LH, et al. A randomised controlled trial of blood pressure self-monitoring in the management of hypertensive pregnancy. OPTIMUM-BP: A feasibility trial. Pregnancy Hypertens 2019;18:141–9.

30. Waugh J, Habiba MA, Bosio P, et al. Patient initiated home blood pressure recordings are accurate in hypertensive pregnant women. Hypertens Pregnancy 2003;22(1):93–7.

31. Marko KI, Krapf JM, Meltzer AC, et al. Testing the feasibility of remote patient monitoring in prenatal care using a mobile app and connected devices: a prospective observational trial. JMIR Res Protoc 2016;5(4):e200.

32. McManus RJ, Mant J, Bray EP, et al. Telemonitoring and self-management in the control of hypertension (TASMINH2): a randomised controlled trial. Lancet 2010;376(9736):163–72.

33. DeNicola N, Ganju N, Marko KI, et al. Evaluation of antepartum and postpartum blood pressure monitoring in low-risk pregnancy. Obstet Gynecol 2019;133:120S.

34. American College of Obstetricians and Gynecologists' Committee on Practice Bulletins-Obstetrics. Gestational hypertension and preeclampsia: ACOG practice bulletin, number 222. Obstet Gynecol 2020;135(6):e237–60.

35. Peahl AF, Turrentine M, Barfield W, et al. Michigan plan for appropriate tailored healthcare in pregnancy prenatal care recommendations: a practical guide for maternity care clinicians. J Womens Health (Larchmt). 2022;31(7):917–25.

36. Eberly LA, Kallan MJ, Julien HM, et al. Patient characteristics associated with telemedicine access for primary and specialty ambulatory care during the COVID-19 pandemic. JAMA Netw Open 2020;3(12):e2031640.

37. Marko KI, Ganju N, Krapf JM, et al. A mobile prenatal care app to reduce in-person visits: prospective controlled trial. JMIR Mhealth Uhealth 2019;7(5):e10520.

38. Hodgkinson JA, Sheppard JP, Heneghan C, et al. Accuracy of ambulatory blood pressure monitors: a systematic review of validation studies. J Hypertens 2013; 31(2):239–50.

39. Stergiou GS, Kario K, Kollias A, et al. Home blood pressure monitoring in the 21st century. J Clin Hypertens 2018;20(7):1116–21.

40. Whelton PK, Carey RM, Aronow WS, et al. 2017 ACC/AHA/AAPA/ABC/ACPM/AGS/APhA/ASH/ASPC/NMA/PCNA Guideline for the Prevention, Detection, Evaluation, and Management of High Blood Pressure in Adults: A Report of the American College of Cardiology/American Heart Association Task Force on Clinical Practice Guidelines. Hypertension 2018;71(6):e13–115.

41. Carlson AL, Martens TW, Johnson L, et al. Continuous glucose monitoring integration for remote diabetes management: virtual diabetes care with case studies. Diabetes Technol Ther 2021;23(S3):S56–65.

42. Majithia AR, Kusiak CM, Armento Lee A, et al. Glycemic outcomes in adults with type 2 diabetes participating in a continuous glucose monitor-driven virtual diabetes clinic: prospective trial. J Med Internet Res 2020;22(8):e21778.

43. Lee JP, Freeman G, Cheng M, et al. Clinical relevance of home monitoring of vital signs and blood glucose levels: a narrative review. Int J Technol Assess Health Care 2019;35(4):334–9.

44. Kalafat E, Benlioglu C, Thilaganathan B, et al. Home blood pressure monitoring in the antenatal and postpartum period: A systematic review meta-analysis. Pregnancy Hypertens 2020;19:44–51.

45. Mhajna M, Schwartz N, Levit-Rosen L, et al. Wireless, remote solution for home fetal and maternal heart rate monitoring. Am J Obstet Gynecol MFM 2020;2(2): 100101.

46. Tucker KL, Mort S, Yu LM, et al. Effect of self-monitoring of blood pressure on diagnosis of hypertension during higher-risk pregnancy: the BUMP 1 randomized clinical trial. JAMA 2022;327(17):1656–65.

47. Chappell LC, Tucker KL, Galal U, et al. Effect of self-monitoring of blood pressure on blood pressure control in pregnant individuals with chronic or gestational hypertension: the BUMP 2 randomized clinical trial. JAMA 2022;327(17):1666–78.

48. Peahl AF, Zahn CM, Turrentine M, et al. The michigan plan for appropriate tailored health care in pregnancy prenatal care recommendations. Obstet Gynecol 2021; 138(4):593–602.

49. World Health Organization. A Conceptual Framework for Action on the Social Determinants of Health. Available at: https://www.who.int/publications/i/item/9789241500852. Accessed November 30, 2022.

50. National Academies of Sciences Engineering and Medicine. Communities in Action: Pathways to Health Equity. Available at: https://nap.nationalacademies.org/catalog/24624/communities-in-action-pathways-to-health-equity. Accessed November 30, 2022.

51. Centers for Disease Control and Prevention. Social Determinants of Health: Know What Affects Health. Available at: https://www.cdc.gov/socialdeterminants/index.htm. Accessed September 26, 2022.

52. Davidson KW, Krist AH, Tseng CW, et al. Incorporation of Social Risk in US Preventive Services Task Force Recommendations and Identification of Key Challenges for Primary Care. JAMA 2021;326(14):1410–5.

53. Booske BC, Athens JK, Kindig DA, Park H, Remington PL, University of Wisconsin Population Health Institute. Different Perspectives for Assigning Weights to Determinants of Health. Available at: https://www.countyhealthrankings.org/sites/default/files/

differentPerspectivesForAssigningWeightsToDeterminantsOfHealth.pdf. Accessed September 28, 2021.

54. County Health Rankings & Roadmaps. Explore Health Rankings. Available at: https://www.countyhealthrankings.org/explore-health-rankings. Accessed November 30, 2022.

55. National Academies of Sciences Engineering and Medicine, Integrating social care into the delivery of health care: moving upstream to improve the nation's health, 2019, National Academies Press. Available at: https://www. nationalacademies.org/our-work/integrating-social-needs-care-into-the-delivery-of-health-care-to-improve-the-nations-health.

56. Reyes AM, Akanyirige PW, Wishart D, et al. Interventions addressing social needs in perinatal care: a systematic review. Health Equity 2021;5(1):100–18.

57. Centers for Medicare & Medicaid Services Office of Minority Health. Utilization of Z Codes for Social Determinants of Health among Medicare Fee-for-Service Beneficiaries, 2019. November 30, 2022. Available at: https://www.cms.gov/files/document/z-codes-data-highlight.pdf. Accessed November 1, 2022.

58. Tong ST, Liaw WR, Kashiri PL, et al. Clinician Experiences with Screening for Social Needs in Primary Care. J Am Board Fam Med 2018;31(3):351–63.

59. De Marchis EH, Hessler D, Fichtenberg C, et al. Assessment of social risk factors and interest in receiving health care-based social assistance among adult patients and adult caregivers of pediatric patients. JAMA Netw Open 2020;3(10): e2021201.

60. McConnell MA, Rokicki S, Ayers S, et al. Effect of an intensive nurse home visiting program on adverse birth outcomes in a medicaid-eligible population: a randomized clinical trial. JAMA 2022;328(1):27–37.

61. Thorland W, Currie DW. Status of birth outcomes in clients of the nurse-family partnership. Matern Child Health J 2017;21(5):995–1001.

62. Catling CJ, Medley N, Foureur M, et al. Group versus conventional antenatal care for women. Cochrane Database Syst Rev 2015;2015(2):CD007622.

63. Peahl AF, Novara A, Heisler M, et al. Patient preferences for prenatal and postpartum care delivery: a survey of postpartum women. Obstet Gynecol 2020; 135(5):1038–46.

64. Williamson PR, Altman DG, Bagley H, et al. The COMET handbook: version 1.0. Trials 2017;18(Suppl 3):280.

65. COMET Initiative. Frequency Of pRenatal CAre viSiTs (FORCAST) - Core Outcome Set. Available at: https://www.comet-initiative.org/Studies/Details/ 2021. Accessed November 30, 2022.

66. Fitch K, Bernstein SJ, Aguilar MD, et al. The RAND/UCLA appropriateness method user's manual, 2001, RAND Corporation. Available at: https://www. rand.org/pubs/monograph_reports/MR1269.html.

67. Rosen MG, National Institutes of Health. Caring for our future: the content of prenatal care. A report of the public health service expert panel on the content of prenatal care. Available at: https://eric.ed.gov/?id=ED334018. Accessed December 6, 2022.

68. Friedman Peahl A, Turrentine M, Barfield W, et al. Designing your patient's prenatal care "PATH". Contemp Ob Gyn 2022;67(1):27–30.

Group Prenatal Care

Sarah Jean Hanson, MD[a,b,*], Katherine Lee, MD[c]

KEYWORDS

• Group prenatal care • Health care equity • Pregnancy outcomes

KEY POINTS

- Group prenatal care (GPC) is an integrated and holistic model of health care for pregnant patients.
- Pregnant patients of similar gestational age, along with support partners, receive both prenatal education as well as physical assessment during facilitated group sessions instead of the traditional one-on-one prenatal care office visit model.
- GPC has benefits in patient care outcomes as well as improved patient and provider satisfaction.
- GPC seeks to improve health care equity and quality.
- Delivery of prenatal care in a group setting is a major divergence from traditional care delivery and takes planning, commitment, and flexibility from the health care system for success.

INTRODUCTION

The goal of prenatal care is prevention and identification of complications of pregnancy, and improved birth outcomes.[1] Traditional one-on-one prenatal care typically includes short visits with a provider, increasing in frequency with advancing gestational age. Health assessments as well as education on a myriad of topics should be discussed during these visits. This load of information inevitably leads to an inadequate amount of time for questions or in-depth discussion of topics. This often inadvertently omits important educational points, identification of risk factors, or appreciation of individual patient values throughout a birthing person's pregnancy journey. Some patients gather additional support and education from childbirth classes, additional community or health care services such as doulas, but these services and education are almost always separated from the medical care of the prenatal visits. This separation can lead to both redundancy as well as gaps in health education

---

[a] Division of Global and Community Health, Department of Obstetrics and Gynecology, Beth Israel Deaconess Medical Center, Harvard Medical School, 330 Brookline Avenue, Kirstein, 3rd Floor, Boston, MA 02215, USA; [b] Department of Obstetrics and Gynaecology, Princess Marina Hospital, University of Botswana, Gaborone; [c] Harbor – UCLA Medical Center, University of California Los Angeles, 1000 West Carson Street, Torrance, CA 90502, USA
* Corresponding author. 330 Brookline Avenue, Kirstein 3rd Floor, Boston, MA 02215.
E-mail address: shanson1@bidmc.harvard.edu

Obstet Gynecol Clin N Am 50 (2023) 457–472
https://doi.org/10.1016/j.ogc.2023.03.003
0889-8545/23/© 2023 Elsevier Inc. All rights reserved.

and wellness interventions. For providers, much of the patient education conversations are repetitive and may not be inherently structured for effective adult learning. There is a need from both patients and providers to restructure prenatal care for more supportive and meaningful health care and educational experiences during pregnancy.[2,3]

BACKGROUND

With the goal of a more integrated and holistic approach through the formation of a supportive birthing community, group prenatal care (GPC) aims to improve prenatal care delivery. GPC is prenatal care in a group setting where both education and routine prenatal care visits are coupled together for pregnant patients of the same gestational age. GPC provides holistic care covering topics ranging from normal physical changes of pregnancy, medical warning signs, birth, breastfeeding, newborn care, emotional health, and wellness. More than a dozen types of GPC have been described, but all of them have similar tenants including physical assessment, facilitated discussion, and self-care activities in the structure of a supportive community.[3,4]

DEFINITIONS

CenteringPregnancy♥ is the most widespread model of GPC. Offering online or in-person facilitator training from their Centering Healthcare Institute (CHI), a 501(c)3 non-profit organization. CHI provides a structured curriculum and resource materials. These include a comprehensive guide for each facilitator with extensive resources and organized content of scheduled sessions, as well as a patient notebook that encourages participation with integrative and interactive activities aligning with the scheduled GPC sessions. Practices utilizing CenteringPregnancy♥ participate in certification and assessment for site licensure.[3]

Some practices and health care systems choose to deliver GPC through self-designed formats. Many of these groups are adaptations of the general structure of CenteringPregnancy♥, while others combine their own baseline childbirth education groups with prenatal visits. Future directions of GPC are likely to include more technological and telehealth integration. For example, "Expect with me," is an adapted GPC model that combines group meetings with a smartphone/computer interface to engage patients in remote monitoring between visits and foster the group dynamic. This is a promising concept in the optimization of GPC still being developed and researched.[3,4]

EDUCATIONAL SCHEDULE

The goals of GPC are to provide health care for pregnant patient and to encourage group learning and patient empowerment through educational discussions. **Tables 1** and **2** outline basic examples of GPC models.

ADVANTAGES

GPC models began originating in the 1990s. From then, GPC has been studied worldwide and has been shown to be effective and possibly superior to individual care for some patients. These observed benefits of GPC are summarized in **Box 1** and discussed below.

- Improved Birth Outcomes and Reduced Pregnancy-Related Complications
  The most compelling outcome from GPC studies is a consistent decrease in preterm birth and low birth weight in both low- and high-risk women, especially

Table 1
Example group prenatal care session timing and topics

Session	Themes	Topics
1 (13–17 weeks)	You are a healthy mom	• Eat and live healthy for you and your baby • Stay active while you are expecting • Maintain healthy weight during pregnancy • Understand routine prenatal testing and emergencies • Know what blood pressure and weight numbers are healthy for you
2 (17–21 weeks)	Staying healthy and strong through change	• How babies grow and develop • Mom's clean teeth = healthier mother and baby • Learn why you are feeling the way you do • Move safely and comfortably while pregnant • Get a good night's sleep • Keep calm and stress-free while expecting • Stay safe at home, work, and play
3 (21–24 weeks)	Breastfeeding = Healthy Babies and Healthy Moms	• Benefits of breastfeeding • Barriers to breastfeeding • Basics of breastfeeding • Choose a pediatric provider (Part 1) • Your support systems (Part 1)
4 (25–29 weeks)	Healthy moms building healthy relationships	• Understand Gestational Diabetes Testing • Build healthy relationships • Prevent STDs including HIV (Part 1) • Choose when to get pregnant (Part 1)
5 (27–31 weeks)	Healthy moms and healthy labor	• Signs of labor • Stages of labor (Part 1) • Fetal heart rate monitoring • Stay comfortable during labor • Understand Cesarean birth
6 (29–33 weeks)	Healthy labor	• Stages of Labor (Part 2) • What happens immediately after delivery

(continued on next page)

Table 1
(continued)

Session	Themes	Topics
		• Labor and delivery decisions • Provider policies and options for labor and delivery • Prevent STDs including HIV (Part 2)
7 (31–35 weeks)	Healthy labor and healthy relationships	• Prepare for hospital stay and return home • Negotiate to build healthy relationships • Understand Group B Strep testing and prevention
8 (33–37 weeks)	Taking care of mom and baby	• Caring for your baby • Choose a pediatric provider (Part 2) • Care for your postpartum body • Set goals to build healthy relationships (Part 1)
9 (35–39 weeks)	Preparing for a Healthy Future	• How to breastfeed • Staying healthy and strong after pregnancy • Signs of postpartum depression • Make sure your home is safe for you and your baby
10 (37+ weeks)	Build a healthy future	• Choosing a daycare provider • Going back to work • Your support systems (Part 2) • Choose when to get pregnant again (Part 2) • Set goals for a healthy relationship (Part 2)

From Cunningham, S.D., Lewis, J.B., Thomas, J.L. et al. Expect With Me: development and evaluation design for an innovative model of group prenatal care to improve perinatal outcomes. BMC Pregnancy Childbirth 17, 147 (2017). https://doi.org/10.1186/s12884-017-1327-3.

Table 2
Centering pregnancy ♥ schedule and session content

Schedule of Meetings	
4 Sessions Every 4 Weeks	16, 20, 24, 28 weeks
5 Sessions Every 2 Weeks	30, 32, 34, 36, 38 weeks
Individual follow-up as needed with the provider	38–39 weeks
Reunion "Baby Shower"	2–6 weeks postpartum
Session Outline	
1	Prenatal Testing, Nutrition, Size Your Servings, Food Diary, Health Lifestyle Choices
2	Body Changes in Pregnancy, Common Discomforts, Taking Care of Your Back, Healthy Gums and Teeth
3	Mental Relaxation, Breastfeeding My Baby, The Family I Want to Have
4	Thinking about My Family, Family Planning, Sexuality, Domestic Violence and Abuse, Fetal Brain Development, Preterm Labor
5	Labor, Birth Facility, Breathing, Medications for Labor and Birth, Early Labor—When to Call
6	The Birth Experience
7	The Newborn's First Days, Planning Pediatric Care, Caring for Your Baby, Circumcision, Brothers and Sisters, Newborn—When to Call
8	Pregnancy to Parenting Transition, Kick Counts, Emotional Adjustments, Postpartum Depression, Pregnancy—When to Call
9	Putting it all together, Newborn Safety, Infant Massage
10	Growth and Development, Home Changes and Family Changes, Mom Postpartum—When to Call

Courtesy of Centering Healthcare Institute, Boston, MA; with permission.

in Black participants. Other evidence-based positive birth outcomes include fewer babies born at low birth weight and fewer neonatal intensive care unit (NICU) admissions. GPC has shown proven benefits for perinatal mental health. Patients in GPC with gestational diabetes have been shown to have better glycemic control, postpartum visit rates, are more likely to get screened for, and less likely to develop type 2 diabetes. Studies have found improvements in other quality measures, including increased vaccination rates, prenatal attendance, hospital-based delivery rate, postpartum contraception uptake, and decreased sexually transmitted diseases for GPC mothers. Finally, GPC mothers have higher breastfeeding initiation and continuation rates. All of these health benefits can also lead to decreased overall health care costs.[2,5–8]

- Health Equity

  Inequity, particularly in racial, socioeconomic, and geographic disparity, is a leading cause of adverse pregnancy outcomes. Social and structural determinants of health impact pregnant patients for issues such as preterm birth, unintended pregnancy, and maternal mortality. Interventions by health care organizations and providers that can reduce inequities by improving

---

Box 1
Advantages of group prenatal care

- Better birth outcomes
  - Decreased preterm birth rates
  - Fewer NICU admissions
  - Fewer babies with low birth weight
- Lower cost
- Increased efficiency
- Higher patient and provider satisfaction
- Improved patient–provider relationships
- Higher rates of breastfeeding
- Improved management of gestational diabetes
- Improved utilization of family planning
- Better attendance at visits
- Fewer emergency visits and calls
- Higher immunization rates
- Better psychosocial outcomes
- Improved health equity and decreased racial disparity

---

communication and engaging community resources are required steps to bring equity to the health care system. GPC research has consistently shown reduction in preterm birth and low birth weight, most significantly in Black patients, who consistently experience significant birth outcome disparities. In GPC, women join based on due date, and the composition of a group brings together women with differing stories–age, parity, race, income, sexual orientation, family structure–with the shared value of caring for their growing family, and a desire to connect. During GPC sessions, time and attention are given to listen to the stories and experiences of patients in a group context. This participatory atmosphere of group facilitation levels the hierarchy of the traditional health care system and elevates the value of voices usually not actively encouraged to share a health care system meant to serve them. This approach, with humility and inquiry, brings increased awareness to the needs of families and the community with the goal toward improved outcomes related to social determinants of health.[5,9,10]

- Patient Satisfaction

  Common concerns from patients regarding prenatal care include a desire for more time with their health care provider, shorter wait times for visits, and more attention to their needs. GPC combines education with health care, allowing patients up to 10 times more contact with their provider, and vastly improving efficiency and quality time. This builds more touchpoints with the patient to identify and treat complications, moreover leading to a deeper provider–patient relationship that fosters trust and understanding. The composition of the GPC is consistent, providing a rare and enjoyable continuity of care throughout the pregnancy journey of the patient and provider. Even during the early part of a GPC visit where some patients are having one-on-ones, no time is wasted. Patients are taking their weight and blood pressure, socializing, and connecting, which builds a supportive community allowing patients to find more joy in their pregnancy journey and health care experience. GPC by its nature encourages participation and discussion, leading to more patient engagement. It is no surprise that GPC is very popular with patients, with studies showing up to 97% of women who have experienced both types of prenatal care prefer the GPC model. Additional studies show GPC significantly improves prenatal care visit attendance due to this active engagement.[3–5,11,12]

- Provider Satisfaction

  Providers delivering GPC find the format more engaging, and efficient and improves work satisfaction as compared to the traditional model that can include many rushed visits and repetitive counseling. Providers have said GPC has helped them find more joy in the practice of medicine, as they have more high-yield time with patients leading to stronger patient relationships. Improved provider satisfaction has shown to lead to less burnout, a current crisis in medicine. GPC is a format that an entire practice can enjoy. GPC encourages a team-based and interdisciplinary approach to care where co-facilitators are engaged at a high level. Tasks are shared which not only helps providers with workload and efficacy, but builds interprofessional respectful relationships, leading to improved team performance and job satisfaction. GPC connects medical colleagues and community resources as guest speakers during groups (**Table 3**). These interactions lead to better relationships with these members of the health care team, encourage outreach, and provide holistic care. Improved communication and interdisciplinary teamwork have been shown time and time again to improve patient safety and outcomes. GPC encourages better resource utilization in other ways as well. Because of more provider contact and better prenatal education, GPC patients are less likely to present for unnecessary triage visits or call after hours with questions. This type of care is highly desirable, but few practices offer it.[3,4]

- Effective Education and Empowerment

  GPC education is much more extensive and in-depth than what can be offered during brief visits. Discussion of topics in a group setting allows for more questions to be addressed and the group gets to share the answers and learning opportunities that otherwise might not have been elicited in a one-on-one visit. The education is more comprehensive because there are expert speakers along with a structured curriculum to be covered, leading to more relevant and less redundant content. The GPC structure also fits better with models for effective adult education. GPC creates an atmosphere of trust, autonomy, participation, and collaboration that allows for true transformational learning. In discussion, everyone is encouraged to share their experiences with the group and process the relevance of the topics to their lives. Patients check in on goals at each visit and are given encouragement from the group. Because partners or birth companions are present, they too are better equipped for their role. GPC studies have shown participants have better prenatal knowledge and are more prepared for delivery, postpartum, and newborn care. Intra and postpartum teams report that patients who have had GPC ask fewer questions and are more prepared for the birth experience than those having traditional care. Many providers report GPC patients needing interventions to have fewer concerns and need less explanation, making consent easier. It has been said that knowledge is power. The GPC health educational model aims to increase

Table 3
Suggested guest speakers for group prenatal care sessions

Medical Providers	Physical Wellness	Nutrition	Birthing	Psychosocial
Pediatrician	Massage Therapist	Dietitian	Doula	Social Worker
Anesthesiologist	Physical Therapist	Diabetes educator	Labor and Delivery Nurse	Mental health counselor
Other members of the obstetric group	Prenatal Yoga Instructor	Lactation Consultant	Childbirth instructor	Behavioral health counselor

patient self-interest and to empower women to take ownership of their health. Studies in the United States and globally have found women have significantly higher empowerment if they are engaged in GPC as compared to individual prenatal care. For example, in high-risk women, GPC participants were less likely to engage in unprotected sex and were more likely to communicate with partners about infection prevention.[2–5,7]

- Attention to Psychosocial Issues

    Mental health issues including anxiety and depression impact many women during pregnancy. Studies have shown social support is protective of mental health and reduces postpartum depression. With increased social isolation, including changes from the coronavirus (COVID) pandemic, the diagnosis of anxiety and depression is increasingly common. GPC provides more social support outside of one's family and therefore offers significant benefits to patients' mental health. The increased time with providers brings more touchpoints and opportunities for screening, discussion, and diagnosis. In research studies, GPC participants reported fewer anxiety and depression symptoms than patients in traditional care. For those hesitant to engage in mental health care due to stigma or lack of comfort, GPC has the advantage of the introduction of behavioral health professionals as guest speakers to the group. The presence of a mental health professional can help to begin a relationship for those hesitant to engage otherwise. Anxiety and depression can be particularly underdiagnosed and undertreated in more vulnerable patient populations. In studies with immigrant patients, for example, GPC participants felt they could share feelings more openly with the support of the GPC group than during one-on-one visits. This increased comfort and engagement led to lowered rates of anxiety and depression in GPC patients, removing this racial disparity and improving care and outcomes.[13–15]

APPLICATION

When surveyed, most women would elect a group care model if given the choice; yet despite improved outcomes, less than 3% of women have this option as a choice or are able to participate. This is likely due to different challenges that face individual health care systems and not due to decreased interest or unwillingness of participants. Therefore, with the knowledge that GPC has the power to improve outcomes, and decrease racial disparities, it is up to health care providers to champion this novel method.[12,16,17]

So how is GPC delivered successfully? We will discuss a generalizable model of delivery of GPC for those looking to establish it in their practice and how to prepare for challenges that may be faced.

Box 2 Outlines the approach to providing GPC including pre-planning as well as a review of the general structure of the GPC sessions.

CONSIDERATIONS

Challenges are expected with major changes, and GPC is no different. Barriers in each system will vary, but by anticipating some of these hurdles, plans can be made to manage and overcome them.

- Provider Logistics

    Multiple providers need time to be trained to allow for adequate coverage of the groups. For chronically multi-tasking obstetric providers who may have call

Box 2
Group prenatal care approach

Session Pre-Planning:
- At the onset of prenatal care, GPC is encouraged and described to the prospective pregnant patient.
- Accepting new obstetric patients are enrolled in the next group based on the month of their due date.
- Eight to 12 patients are enrolled in the group, and partners or birth companions are also invited.
- Before their first session, new group members are given information about GPC and commit to attend.
- The schedule for the group is set: 1 to 2 hours per session, roughly 10 visits, monthly for 4 months, then every 2 weeks until delivery, then once postpartum.
- The group members stay consistent throughout the sessions, including patients, companions, the provider, and co-facilitator (rare facilitator substitution, if need be, is planned in advance).
- Two facilitators are present for each session: a provider (MD, CNM, or Family Medicine) along with a co-facilitator (Nurse, Nurse Practitioner, Physician Assistant, Doula, Medical Assistant, Community Health worker); ideally the same two facilitators are present for all sessions for consistency.
- Additional guests who will visit the group are contacted and scheduled (see **Table 3**).
- Before each session, providers briefly review patient charts and planned topics.
- The co-facilitator assists in preparation, compiling a brief list of group members that is updated for each visit with basic relevant information (gestational age, parity, high-risk issues, and tests or screenings due) as well as preparation of items needed for the visits (eg, Doppler, tape measure, BP cuff, scale, educational items, vaccines, testing materials, and health screening questionnaires).

Session Structure:
1. Patients arrive at the group meeting space at the scheduled time.
2. Upon arrival, patients undergo a brief health screening at the door for symptoms of acute illness.
3. After checking in, patients are involved in self-care activities: after basic instruction from the co-facilitator, patients take and record their own blood pressure and weight, and log these data for review.
4. In the first 30 minutes of the session, brief (5 minutes or less) individual health assessments with the provider are performed. Patients are pulled aside one-by-one for short examination of maternal and fetal well-being, and review of logged information.
5. Brief or personal questions or issues that arise during these one-on-ones are addressed; anything generalizable is deferred to discussion with the group. If urgent issues are identified, patients are referred to triage; non-urgent issues needing follow-up (mild blood pressure elevation, complaints of vaginal discharge, issues needing other referral services) are readdressed after the end of the session.
6. Documentation is concurrent with the short one-on-one sessions (some providers only do basics, eg, filling in data on the prenatal visit flowsheet; while others complete all charting).
7. During this early part of the group, while individual exams are taking place, participants are encouraged to have casual socialization; they also have time to review logs or journals from sessions, and complete health screening questionnaires, or other paperwork such as breast pump order forms.
8. After the completion of the individual visits, patients and the facilitators come together in a circle to begin the facilitated group portion of the visit.
9. Using group facilitation skills, the planned topics of education for that session are discussed (see **Tables 1** and **2**). Engagement activities such as reflective writing and interactive games encourage each member to share. Relaxation and mindfulness techniques and goals are set during this time to reinforce the health education of the session for individuals, and for future reference for other visits and for birthing.
10. Visits from frequent guest speakers add to the education with ample time for questions.

11. The group concludes with a review of the topics covered during the session, discussion of the patient's health goals, and plans for the next session.
12. The session ends on time with everyone dismissed together. If individuals need specific follow-up plans, these are organized as needed.
13. The provider completes chart documentation while the co-facilitator reorganizes.
14. The co-facilitators debrief and plan for the next session.

or covering responsibilities at the same time as scheduled office patients, GPC causes conflict. Rather than a small number of patients who may be in jeopardy of being rescheduled if a provider on-call is pulled away for a clinical emergency, GPC has a large cohort of patients scheduled at a very specific time that cannot be rebooked easily due to the logistics involved in the group planning. The practice must have adequate staffing to give the GPC provider protected time for the group and charting, usually at least 2 hours, without any conflicting responsibilities. Thoughtful planning with practice management and leadership can help anticipate and plan for these logistical issues in the provider schedule.

- Physical Space and Infrastructure

    Finding an area large enough to fit a group of more than 20 people (patients, partners, and providers) may take planning. Additional space considerations include planning for an area aside from this large space for individual exams. If no smaller rooms are nearby, then utilizing a privacy screen or curtain to create this area can be successful. Those with complaints necessitating a pelvic examination may need to be examined in another location. Finally, if the space for GPC meetings is away from the typical clinical setting, then preparation must be undertaken to organize needed resources at the GPC site. This may include testing supplies (eg, group b streptococcus [GBS] swabs, glucola bottles), medications (eg, vaccines, RhoGAM), etc. Again, team organization and anticipation of needs before sessions are key to success.

- Scheduling

    One common reason patients who desire GPC do not choose the model if given the opportunity is based on difficulties with scheduling. Patients must commit to a group at the same time and place every 2 to 4 weeks for up to 2 hours at a time. Due to transportation, work conflicts, and childcare responsibilities, this lack of scheduling flexibility and length of visit times may be a deterrent to attendance. Some practices have overcome this barrier by offering times more suitable to working women (evening or weekend groups) or by offering childcare. These solutions cause their own dilemmas, however, with providers then asked to work out of normal office hours, and referral options more limited for urgent needs if they arise during the session. Providers can have more schedule flexibility these days (mornings off if working in the evening for a GPC session), but this still may not be desirable to some practice models or providers unless large scheduling or group changes occur. Childcare options exist for some GPC sites, but with an associated cost that must be part of the program budget. Ongoing conversations with the health care team including scheduling will need to occur to address these possible needs.[3,12]

- Costs

    GPC start-up expenses mostly lie in the cost of training and materials, if practices choose to use the CenteringPregnancy♥ model (facilitator training

$995, facilitators guide $75, patient log books $22). Additional on-going costs are variable and may include salary of a program coordinator, and annual fees for a site license for continued operation using the CenteringPregnancy♥ name for sites with this format, or nominal accrued needs such as a budget for snacks. As GPC enrollment increases, then these costs will be recouped in time. Planning with management and marketing is key for successful budget planning.[3]

- Reimbursement

GPC has been shown to reduce overall health care costs in some studies; nonetheless, on the provider or practice level, compensation may be an issue. For example, providers who meet a new obstetric (OB) patient may have to hand over their patient to another provider based on due date or availability, although this should even out between providers. Additionally, if the time given to the GPC session would be more than what a provider would usually be able to bill during an equivalent time in the office, revenue may be lost. GPC payment-related barriers can possibly be overcome by linking care with value-based payment systems, which reward improved health care outcomes; alternate options are enhanced payments for visits based on time and education provided. Again, team collaboration including the billing department before initiating care can help with planning for financial-related issues.[3,5,6]

- High-risk patients

Trouble-shooting when low-risk prenatal care patients change their risk based on complications that arise during pregnancy is important when initiating GPC. Two common acquired health conditions during pregnancy include gestational diabetes and gestational hypertension. Managing a new gestational diabetes diagnosis could include continuing GPC with the addition of a separate group or private diabetes education with additional appointments with providers to address diabetes management. Some data support group-based diabetes management as more cost-effective and successful for lifestyle behavioral changes, such as diet and exercise. Patients in group diabetes management find the group setting creates a supportive environment, helps them build friendships, and improves accountability by sharing goals. Similarly, with a new gestational hypertension diagnosis, these patients can have increased monitoring as indicated while continuing with normal prenatal care sessions (eg, BP checks, lab testing). Patients who already begin as higher-risk pregnancies should be considered for GPC as well, based on individual health assessments by providers. Group discussion and educational topics are likely universal regardless of risk, but attending GPC should not be taking away from needed specialist time for high-risk conditions. Management of high-risk patients should likely continue with individualized care as GPC pilots at an institution, but consider adding high-risk patients to GPC after implementation is successful.[2]

- Special circumstances

Very private or introverted patients or those with personal or sensitive issues may be hesitant to join a group care model. Although they may find GPC overwhelming, with good facilitation, the willing but more quiet patients can be drawn out. Patients with conditions that are often stigmatized socially like mental illness, marked obesity, or infectious disease may be reluctant to share; however, in the safety of the group, they may slowly open-up and share about their personal journey. Discussion of topics such as intimate partner violence and substance use disorders may be triggering to some patients, and difficult to disclose for others due to concerns about social acceptability of behaviors. Careful navigation of these topics in a group setting can lead to empowerment and reduced stigma. A mitigating factor may be that all groups agree to confidentiality at the first meeting. Finally, in patients with a language barrier or significant disability, an additional support person may be needed to help facilitate the GPC participation. Practices should consider a language-specific GPC cohort or a bilingual co-facilitator if there are many of these patients in the community served.[2,13]

- COVID

The pandemic has influenced almost everything in society, significantly in the health care system. Restrictions of group events particularly impact the core nature of GPC–social gathering. GPC was on a moratorium or halted altogether at many sites post-pandemic, sadly with some still not resuming. However, with the strong desire for continued social interactions among expecting mothers, many GPC practices found creative solutions to keep groups running, even early in the pandemic. With the encouragement of more individualized prenatal care and telehealth expansion, groups that are temporarily closed due to gathering restrictions can still have tele-med visits through secure systems on virtual meeting platforms. GPC providers should have plans for illness screening, testing policies, and vaccination education to resume in-person sessions at the soonest possible safe date.[13]

- Change

A myriad of anticipated logistical challenges may face a practice newly implementing GPC. Change itself takes advocacy and a general willingness to do something differently that may not at first be easy. Providers need to gain comfort with facilitation and find a workflow to integrate charting with the

---

Box 3
Disadvantages of group prenatal care

- Providers must be trained in and master group facilitation
- Requires a major system change
- May not suit some patients based on:
  - Risk factors
  - Individual needs
  - Personal preferences
- Does not allow for schedule flexibility
- Significant time commitment
- Requires a large group meeting space
- Requires provider to focus on a limited group of patients
- Providers cannot have competing responsibilities
- Discussion of sensitive topics may pose a challenge
- Cost barriers:
  - Start-up
  - Maintenance
  - Reimbursement issues

Box 4
Implementation considerations for initiation of group prenatal care

- Identify team of champions
- Choose model of care
- Assess start-up costs and on-going costs
- Engage key stakeholders
  ○ Administrators, managers, billing, marketing, scheduling, patients, community
- Acquire a space—includes area for group discussion as well as individual assessments
- Recruit program coordinator
- Train health care providers to facilitate sessions
- Make roll-out plan, including start date for enrollment of the first groups
- Advertise and encourage
  ○ Place posters in waiting areas and exam rooms
  ○ Website and social media posts
  ○ Recommend by all providers and staff at intake visits, calls for new obstetric appointments, and first exam visits
- Continuous reassessment

Adapted from Smith J. Redesigning health care. BMJ. 2001;322(7297):1257-1258. https://doi.org/10.1136/bmj.322.7297.1257; with permission.

---

group session visits. Once the groups have started, most providers overcome the initial adjustments with practice and find their workflow by collaborating with their co-facilitator. Despite perceived difficulties at the onset, some of the most successful GPC facilitators are those experienced and late-career providers who are completely new to group care, health education, or multi-dimensional care models. These providers bring trust and wisdom to the group, and to whom the group brings a renewed interest in energy to patient care relationships.

GPC will not be for everyone. For some, GPC will pose significant challenges without easy solutions that can be overcome to make this model viable for their practice. **Box 3** summarizes these considerations.

DISCUSSION

The initiation and integration of GPC will come with new challenges for an existing health system. With any radical change, especially to complex systems like health care, planning is key to success. The ideal incorporation of GPC will vary based on the unique resources and barriers in the existing practice. A generalized guide of considerations in planning for implementation of GPC is outlined in **Box 4** based on successful health system change concepts. GPC may not be for everyone as its initiation will pose challenges to individual sites with or without easy solutions that can make this model viable for practice. However, given the advantages GPC can bring to a practice and patient care, integration should be explored.

SUMMARY

Pregnant patients are more empowered and knowledgeable than ever. They are requesting integrated health care models that are more modern, provide better education, and focus on wellness. GPC replaces the traditional model of individual prenatal care visits with a more holistic group care model including more comprehensive education coupled with medical care. GPC patients of similar gestational age meet at scheduled intervals and are led through interactive facilitated discussions about pregnancy, birth, and postpartum and contact multiple health care and community services. GPC can help to improve health equity by improving outcomes, including for women who have traditionally experienced poor outcomes due to institutional racism in our health care systems. Thoughtful planning is needed by the health care system, providers, and patients for implementation with an on-going commitment to continued success. With its improved outcomes and patient-centered care model, patients will increasingly request we provide GPC as an option for care. Those of us who successfully integrate GPC enjoy overwhelming benefits to our patients, our practice, and the obstetric communities we serve.

CLINICS CARE POINTS

- GPC is highly desired by patients, but vastly underutilized with less than 3% of women receiving prenatal care through this model.
- In GPC, 8 to 12 pregnant patients of similar gestational age, along with support partners, receive both facilitated prenatal education as well as health care during approximately 10 scheduled, structured 1 to 2 hour group sessions, instead of traditional brief one-on-one visits.
- GPC may help to improve health equity and birth outcomes by delivering more comprehensive and holistic patient-centered prenatal care.
- Both low- and high-risk pregnancies can receive care through GPC models, although very high-risk women may need additional visits.
- GPC requires a willingness to change and a commitment from the practice, providers, and patients to be successful.

DISCLOSURE

Authors have no disclosures.

REFERENCES

1. Rousseau DM, ten Have S. Evidence-based change management. Organ Dynam 2022;51(3):100899.
2. Byerley BM, Haas DM. A systematic overview of the literature regarding group prenatal care for high-risk pregnant women. BMC Pregnancy Childbirth 2017; 17:329.
3. "Centeringpregnancy." centering healthcare Institute, copyright © 2009–2022. Centering Healthcare Institute Inc. Available at: https://centeringhealthcare.org/what-we-do/centering-pregnancy. Accessed November 11, 2022.
4. Cunningham SD, Lewis JB, Thomas JL, et al. Expect With Me: development and evaluation design for an innovative model of group prenatal care to improve perinatal outcomes. BMC Pregnancy Childbirth 2017;17:147 (Table 1).
5. Ickovics JR, Kershaw TS, Westdahl C, et al. Group prenatal care and perinatal outcomes: a randomized controlled trial. Obstet Gynecol 2007;110:330–9, published erratum appears in Obstet Gynecol 2007;110:937.

6. Ickovics JR, Kershaw TS, Westdahl C, et al. Group prenatal care and preterm birth weight: Results from a matched cohort study at public clinics. Obstet Gynecol 2003;102(5, Pt. 1):1051–7.

7. Kershaw TS, Magriples U, Westdahl C, et al. Pregnancy as a window of opportunity for HIV prevention: Effects of an HIV intervention delivered within prenatal care. Am J Public Health 2009;99(11):2079–86.

8. Grenier L. Impact of Group Antenatal Care (G-ANC) versus Individual Antenatal Care (ANC) on Quality of Care, ANC Attendance and Facility-Based Delivery: a pragmatic cluster-randomized controlled trial in kenya and nigeria. PLoS One 2019;14(10).

9. Importance of social determinants of health and cultural awareness in the delivery of reproductive health care. ACOG Committee Opinion No. 729. American College of Obstetricians and Gynecologists. Obstet Gynecol 2018;131:e43–8.

10. Racism in Obstetrics and Gynecology. ACOG Policy and Position Statements. American College of Obstetricians and Gynecologists, *Obstet Gynecol*, 2022. Available at: https://www.acog.org/clinical-information/policy-and-position-statements/statements-of-policy/2022/racism-in-obstetrics-gynecology. Accessed November 11, 2022.

11. Group prenatal care. ACOG Committee Opinion No. 731. American College of Obstetricians and Gynecologists. Obstet Gynecol 2018;131:e104–8.

12. Declercq ER, Sakala C, Corry MP, et al. Listening to mothers III: pregnancy and birth. New York: Childbirth Connection; 2013.

13. Filippetti ML, Clarke ADF, Rigato S. The mental health crisis of expectant women in the UK: effects of the COVID-19 pandemic on prenatal mental health, antenatal attachment and social support. BMC Pregnancy Childbirth 2022;22:68.

14. Buultjens M, Farouque A, Karimi L, et al. The contribution of group prenatal care to maternal psychological health outcomes: a systematic review. Women Birth 2021;34(6):e631–42.

15. Screening for perinatal depression. ACOG Committee Opinion No. 757. American College of Obstetricians and Gynecologists. Obstet Gynecol 2018;132:e208–12.

16. Sharon S. Rising. CENTERING PREGNANCY: an interdisciplinary model of empowerment. J Nurse Midwifery 1998;43(1):46–54.

17. Smith J. Redesigning health care: radical redesign is a way to radically improve. Br Med J 2001;322:1257–8.

Vaginal Bleeding Before 20 Weeks Gestation

Brenna Banwarth-Kuhn, BS[a], Miriam McQuade, MD[b],
Jamie W. Krashin, MD, MSCR[c],*

KEYWORDS

- Pregnancy loss • Miscarriage • Ectopic pregnancy • Molar pregnancy
- Septic abortion

KEY POINTS

- The most common early pregnancy conditions that present with vaginal bleeding and are associated with morbidity and mortality before 20 weeks gestation are pregnancy loss, ectopic pregnancy, and molar pregnancy.
- Determine if a bleeding patient is stable while establishing a diagnosis.
- Clinically unstable patients require prompt procedural management.
- Mifepristone pretreatment before misoprostol is more effective than misoprostol alone for medication management of pregnancy loss.
- Evidence around the necessity for prophylaxis against Rh(D) allo-immunization and remote follow-up are evolving for early pregnancy loss.

INTRODUCTION

Bleeding in the first 20 weeks of pregnancy can be a sign of anything from benign implantation bleeding to life-threating conditions. This article aims to provide connections between and resources for the most common early pregnancy complications that often present with bleeding in the first half of pregnancy: pregnancy loss, ectopic pregnancy, and molar pregnancy. Some of these conditions have been recently presented in the Emergencies in Obstetrics and Gynecology issue of this journal (Volume 49, Issue 3) and can be referenced for additional details on epidemiology, risk factors, diagnosis, and treatment regimens: First Trimester Miscarriage and Ectopic Pregnancy Miscarriage[1,2] No matter which condition is present, the first steps in evaluating bleeding in the first 20 weeks of pregnancy will always include assessing patient stability and establishing whether the pregnancy is intrauterine.

[a] University of New Mexico School of Medicine; [b] University of New Mexico Health Sciences Center; [c] Department of Obstetrics & Gynecology, University of New Mexico Health Sciences Center, MSC 10 5580, 1 University of New Mexico, Albuquerque, NM 87131-0001, USA
* Corresponding author.
E-mail address: jkrashin@salud.unm.edu

Obstet Gynecol Clin N Am 50 (2023) 473–492
https://doi.org/10.1016/j.ogc.2023.03.004
0889-8545/23/© 2023 Elsevier Inc. All rights reserved.

obgyn.theclinics.com

FIRST AND SECOND TRIMESTER PREGNANCY LOSS

Pregnancy loss or miscarriage is an intrauterine embryonic or fetal demine before 20 weeks gestation.[3] Early pregnancy loss (EPL) is the most common type of pregnancy loss and is defined by the American College of Obstetricians and Gynecologists as a nonviable intrauterine pregnancy before 13 weeks gestation with ultrasound showing an empty gestational sac or a gestational sac containing an embryo without fetal cardiac activity.[4]

Pregnancy loss can present at different stages, the names of which will be used throughout the article. When the pregnancy tissue is still inside the uterus, the cervix can be closed (missed abortion) or open (inevitable abortion). When the pregnancy tissue has all passed (complete abortion), the cervix may be open or closed. When some tissue has passed (incomplete abortion), the cervix is generally still open. The patient may or may not present with bleeding. Concerning bleeding is often considered saturating more than two pads per hour for 2 hours in a row or bleeding at a rate anticipated to exceed this volume.[2,5] Concerning bleeding, signs or symptoms of infection, abnormal vital signs, and/or abnormal laboratory values indicate clinical instability and require urgent procedural management.

Epidemiology

Approximately 10% of clinically identified pregnancies and one-third of all pregnancies end in pregnancy loss.[4,6,7] Increasing age and prior pregnancy loss are common risk factors for EPL.[4,8,9] Disparities exist in pregnancy loss: Black patients experience higher rates of miscarriage compared with White patients and Black and Hispanic patients are more likely to present to emergency departments (ED) for vaginal bleeding in early pregnancy than non-early pregnancy issues, potential indicators of inequitable social and structural determinants of health.[10–12]

Evaluation

Pregnancy loss is diagnosed primarily by ultrasound. According to the Society of Radiologists' guidelines, EPL can be definitively diagnosed by any of four specific ultrasound findings: (1) crown-rump (CRL) length of 7 mm or greater and no cardiac motion, (2) mean sac diameter (MSD) of 25 mm or greater and no embryo, (3) absence of embryonic cardiac motion 2 weeks or more after a scan showing a gestational sac without a yolk sac, or (4) the absence of embryonic cardiac motion 11 days or more after a scan showing a gestational sac with a yolk sac[13] The guidelines also stipulate findings suspicious for, but not diagnostic of, pregnancy loss: (1) CRL <7 mm and no cardiac motion, (2) MSD 16 to 24 mm and no embryo, (3) absence of embryonic cardiac motion 7 to 13 days after a scan that showed a gestational sac without a yolk sac, (4) absence of embryonic cardiac motion 7 to 10 days after a scan that showed a gestational sac with a yolk sac, (5) absence of an embryo ≥6 weeks after last menstrual period, (6) empty amnion, (7) enlarged yolk sac (>7 mm), (8) small gestational sac in relation to the size of the embryo (<5 mm difference between MSD and CRL).[13] Some patients prefer to start management after meeting "suspicious for" pregnancy loss criteria rather than waiting for an additional ultrasound to meet definitive criteria; patient-centered counseling allows providers to provide care according to the patient's preferred timeline.[4,13]

Patient history, laboratory confirmation of recent pregnancy, or available products of conception can help diagnose a complete abortion when ultrasound shows no gestational sac and low concern for ectopic pregnancy.[4] For example, a patient may report positive pregnancy test one week ago followed by heavy bleeding and a negative pregnancy test in the clinic. They may present with resolving bleeding, no gestational sac, and no obvious signs of ectopic pregnancy on ultrasound, and a positive pregnancy test. Some patients may bring products of conception with an obvious gestational sac and villi. If the clinical picture is not clear, trending serum human chorionic gonadotrophin (hCG) levels and/or repeating an ultrasound are needed for resolution of pregnancy of unknown location.[4,14]

Management

Early pregnancy loss
There are three management options for EPL: (1) expectant, (2) medication, or (3) procedural.

Clinically stable patients can choose any of the three options; those who receive their preferred options report higher satisfaction with care.[4,15–17] See **Table 1** for management overview. Unstable patients require prompt procedural management via uterine aspiration.[4,18]

Expectant management involves the patient waiting for the pregnancy tissue to pass without intervention. Expectant management was successful within 14 days for 84% of patients with incomplete abortion and approximately half of the patients with missed abortion and anembryonic pregnancies.[19] Waiting 7 weeks resulted in 91%, 76%, and 66% success for incomplete abortions, missed abortions, and anembryonic pregnancies, respectively.[19] Complications are rare at ~1% for patients opting for expectant management, with no major differences in pelvic infection by 8 weeks and higher, but still rare, risk of the need for transfusion compared with patients choosing procedural management.[20] Expectant management is less expensive than procedural management.[20,21]

Medication management expedites EPL resolution for patients who wish to avoid a procedure. Although misoprostol had been the standard medication regimen for years, in 2018, a randomized controlled trial of patients 5 weeks to 12 weeks 6 days with a closed cervix demonstrated a large improvement in treatment success when mifepristone—a steroid that competitively antagonizes progesterone and glucocorticoid receptors and is approved by the Food and Drug Administration for induced abortion and treatment of Cushing's Syndrome—was administered before misoprostol.[22–25] Eighty-four percent of patients who received mifepristone 200 mg orally followed by misoprostol 800 mcg vaginally had successful treatment of their miscarriage within 2 days compared to 67% of patients who received misoprostol alone.[22] Thirty days after treatment, only 9% of patients in the mifepristone group needed procedural management compared with 24% in the misoprostol-only group.[22] Side effects were similar between groups.[22] The optimal timing between mifepristone and misoprostol is likely 6 to 20 hours, but still effective through 48 hours.[26] Mifepristone and misoprostol are cost-effective compared with procedural management.[27,28] American College of Obstetricians & Gynecologists (ACOG) recommends mifepristone before misoprostol, but if mifepristone is not available, then misoprostol 800 mcg be administered vaginally with one repeat dose between 3 hours and 7 days later if needed.[4,29] For incomplete abortion, misoprostol is not clearly superior to expectant management.[30]

Patients choosing expectant or medication management can be counseled about managing symptoms at home, reasons to present for urgent care, and how to ensure their miscarriage is complete. Vaginal bleeding that is heavier than menses and intense cramping are normal.[22,31] There have not been studies about pain management during expectant management of miscarriage, however, literature for medication induced abortion reports decrease in pain with administration of ibuprofen after cramping begins.[32] An easy reference for patients regarding when to seek medical attention for

Table 1
Management options for early pregnancy conditions that often present with vaginal bleeding

Early Pregnancy Condition	Management Options		
	Expectant	Medication	Procedural
Pregnancy loss <13 weeks (EPL)	Can wait until 8 weeks but likely diminishing returns with increasing time At home	Mifepristone 200 mg PO + Misoprostol 800 mcg PV In clinic → at home At home[a] *Antibiotics not recommended*	Uterine aspiration In clinic In operating roomIn ED or L&D *Antibiotics recommended*
Pregnancy loss 13–20 weeks	n/a	Mifepristone 200 mg PO + Serial misoprostol 800 mcg PV On Labor & Delivery	Uterine aspiration or Dilation & evacuation In clinicIn operating roomIn ED or L&D *Antibiotics recommended*
Ectopic pregnancy	Limited circumstances	Methotrexate	Salpingectomy or salpingostomy In operating room
Molar pregnancy	n/a	Rarely used	Uterine aspiration or hysterectomy *Antibiotics* In operating room *Antibiotics recommended*
Septic abortion	n/a	n/a	Uterine aspiration or Dilation & Evacuation Intravenous fluids In operating roomIn ED or L&D *Intravenous followed by po antibiotics recommended*

Abbreviations: ED, emergency department; EPL, early pregnancy loss; L&D, labor & delivery; n/a, not applicable; PO, per os; PV, per vagina.
[a] Medication management of EPL may involve home care currently or in the future, based on growing experience with the same medications in self-managed abortion.

bleeding is soaking two maxi pads per hour for two consecutive hours or bleeding at a rate that will likely exceed that amount.[2,5] The Reproductive Health Access Project and University of Washington's Training, Education, & Advocacy in Miscarriage Management (TEAMM) have helpful patient handouts for counseling and home management (see Resources section).[33,34] Follow-up ultrasound showing lack of a gestational sac confirms successful treatment.[22] The thickness of the endometrial stripe does not determine treatment success.[35] Where ultrasound is not available, follow-up calls, urine pregnancy tests, and serial quantitative serum β-hCG measurements may be used to confirm completion, although most of the data on these follow-up options are extrapolated from medication-induced abortion.[4,36–38]

Uterine aspiration is the preferred procedural management and is used for patients who prefer to have a procedure or who are not candidates for expectant or medication management. Uterine aspiration is also known as suction dilation and curettage. ACOG and the World Health Organization recommend against sharp curettage based on studies showing its associated adverse effects.[4,39,40] Uterine aspiration can be completed in clinic or in an operating room with manual vacuum aspiration or electric vacuum aspiration. Clinic aspiration is cost- and time-saving compared with aspiration in the operating room, and patients report high satisfaction with both options.[41] Unlike expectant or medication management, antibiotic prophylaxis is recommended, although data are less conclusive for pregnancy loss than for induced abortion.[42–46] Common regimens are a single pre-procedural dose of doxycycline 200 mg, metronidazole 500 mg, or azithromycin 500 mg.[42,43,47]

Second trimester pregnancy loss until 20 weeks

Because second trimester pregnancy loss is less common and less frequently studied, its management is based on the existing literature on second trimester induced abortion.[48] Given the risk of hemorrhage for second trimester pregnancy loss, expectant management is not recommended.[4] Medication management with labor induction is 97% effective within 24 hours when mifepristone 200 mg oral is administered 36 to 48 hours before a loading dose of misoprostol 800 mcg vaginal and then 400 mcg every 3 hours.[39,43,49–52] Different regimens that alter the mifepristone pretreatment interval and misoprostol dosing and route are also highly effective.[49] Mifepristone and misoprostol are cost-effective compared to misoprostol alone.[53] Misoprostol alone results in longer induction times, but is faster than high-dose oxytocin, which can be used in the absence of misoprostol.[49,54,55] The risk of rupture is estimated to be 0.04% for unscarred uteri and 0.28% for one prior cesarean delivery.[49,56] Patients can receive the same analgesic options as for term labor inductions as well as also patient-controlled analgesia. Labor induction typically occurs in hospitals in North America.[49]

Procedural management of second trimester loss includes uterine aspiration through 14 to 16 weeks and dilation and evacuation (D&E) thereafter, similar to how induced abortion is performed.[57] Cervical preparation with misoprostol, osmotic dilators, and/or mifepristone reduces the risk of cervical laceration and uterine perforation in the late first and throughout the second trimester.[58,59] The same pre-procedural antibiotic prophylaxis can be used in the first or second trimester.[42,43,60] Although prevalence data are limited, potential complications such as disseminated intravascular coagulation, amniotic fluid embolism, hemorrhage, and infection may make the operating room an appropriate setting when available for second trimester loss D&E.[61–67]

Potential Complications

Pregnancy loss is associated with psychological and physical complications. Pregnancy loss can be a significantly distressing event with almost half of the people experiencing persistent and enduring psychological morbidity including depression, anxiety, and grief. Depressive disorders after miscarriage have the same incidence and prevalence as postpartum depression, but often are not screened for or treated.[68–73] Patients' partners may also suffer depression, anxiety, or post-traumatic stress disorder symptoms after pregnancy loss.[74,75] Again, disparities exist: Black patients have twice the risk of major depression after EPL compared with White patients.[76]

Minor physical complications include side effects of medication management — nausea, vomiting, diarrhea, and cramping pain.[22] Retained products of conception can occur with any management option and can be treated with misoprostol or uterine aspiration. Cervical laceration after a procedure can be managed with pressure or suturing.

Hemorrhage that requires hospitalization or blood transfusion occurs no more than 1% of the time with any treatment options and can often be managed with immediate uterine aspiration, uterotonics, and blood transfusion as needed.[4,29,77] We have seen disseminated intravascular coagulation and amniotic fluid embolism in our practice, but these complications are rare.

Maternal sepsis is responsible for 10% of maternal deaths worldwide.[78] Septic abortion is infected products of conception, endometritis, or parametritis during a current or following a recent pregnancy before 20 weeks gestation.[78,79] Importantly, septic abortion accounts for two-thirds of deaths from miscarriage.[61] Septic abortion presents with numerous different symptoms, however, most likely are uterine tenderness and foul smelling discharge and mild fever.[79] Patients with septic abortions require immediate uterine evacuation, broad-spectrum intravenous antibiotics, intravenous fluids, and, depending indicated depending on the severity, intensive care unit admission.[78,79] Expectant and medication management are contraindicated.

Several guidelines exist for managing labor induction and procedural management that are applicable to pregnancy loss care, including ACOG's Early Pregnancy Loss, Society of Family Planning's (SFP) Clinical Guidance, the National Abortion Federation's Clinical Policy Guidelines, Ipas' Clinical Updates in Reproductive Health, and the World Health Organization's Abortion Care Guidelines (see Resources).[4,39,47,80,81] These guidelines discuss the prevention and management of complications.

Counseling Patients After Pregnancy Loss

Many patients have historically felt as though they had a lack of information or support; we do not yet know if the recent media attention from celebrities sharing their personal stories will change this.[82–84] It may be helpful to share that more than half of miscarriages are due to genetic causes that are unlikely to happen again, rather than something the patient felt they did wrong.[85] First-time miscarriages usually do not require evaluation for a cause and most patients will have a baby in their next pregnancy.[86] Patients who want to conceive again should continue folic acid supplementation. Waiting beyond 1 to 2 weeks, when theoretically the cervix should be closed and infection risk decreased, does not improve the likelihood of having a baby in their next pregnancy.[87] Patients who wish to avoid pregnancy can start any method of contraception after pregnancy loss, except that intrauterine contraception is contraindicated after septic abortion.[88] Please see additional considerations for psychological care after all conditions below.

Rh(D) Immunoglobulin for Allo-Immunization Prophylaxis

ACOG recommends administering Rh(D) immunoglobulin (RhIG) for EPL (evidence level C).[4] SFP recommends against RhIG before 12 weeks gestation for uterine aspiration, 100 mcg/500 IU for 13 to 17 completed weeks gestation, and 300 mcg/1500 IU dose starting at 18 weeks.[89] If sharp curettage is the only option available, then 50 mcg/250 IU should be given before 12 weeks.[89]

ECTOPIC PREGNANCY

Ectopic pregnancy occurs when an embryo implants outside the endometrial cavity. The fallopian tube is the most common ectopic site.[14] Other locations include the abdomen, cervix, ovary, or cesarean scar.[1] Cesarean scar ectopics may be increasing in frequency along with the increasing incidence of cesarean delivery and can appear similar to EPL or low viable pregnancies, leading to delayed diagnosis.[90]

Epidemiology

At least 2% of all reported pregnancies are likely ectopic.[14,91] Hemorrhage from ruptured ectopics is the main cause of first trimester pregnancy-related mortality.[14] The most common risk factors are a history of prior ectopic(s), fallopian tube injury, and having an intrauterine device in place when pregnant; however, half of the patients lack risk factors.[14] Again, disparities exist that are likely related to social and structural determinants of health: the mortality rate from ectopic complications is a disturbing 6.8 times higher in Black patients compared with White patients in the United States and is 3.5 times higher for people over the age of 35 years.[14,92]

Evaluation

Any reproductive-age patient with female sex reproductive organs and vaginal bleeding should be evaluated for ectopic pregnancy. Suspected ectopic pregnancy requires confirmation of pregnancy with urine or serum hCG. Ultrasound evaluation of the endometrial cavity, cervix, and adnexa can establish any concerning masses, particularly an ectopic gestational sac with yolk sac. Significant free fluid in the posterior cul-de-sac deserves evaluation of intraperitoneal bleeding from rupture. Clinically unstable patients with high suspicion of ectopic pregnancy need immediate surgical evaluation.[14]

However, patients with early vaginal bleeding do not always have obvious intrauterine or ectopic pregnancies on ultrasound. Therefore these pregnancies of unknown location require clinical judgment regarding whether to proceed with diagnostic laparoscopy or to follow closely by trending hCG values and ultrasound. If hCG levels are used, clinical judgment still needs to be applied because the discriminatory zone—the hCG level at which an intrauterine pregnancy should be seen—may misclassify multiple gestations and overlap exists in the hCG trends between viable intrauterine pregnancies, EPL, and ectopics.[93] Additionally, a patient's pregnancy desires should guide treatment. For example, management can be expedited for clinically stable patients with undesired pregnancies via uterine aspiration and/or methotrexate, but a highly desired pregnancy in a stable patient may follow a longer hCG trend.[94] A helpful algorithm for this patient-centered approach exists.[94]

Management

Once ectopic pregnancy is diagnosed, three management options can be offered: (1) expectant, (2) medication, (3) surgical. Similar to pregnancy loss, unstable patients require urgent surgical management.

Expectant management of ectopic pregnancies is rare. This management option may be considered for asymptomatic patients whose ectopic pregnancies are likely resolving spontaneously. Indications of resolving ectopic pregnancy include low and decreasing hCG levels, no evidence or concerning findings for ectopic on ultrasound, and the ability to follow-up.[95]

Intramuscular methotrexate—a folate antagonist—is currently the only recommended medical treatment of ectopic pregnancy.[14] Before administering methotrexate, patients should have blood count, liver function, and renal function evaluated to determine any contraindications. Absolute contraindications include hemodynamic instability, intrauterine pregnancy, suspected ruptured ectopic pregnancy, severe anemia/leukopenia/neutropenia, active pulmonary or peptic ulcer disease, significant hepatic or renal dysfunction, breastfeeding, and allergy to methotrexate.[14] Relative contraindications to methotrexate use are related to the increased risk of methotrexate failure with higher hCG levels, increased CRL, and presence of embryonic cardiac motion.[14,96] For example, the risk of failure is almost four times as high with hCG levels above 5000 than below 5000.[97] Single- and multiple-dose regimens exist and the decision for which to use may be guided by the risk of failure and facility logistics.[14] For example, the two-dose regimen may be more effective when hCG levels are higher.[98] Alternative management should be considered for non-tubal ectopics, including intra-sac injection of methotrexate or potassium chloride with or without adjunctive systemic methotrexate, uterine aspiration, or surgical excision, depending on the location.[90,96,99–101] During management with methotrexate, hCG follow-up is necessary to monitor the treatment effect.[96] Patients treated with methotrexate should be educated about symptoms of tubal rupture versus tubal abortion, and the need for immediate medical attention if symptoms of rupture occur. Patients should also be advised to avoid folic acid supplements, foods that contain folic acid, nonsteroidal anti-inflammatory drugs, sexual intercourse, and sun exposure during therapy because these products may decrease the efficacy of methotrexate, increase side effects, or cause tubal rupture.[14,96]

Surgical management is indicated for clinically unstable patients, patients with absolute contraindication to methotrexate or failed medical management, concerns about follow-up, or patient preference.[14] Surgical management of ectopic pregnancy is usually performed using laparoscopic salpingectomy or salpingostomy. Salpingostomy allows for future fertility in patients with an absent or badly damaged contralateral tube.[14] Consider trending hCGs after salpingostomy and potentially giving a dose of methotrexate if a complete resection was not achieved.[14]

Rh(D) Immunoglobulin for Allo-Immunization Prophylaxis

ACOG and SFP recommend administering Rh(D) immunoglobulin (RhIG) for ectopic pregnancy.[89,102]

MOLAR PREGNANCY

Molar pregnancies, or hydatidiform moles, are caused by abnormal growth of pre-placental cells. Complete molar pregnancies have a diploid karyotype, no fetal tissue, and a 15% to 20% risk of progression to gestational trophoblastic neoplasia (GTN).[103] Partial moles are triploid, may have fetal tissue, and have a 1% to 5% risk of progression to GTN.[103]

Epidemiology

The incidence of molar pregnancy is difficult to know because it is rare. Recent data are limited, but older studies reveal North American and European countries report rates of 66 to 121 per 100,000 pregnancies, compared to Latin American, Asian, and Middle Eastern countries reporting rates as high as 1299 per 100,000 pregnancies.[104] Older and younger patients have higher risks of molar pregnancy.[105]

Evaluation

Molar pregnancy often initially presents with signs and symptoms of early pregnancy complications, including vaginal bleeding, pelvic or abdominal pain, uterus enlargement greater than expected for gestational age, hyperthyroid, pre-eclampsia, and hyperemesis gravidarum.[106] Quantitative serum hCG should be measured, as molar pregnancy usually has higher than expected levels than viable intrauterine pregnancy or ectopic pregnancy. Initial hCG level can be higher than 100,000 mIU/mL and should be followed with a transvaginal ultrasound to exclude twin pregnancy or coexistence of singleton pregnancy and molar pregnancy.[104,106] Transvaginal ultrasound findings suggestive of complete mole include absence of an embryo or fetus, absence of amniotic fluid, central heterogeneous mass with numerous discrete anechoic spaces or what has been described as a "snowstorm pattern", which indicates hydropic villi, and theca lutein cysts.[103] Ultrasound findings for partial mole may include identification of a growth-restricted fetus, oligohydramnios, placental enlargement and cysts, chorionic villi echogenicity, sac diameter, and absence of theca lutein cysts.[103] Partial mole ultrasound findings can be more difficult to interpret and are often misdiagnosed as EPL in up to 60% of cases.[107] When concerned about potential molar pregnancy, ask for pathology to perform p57 staining and ploidy.[103]

Management

Surgical removal of molar pregnancy is the mainstay of treatment. Uterine evacuation in the operating room is the preferred method, as it is effective and preserves childbearing capacity.[108] Hysterectomy may be appropriate for patients who do not wish to have any more children or have signs of trophoblastic proliferation and GTN.[109]

Complications

As diagnosis and management are occurring earlier in pregnancy, complications associated with molar pregnancy are less, however, there is still risks of hemorrhage or cardiopulmonary compromise.[103]

Additionally, there is a risk of development of GTN. This is less common due to earlier detection and intervention, however, even after uterine aspiration or hysterectomy, there is still a risk of development of GTN so it is recommended to follow hCG for 3 months after complete moles and 1 month after partial moles.[103]

Rh(D) Immunoglobulin for Allo-Immunization Prophylaxis

The Society of Gynecologic Oncology recommends administering Rh(D) immunoglobulin (RhIG) for molar pregnancy.[103]

PSYCHOLOGICAL CARE

Along with those experiencing miscarriage, patients with ectopic or molar pregnancies may also grieve. In a recent opinion editorial, a mother describes seeking care for ectopic pregnancy and the importance of her surgeon listening to her, taking her desire to bury her baby seriously, and caring for both her and her lost baby.[110] Some questions for all of us when helping our patients are listed in **Box 1**.

The TEAMM Project has a list of emotional support resources for EPL (see under Resources in **Box 2**).[33]

Box 1
Potential questions for clinicians when considering psychological care of patients with early pregnancy complications

- Does our health care organization offer chaplaincy services?

- What are our state laws and organizational policies regarding disposal of remains?

- Do these laws and policies accommodate patients with a diverse range of belief systems related to burial and cremation?

- Are we near a volunteer organization that offers professional photography for patients experiencing pregnancy loss, fetal demise, or stillbirth?[111]

- What words do we use in our clinical notes?

- Do we screen for depression?

- To whom in our clinics, hospitals, or communities can we send patients who need counseling or medication management for mood disorders following pregnancy loss?

- Are there support groups locally?

EARLY PREGNANCY ASSESSMENT CENTERS

Early pregnancy assessment centers (EPAC) or Early Pregnancy Units are clinics where patients can seek care for first trimester complications. Early pregnancy assessment services or units were started in the United Kingdom in the 1990s to improve care quality and to divert patients with first trimester bleeding and pain away from EDs.[112] In the United States, approximately 900,000 ED visits annually are for vaginal bleeding in early pregnancy, of which roughly 250,000 likely carry a diagnosis of EPL.[11] This represents a substantial burden on EDs and hundreds of thousands of patients who might prefer to receive care in a clinic. Hundreds of Early Pregnancy Units and clinics exist in the United Kingdom, Australia, New Zealand, and Canada.[113] Though not always called by the same name, similar clinics exist in the United States. EPACs can provide a range of services or referrals before most patients typically initiate prenatal care, including ultrasound; diagnosis and management of EPL, ectopic pregnancy, molar pregnancy, and induced abortion; and contraceptive services. Protocols drive evidence-based care, and clinicians and staff are trained in the emotional aspect of early pregnancy care. In the United States, EPACs have been proposed as an opportunity to improve health equity by providing high-value, efficient, and patient-centered care to historically marginalized groups that often disproportionately present to EDs with vaginal bleeding in early pregnancy.[12]

ADDITIONAL CONSIDERATIONS IN EARLY PREGNANCY
Barriers to Mifepristone Access

Although proven safe to use among millions of women since 2000, mifepristone has only been available with the Risk Evaluation and Mitigation Strategy (REMS) restrictions. The REMS required in-person dispensing (no prescriptions to retail pharmacies), signed Patient Agreement Forms, Prescriber Agreement Forms, and that mifepristone be ordered, prescribed, and dispensed by or under the supervisor of a provider who meets certain qualifications.[114] Qualitative research shows that providers were interested in using mifepristone for EPL management but the REMS restrictions were barriers to use.[115,116] ACOG has advocated for removing the REMS to improve access to mifepristone for EPL and induce abortion since 2018.[117] Due to the COVID-19 pandemic, there was a push to remove the in-person dispensing requirement of the

---

Box 2
Resources

Clinical and Patient Education

Reproductive Health Access Project: https://www.reproductiveaccess.org/miscarriage/

The TEAMM: https://www.miscarriagemanagement.org/resources

Clinical guidance
American College of Obstetricians & Gynecologists (ACOG): https://www.acog.org/clinical
  • EPL
  • Tubal ectopic pregnancy
Society of Family Planning (SFP): https://societyfp.org/clinical-guidance/
  • Rh testing in early pregnancy
  • Cesarean scar ectopic pregnancy
  • Cervical preparation in the first trimester and before 20 weeks
  • Labor induction in the second trimester
  • Management of postabortion hemorrhage
  • Multiple guidelines on procedural and medication management considerations for abortion that are applicable to pregnancy loss management as well as policy statements about access to women's health care
Society of Maternal Fetal Medicine: https://www.smfm.org/publications
  • Cesarean scar ectopic pregnancy (endorsed by SFP)
  • Clinical considerations for management of severe complications when abortion care is restricted (endorsed by SFP)
  • Checklist for initial management of amniotic fluid embolism
Society of Gynecologic Oncologists: https://www.sgo.org/practice-management/statements-and-recommendations/
  • Gestational trophoblastic disease (endorsed by ACOG)
National Abortion Federation: https://prochoice.org/store/clinical-policy-guidelines/
  • Clinical Policy Guidelines
Ipas: https://www.ipas.org/resource/clinical-updates-in-reproductive-health/
  • Clinical Updates in Reproductive Health
World Health Organization
  • Abortion Care Guideline: https://www.who.int/publications/i/item/9789240039483

REMs for miscarriage and abortion management.[118] In December 2021, the FDA removed (1) the in-person dispensing requirement but still required a certified provider and (2) the prohibition against dispensing in retail pharmacies.[114] The certification process for retail pharmacies has yet to be established.[119] Although the availability to send prescriptions to retail pharmacies will hopefully improve access to mifepristone, implementation will take time and the other REMS barriers remain. At time of the final proof for this article, the future status of mifepristone availability in the United States is unknown.[120–122]

Potential Consequences of Restrictive Abortion Bans on Early Pregnancy Conditions

Managing these early pregnancy conditions overlaps with induced abortion care. Ectopic and molar pregnancies, septic abortions, and inevitable miscarriages may have cardiac activity and yet need prompt termination of the pregnancy to avoid maternal morbidity and mortality.[4,14,78] Uterine aspiration is the procedure used for induced abortion as well as EPL and molar pregnancies; it can be used in the diagnosis of ectopic pregnancy.[14,94] D&E and labor induction are used for second trimester pregnancy loss and for induced abortion.[48,123] The medication management of EPL is almost the same as for induced abortion, with mifepristone and misoprostol.[4,124] Patients residing in states with strict abortion regulations may face barriers to obtaining early abnormal pregnancy care if embryonic or fetal cardiac activity is present or if states ban medications and procedures also used for induced abortion care.[125,126]

The risks associated with restricting access to care that is associated with induced abortion techniques or delaying management in the setting of fetal cardiac motion have been shown in two studies of expectantly managementing pre- or peri-viable rupture of membranes (ROM). In both studies, expectant management was associated with increased maternal morbidity and poor neonatal outcomes.[127,128] One retrospective cohort study in three institutions over seven years compared patients who opted for expect management with pregnancy termination in the setting of second trimester ROM. Women who chose expectant management had four times the odds of developing an infection, more than twice the odds of hemorrhaging, and were the only patients to be admitted to the intensive care unit or receive a hysterectomy.[127] Only 16% of women expectantly managed did not experience any morbidity and also had a neonate that survived hospital discharge.[127] The second study described outcomes in two large Dallas hospitals after passage of statewide restrictive abortion bans in September 2021 Both hospitals stopped offering labor induction for patients with pre-viable ROM and fetal cardiac motions. Expectant management in this setting resulted in rare neonatal survival (1/28 (4%): the neonate was admitted to the neonatal intensive care unit with multiple severe comorbidities at time of publication), and an increased proportion of severe maternal morbidity (57%) compared with historical controls who had received labor induction (33%).[128] Following the *Dobbs v Jackson Women's Health Organization* decision, the secretary of Health and Human Services wrote a letter to health care providers that the Emergency Medical Treatment and Active Labor Act statute preempts any state laws that might otherwise limit stabilizing management, including "abortion, removal of one … fallopian tube, anti-hypertensive therapy, methotrexate therapy" deemed necessary by a "physician or other qualified medical personal".[129,130]

KNOWLEDGE GAPS

- What are the sensitivity, specificity, position, and negative predictive values of remote EPL follow-up in a generalizable group of patients?
- What are the optimal ways to manage early pregnancy complications in rural settings? Are cost-effectiveness models developed in urban academic centers generalizable to rural hospitals and clinics? Do patients living in rural areas present differently or need different follow-up than their urban counterparts? Are the prevalence or complications of these conditions different in rural areas compared to urban areas?
- What additional disparities exist in the epidemiology, management, or outcomes of these conditions? If disparities are identified, how can they be addressed?
- What is the incidence of complications from second trimester pregnancy loss management?
- How can health care systems support self-management for people experiencing EPL in a safe and effective manner?
- What are the incidences of complications from these conditions?
- How can we improve the psychological aspect of pregnancy loss, ectopic pregnancy, and molar pregnancy care?
- Do strict abortion bans affect pregnancy loss, ectopic pregnancy, and molar pregnancy outcomes? Have morbidity and mortality related to septic abortion increased since these bans went into effect?

CLINICS CARE POINTS

- The most common early pregnancy conditions that present with vaginal bleeding and are associated with morbidity and mortality before 20 weeks gestation are pregnancy loss, ectopic pregnancy, and molar pregnancy.
- Determine if a bleeding patient is stable while establishing a diagnosis.
- Clinically unstable patients require prompt procedural management.
- Mifepristone pretreatment to misoprostol is more effective than misoprostol alone for EPL up to 12 weeks 6 days gestation.
- Evidence around the necessity for prophylaxis against Rh(D) allo-immunization and remote follow-up is evolving for EPL.
- The table shows management options for each early pregnancy condition included in this article.

FINANCIAL DISCLOSURE

None.

DISCLOSURE OF FUNDING

J.W. Krashin receives salary support through University of New Mexico, United States Health Sciences Center's KL2 program: NCATS, United States UL1TR001449.

REFERENCES

1. Tonick S, Conageski C. Ectopic Pregnancy. Obstet Gynecol Clin North Am 2022; 49(3):537–49.
2. Shaker M, Smith A. First Trimester Miscarriage. Obstet Gynecol Clin N Am 2022; 49:623–35.
3. CDC. Pregnancy and Infant Loss | CDC. Centers for Disease Control and Prevention. Published August 13, 2020. Accessed 17 December, 2022. Available at: https://www.cdc.gov/ncbddd/stillbirth/features/pregnancy-infant-loss.html.
4. ACOG Practice Bulletin No. 200: early pregnancy loss. Obstet Gynecol 2018; 132(5):e197.
5. Early Pregnancy Loss (Miscarriage) Treatment: Letting Nature Take Its Course. Reproductive Health Access Project. Accessed 2 January, 2023. Available at: https://www.reproductiveaccess.org/resource/miscarriage-treatment-letting-nature-take-its-course/.
6. Zinaman MJ, Clegg ED, Brown CC, et al. Estimates of human fertility and pregnancy loss. Fertil Steril 1996;65(3):503–9.
7. Wilcox AJ, Weinberg CR, O'Connor JF, et al. Incidence of early loss of pregnancy. N Engl J Med 1988;319(4):189–94.
8. Evaluation and treatment of recurrent pregnancy loss: a committee opinion. Fertil Steril 2012;98(5):1103–11.
9. Andersen AMN, Wohlfahrt J, Christens P, et al. Maternal age and fetal loss: population based register linkage study. BMJ 2000;320(7251):1708–12.
10. Mukherjee S, Velez Edwards DR, Baird DD, et al. Risk of miscarriage among black women and white women in a US prospective cohort study. Am J Epidemiol 2013;177(11):1271–8.

11. Benson LS, Magnusson SL, Gray KE, et al. Early pregnancy loss in the emergency department, 2006–2016. J Am Coll Emerg Physicians Open 2021;2(6): e12549. https://doi.org/10.1002/emp2.12549.

12. Shorter JM, Pymar H, Prager S, et al. Early pregnancy care in North America: a proposal for high-value care that can level health disparities. Contraception 2021;104(2):128–31.

13. Doublet PM, Benson CB, Bourne T, et al. Diagnostic criteria for nonviable pregnancy early in the first trimester. N Engl J Med 2013;369(15):1443–51.

14. ACOG Practice Bulletin No. 193: tubal ectopic pregnancy. Obstet Gynecol 2018;131(3):e91.

15. Wallace RR, Goodman S, Freedman LR, et al. Counseling women with early pregnancy failure: utilizing evidence, preserving preference. Patient Educ Couns 2010;81(3):454–61.

16. Schreiber CA, Chavez V, Whittaker PG, et al. Treatment decisions at the time of miscarriage diagnosis. Obstet Gynecol 2016;128(6):1347–56.

17. Geller PA, Psaros C, Kornfield SL. Satisfaction with pregnancy loss aftercare: are women getting what they want? Arch Womens Ment Health 2010;13(2): 111–24.

18. Herbert M, Cardy V. June 2017 - Rural Medicine: Catastrophic Vaginal Bleeding - Don't Fear The Stink! | EM:RAP. Accessed 27 May, 2020. Available at: https://www.emrap.org/episode/dontfearthe/ruralmedicine.

19. Luise C, Jermy K, Collins WP, et al. Expectant management of incomplete, spontaneous first-trimester miscarriage: outcome according to initial ultrasound criteria and value of follow-up visits. Ultrasound Obstet Gynecol 2002;19(6): 580–2.

20. Nanda K, Lopez LM, Grimes DA, et al. Expectant care versus surgical treatment for miscarriage. Cochrane Database Syst Rev 2012;2012(3):CD003518.

21. You JHS, Chung TKH. Expectant, medical or surgical treatment for spontaneous abortion in first trimester of pregnancy: a cost analysis. Hum Reprod 2005; 20(10):2873–8.

22. Schreiber CA, Creinin MD, Atrio J, et al. Mifepristone pretreatment for the medical management of early pregnancy loss. N Engl J Med 2018;378(23):2161–70.

23. Baulieu EE. RU 486 (mifepristone). A short overview of its mechanisms of action and clinical uses at the end of 1996. Ann N Y Acad Sci 1997;828:47–58.

24. FDA. Accessed 1 January, 2023. Available at: https://www.accessdata.fda.gov/drugsatfda_docs/label/2016/020687s020lbl.pdf.

25. FDA. Accessed January 1, 2023. Available at: https://www.accessdata.fda.gov/drugsatfda_docs/label/2012/202107s000lbl.pdf.

26. Flynn AN, Roe AH, Koelper N, et al. Timing and efficacy of mifepristone pretreatment for medical management of early pregnancy loss. Contraception 2021; 103(6):404–7.

27. Nagendra D, Gutman SM, Koelper NC, et al. Medical management of early pregnancy loss is cost-effective compared with office uterine aspiration. Am J Obstet Gynecol 2022. https://doi.org/10.1016/j.ajog.2022.06.054. S0002-9378(22)00530-0.

28. Nagendra D, Koelper N, Loza-Avalos SE, et al. Cost-effectiveness of mifepristone pretreatment for the medical management of nonviable early pregnancy: secondary analysis of a randomized clinical trial. JAMA Netw Open 2020;3(3): e201594.

29. Zhang J, Gilles JM, Barnhart K, et al. A comparison of medical management with misoprostol and surgical management for early pregnancy failure. N Engl J Med 2005;353(8):761–9.

30. Lemmers M, Verschoor MAC, Kim BV, Hickey M, Vazquez JC, Mol BWJ, et al. Medical treatment for early fetal death (less than 24 weeks). Cochrane Database Systm Rev 2019;2019(6). https://doi.org/10.1002/14651858.CD002253.pub4.

31. Hasan R, Baird DD, Herring AH, et al. Association between first-trimester vaginal bleeding and miscarriage. Obstet Gynecol 2009;114(4):860–7.

32. Jackson E, Kapp N. Pain control in first-trimester and second-trimester medical termination of pregnancy: a systematic review. Contraception 2011;83(2):116–26.

33. General Resources — The TEAMM Project. Accessed 2 January, 2023. Available at: https://www.miscarriagemanagement.org/resources.

34. Reproductive Health Access Project | Miscarriage - Reproductive Health Access Project. Accessed 2 January, 2023. Available at: https://www.reproductiveaccess.org/miscarriage/.

35. Creinin MD, Harwood B, Guido RS, et al. NICHD Management of Early Pregnancy Failure Trial. Endometrial thickness after misoprostol use for early pregnancy failure. Int J Gynaecol Obstet Off Organ Int Fed Gynaecol Obstet 2004;86(1):22–6.

36. Perriera LK, Reeves MF, Chen BA, et al. Feasibility of telephone follow-up after medical abortion. Contraception 2010;81(2):143–9.

37. Chen M, Rounds K, Creinin M, et al. Comparing office and telephone follow-up after medical abortion. Contraception 2016;94(2). https://doi.org/10.1016/j.contraception.2016.04.007.

38. Roe AH, Abernathy A, Flynn AN, et al. Utility and limitations of human chorionic gonadotropin levels for remote follow-up after medical management of early pregnancy loss. Obstet Gynecol 2022;139(6):1149.

39. World Health Organization. Abortion care guideline. Accessed 25 December, 2022. Available at" https://www.who.int/publications-detail-redirect/9789240039483.

40. Kakinuma T, Kakinuma K, Sakamoto Y, et al. Safety and efficacy of manual vacuum suction compared with conventional dilatation and sharp curettage and electric vacuum aspiration in surgical treatment of miscarriage: a randomized controlled trial. BMC Pregnancy Childbirth 2020;20(1). https://doi.org/10.1186/s12884-020-03362-4.

41. Dalton VK, Harris L, Weisman CS, et al. Patient Preferences, Satisfaction, and Resource Use in Office Evacuation of Early Pregnancy Failure. Obstet Gynecol 2006;108(1):103.

42. ACOG Practice Bulletin No. 195: prevention of infection after gynecologic procedures. Obstet Gynecol 2018;131(6):e172.

43. Achilles SL, Reeves MF. Prevention of infection after induced abortion. Contraception 2011;83(4):295–309.

44. Sawaga GF, Grady D, Kerlikowske K, et al. Antibiotics at the time of induced abortion: the case for universal prophylaxis based on a meta-analysis. Obstet Gynecol 1996;87(5 Part 2):884.

45. Goranitis I, Lissauer DM, Coomarasamy A, et al. Antibiotic prophylaxis in the surgical management of miscarriage in low-income countries: a cost-effectiveness analysis of the AIMS trial. Lancet Glob Health 2019;7(9):e1280–6.

46. Lissauer D, Wilson A, Hewitt CA, et al. A randomized trial of prophylactic antibiotics for miscarriage surgery. N Engl J Med 2019;380(11):1012–21.

47. Ipas. Clinical updates in reproductive health. Ipas. Accessed 1 January, 2023. Available at: https://www.ipas.org/resource/clinical-updates-in-reproductive-health/.

48. Niinimäki M, Mentula M, Jahangiri R, et al. Medical treatment of second-trimester fetal miscarriage; A retrospective analysis. PLoS One 2017;12(7): e0182198.

49. Borgatta L, Kapp N. Labor induction abortion in the second trimester. Contraception 2011;84(1):4–18.

50. Mentula M, Suhonen S, Heikinheimo O. One- and two-day dosing intervals between mifepristone and misoprostol in second trimester medical termination of pregnancy—a randomized trial. Hum Reprod 2011;26(10):2690–7.

51. Elami-Suzin M, Freeman MD, Porat N, et al. Mifepristone followed by misoprostol or oxytocin for second-trimester abortion: a randomized controlled trial. Obstet Gynecol 2013;122(4):815.

52. Allanson ER, Copson S, Spilsbury K, et al. Pretreatment with mifepristone compared with misoprostol alone for delivery after fetal death between 14 and 28 weeks of gestation: a randomized controlled trial. Obstet Gynecol 2021; 137(5):801.

53. Berkley HH, Greene HL, Wittenberger MD. Mifepristone combination therapy compared with misoprostol monotherapy for the management of miscarriage: a cost-effectiveness analysis. Obstet Gynecol 2020;136(4):774.

54. Ramin KD, Ogburn PL, Danilenko DR, et al. High-dose oral misoprostol for mid-trimester pregnancy interruption. Gynecol Obstet Invest 2002;54(3):176–9.

55. Nuthalapaty F, Ramsey P, Biggio J, et al. High-dose vaginal misoprostol versus concentrated oxytocin plus low-dose vaginal misoprostol for midtrimester labor induction: a randomized trial. Am J Obstet Gynecol 2005;193(3 Pt 2). https://doi.org/10.1016/j.ajog.2005.05.087.

56. Goyal V. Uterine rupture in second-trimester misoprostol-induced abortion after cesarean delivery: a systematic review. Obstet Gynecol 2009;113(5):1117–23.

57. Stubblefield PG, Carr-Ellis S, Borgatta L. Methods for Induced Abortion. Obstet Gynecol 2004;104(1):174.

58. Allen RH, Goldberg AB. Cervical dilation before first-trimester surgical abortion (<14 weeks' gestation). Contraception 2016;93(4):277–91.

59. Fox MC, Krajewski CM. Cervical preparation for second-trimester surgical abortion prior to 20 weeks' gestation. Contraception 2014;89(2):75–84.

60. Royal College of Obstetricians and Gynaecologists. Accessed 1 January, 2023. Available at: https://www.rcog.org.uk/media/nwcjrf0o/abortion-guideline_web_1.pdf.

61. Saraiya M, Green CA, Berg CJ, et al. Spontaneous abortion-related deaths among women in the United States–1981-1991. Obstet Gynecol 1999;94(2): 172–6.

62. Grimes DA. Estimation of pregnancy-related mortality risk by pregnancy outcome, United States, 1991 to 1999. Am J Obstet Gynecol 2006;194(1):92–4.

63. Maslow AD, Breen TW, Sarna MC, et al. Prevalence of coagulation abnormalities associated with intrauterine fetal death. Can J Anaesth 1996;43(12):1237–43.

64. Ray BK, Vallejo MC, Creinin MD, et al. Amniotic fluid embolism with second trimester pregnancy termination: a case report. Can J Anesth 2004;51(2): 139–44.

65. Mainprize TC, Maltby JR. Amniotic fluid embolism: a report of four probable cases. Can Anaesth Soc J 1986;33(3):382–7.

66. Edlow AG, Hou MY, Maurer R, et al. Uterine evacuation for second-trimester fetal death and maternal morbidity. Obstet Gynecol 2011;117(2 Part 1):307.
67. Kerns JL, Ti A, Aksel S, et al. Disseminated intravascular coagulation and hemorrhage after dilation and evacuation abortion for fetal death. Obstet Gynecol 2019;134(4):708.
68. Athey J, Spielvogel A. Risk factors and interventions for psychological sequelae in women after miscarriage. Prim Care Update OB/GYNS 2000;7(2):64–9.
69. Nikcevic AV, Snijders R, Nicolaides KH, et al. Some psychometric properties of the Texas Grief Inventory adjusted for miscarriage. Br J Med Psychol 1999;72(Pt 2):171–8.
70. Prettyman RJ, Cordle CJ, Cook GD. A three-month follow-up of psychological morbidity after early miscarriage. Br J Med Psychol 1993;66(Pt 4):363–72.
71. Lok IH, Yip ASK, Lee DTS, et al. A 1-year longitudinal study of psychological morbidity after miscarriage. Fertil Steril 2010;93(6):1966–75.
72. Lok IH, Neugebauer R. Psychological morbidity following miscarriage. Best Pract Res Clin Obstet Gynaecol 2007;21(2):229–47.
73. Farren J, Jalmbrant M, Falconieri N, et al. Posttraumatic stress, anxiety and depression following miscarriage and ectopic pregnancy: a multicenter, prospective, cohort study. Am J Obstet Gynecol 2020;222(4):367.
74. Volgsten H, Jansson C, Svanberg AS, et al. Longitudinal study of emotional experiences, grief and depressive symptoms in women and men after miscarriage. Midwifery 2018;64:23–8.
75. Farren J, Mitchell-Jones N, Verbakel JY, et al. The psychological impact of early pregnancy loss. Hum Reprod Update 2018;24(6):731–49.
76. Shorter JM, Koelper N, Sonalkar S, et al. Racial disparities in mental health outcomes among women with early pregnancy loss. Obstet Gynecol 2021;137(1): 156–63.
77. Davis AR, Hendlish SK, Westhoff C, et al. Bleeding patterns after misoprostol vs surgical treatment of early pregnancy failure: results from a randomized trial. Am J Obstet Gynecol 2007;196(1):31.e1–7.
78. Eschenbach DA. Treating spontaneous and induced septic abortions. Obstet Gynecol 2015;125(5):1042–8.
79. Stubblefield PG, Grimes DA. Septic abortion. N Engl J Med 1994;331(5):310–4.
80. Clinical Guidance. Society of Family Planning. Accessed 1 January, 2023. Available at: https://www.societyfp.org/clinical-guidance/.
81. National Abortion Federation. Accessed 1 January, 2023. Available at: https://prochoice.org/wp-content/uploads/2020_CPGs.pdf.
82. Baird S, Gagnon MD, deFiebre G, et al. Women's experiences with early pregnancy loss in the emergency room: A qualitative study. Sex Reprod Healthc Off J Swed Assoc Midwives 2018;16:113–7.
83. 50 Celebrities Who Opened Up About Their Miscarriages | HuffPost Life. Accessed 8 April, 2021. Available at: https://www.huffpost.com/entry/50-celebrities-who-opened-up-about-their-miscarriages_n_59de72a2e4b0fdad73b1b117.
84. Analysis | Michelle Obama is one of millions who struggled with infertility. Here's why her broken silence could matter. Washington Post. Available at: https://www.washingtonpost.com/politics/2018/11/09/michelle-obama-is-one-millions-who-silently-struggled-with-infertility-heres-why-her-broken-silence-could-matter/. Accessed October 21, 2022.
85. Soler A, Morales C, Mademont-Soler I, et al. Overview of Chromosome Abnormalities in First Trimester Miscarriages: A Series of 1,011 Consecutive Chorionic Villi Sample Karyotypes. Cytogenet Genome Res 2017;152(2):81–9.

86. Cohain JS, Buxbaum RE, Mankuta D. Spontaneous first trimester miscarriage rates per woman among parous women with 1 or more pregnancies of 24 weeks or more. BMC Pregnancy Childbirth 2017;17(1):437.
87. Schliep KC, Mitchell EM, Mumford SL, et al. Trying to conceive after an early pregnancy loss: an assessment on how long couples should wait. Obstet Gynecol 2016;127(2):204–12.
88. Curtis KM, Tepper NK, Jatlaoui TC, et al. U.S. Medical eligibility criteria for contraceptive use, 2016. MMWR Recomm Rep Morb Mortal Wkly Rep Recomm Rep 2016;65(3):1–103.
89. Horvath S, Goyal V, Traxler S, et al. Society of family planning committee consensus on Rh testing in early pregnancy. Contraception 2022;114:1–5.
90. Miller R, Gyamfi-Bannerman C. Society for maternal-fetal medicine consult series #63: cesarean scar ectopic pregnancy. Am J Obstet Gynecol 2022;227(3):B9–20.
91. Current Trends Ectopic Pregnancy – United States, 1990-1992. Accessed 2 January, 2023. Available at: https://www.cdc.gov/mmwr/preview/mmwrhtml/000 35709.htm.
92. Creanga AA, Shapiro-Mendoza CK, Bish CL, et al. Trends in ectopic pregnancy mortality in the United States: 1980–2007. Obstet Gynecol 2011;117(4):837.
93. Morse CB, Sammel MD, Shaunik A, et al. Performance of human chorionic gonadotropin curves in women at risk for ectopic pregnancy: exceptions to the rules. Fertil Steril 2012;97(1):101–6.e2.
94. Flynn AN, Schreiber CA, Roe A, et al. Prioritizing desiredness in pregnancy of unknown location: an algorithm for patient-centered care. Obstet Gynecol 2020;136(5):1001–5.
95. Webster K, Eadon H, Fishburn S, et al. Ectopic pregnancy and miscarriage: diagnosis and initial management: summary of updated NICE guidance. BMJ 2019;367:l6283.
96. Practice Committee of American Society for Reproductive Medicine. Medical treatment of ectopic pregnancy: a committee opinion. Fertil Steril 2013;100(3): 638–44.
97. Menon S, Colins J, Barnhart KT. Establishing a human chorionic gonadotropin cutoff to guide methotrexate treatment of ectopic pregnancy: a systematic review. Fertil Steril 2007;87(3):481–4.
98. Hamed HO, Ahmed SR, Alghasham AA. Comparison of double- and single-dose methotrexate protocols for treatment of ectopic pregnancy. Int J Gynaecol Obstet Off Organ Int Fed Gynaecol Obstet 2012;116(1):67–71.
99. Gilbert S, Alvero R, Roth L, Polotsky A. Direct Methotrexate Injection into the Gestational Sac for Nontubal Ectopic Pregnancy: A Review of Efficacy and Outcomes from a Single Institution - PubMed. Accessed 2 January, 2023. Available at: https://pubmed-ncbi-nlm-nih-gov.libproxy.unm.edu/30930212/.
100. Brincat M, Bryant-Smith A, Holland TK. The diagnosis and management of interstitial ectopic pregnancies: a review. Gynecol Surg 2019;16(1):2.
101. Ramkrishna J, Kan G, Reidy K, et al. Comparison of management regimens following ultrasound diagnosis of nontubal ectopic pregnancies: a retrospective cohort study. BJOG An Int J Obstet Gynaecol 2018;125(5):567–75.
102. ACOG Practice Bulletin No. 181: Prevention of Rh D Alloimmunization. Obstet Gynecol 2017;130(2):e57.
103. Horowitz NS, Eskander RN, Adelman MR, et al. Epidemiology, diagnosis, and treatment of gestational trophoblastic disease: a society of gynecologic oncology evidenced-based review and recommendation. Gynecol Oncol 2021;163(3): 605–13.

104. Berkowitz RS, Goldstein DP. Clinical practice. Molar pregnancy. N Engl J Med 2009;360(16):1639–45.

105. Sebire NJ, Foskett M, Fisher RA, et al. Risk of partial and complete hydatidiform molar pregnancy in relation to maternal age. BJOG An Int J Obstet Gynaecol 2002;109(1):99–102.

106. Soto-Wright V, Bernstein M, Goldstein DP, et al. The changing clinical presentation of complete molar pregnancy. Obstet Gynecol 1995;86(5):775–9.

107. Fowler DJ, Lindsay I, Seckl MJ, et al. Routine pre-evacuation ultrasound diagnosis of hydatidiform mole: experience of more than 1000 cases from a regional referral center. Ultrasound Obstet Gynecol 2006;27(1):56–60.

108. Ngan HYS, Seckl MJ, Berkowitz RS, et al. Update on the diagnosis and management of gestational trophoblastic disease. Int J Gynaecol Obstet Off Organ Int Fed Gynaecol Obstet 2018;143(Suppl 2):79–85.

109. Zhao P, Lu Y, Huang W, et al. Total hysterectomy versus uterine evacuation for preventing post-molar gestational trophoblastic neoplasia in patients who are at least 40 years old: a systematic review and meta-analysis. BMC Cancer 2019;19(1):13.

110. Sargeant LL. Opinion | in a post-roe World, we can avoid pitting mothers against babies. The New York Times; 2022. Available at: https://www.nytimes.com/2022/07/04/opinion/ectopic-pregnancy-roe-abortion.html. Accessed January 2, 2023.

111. Now I Lay Me Down to Sleep. Now I Lay Me Down To Sleep. Accessed 2 January, 2023. Available at: https://www.nowilaymedowntosleep.org/.

112. Bigrigg MA, Read MD. Management of women referred to early pregnancy assessment unit: care and cost effectiveness. Br Med J 1991;302(6776):577–9.

113. The Association of Early Prenancy Units. Accessed 2 January, 2023. Available at: https://www.aepu.org.uk/.

114. Research C for DE and. Questions and Answers on Mifeprex. FDA. Published online December 16, 2021. Accessed 2 January, 2023. Available at: https://www.fda.gov/drugs/postmarket-drug-safety-information-patients-and-providers/questions-and-answers-mifeprex.

115. Neill S, Goldberg A, Janiak E. Medication management of early pregnancy loss: the impact of the U.S. food and drug administration risk evaluation and mitigation strategy [A289]. Obstet Gynecol 2022;139:83S.

116. Flynn AN, Shorter JM, Roe AH, et al. The burden of the Risk Evaluation and Mitigation Strategy (REMS) on providers and patients experiencing early pregnancy loss: A commentary. Contraception 2021;104(1):29–30.

117. Improving Access to Mifepristone for Reproductive Health Indications. Accessed 13 January, 2022. Available at: https://www.acog.org/en/clinical-information/policy-and-position-statements/position-statements/2018/improving-access-to-mifepristone-for-reproductive-health-indications.

118. ACOG Applauds the FDA for its Action on Mifepristone Access During the COVID-19 Pandemic. Accessed 13 January, 2022. Available at: https://www.acog.org/en/news/news-releases/2021/04/acog-applauds-fda-action-on-mifepristone-access-during-covid-19-pandemic.

119. Understanding the Practical Implications of the FDA's December 2021 Mifepristone REMS Decision: A Q&A with Dr. Nisha Verma and Vanessa Wellbery. Accessed 1 January, 2023. Available at: https://www.acog.org/en/news/news-articles/2022/03/understanding-the-practical-implications-of-the-fdas-december-2021-mifepristone-rems-decision.

120. Alliance for Hippocratic Medicine vs. U.S. Food and Drug Administration (Northern District of Texas, #2:22-cv-00223, April 7).

121. Ferguson vs. U.S. Food and Drug Adminstration (Eastern District of Washington, #1:23-cv-03026, April 7).

122. Alliance for Hippocratic Medicien vs. U.S. Food and Drug Administration (Fifth Circuit, #23-10362, April 12, 2023).

123. ACOG Practice Bulletin No. 135: second-trimester abortion. Obstet Gynecol 2013;121(6):1394.

124. Creinin MD, Grossman DA. Planning C on PBG of F. Medication abortion Up to 70 Days of Gestation: ACOG Practice Bulletin, Number 225. Obstet Gynecol 2020;136(4):e31.

125. Perritt J, Grossman D. The health consequences of restrictive abortion laws. JAMA Intern Med 2021;181(5):713–4.

126. Grossman D, Perritt J, Grady D. The impending crisis of access to safe abortion care in the US. JAMA Intern Med 2022;182(8):793–5.

127. Sklar A, Sheeder J, Davis AR, et al. Maternal morbidity after preterm premature rupture of membranes at <24 weeks' gestation. Am J Obstet Gynecol 2022; 226(4):558.e1–11.

128. Nambiar A, Patel S, Santiago-Munoz P, et al. Maternal morbidity and fetal outcomes among pregnant women at 22 weeks' gestation or less with complications in 2 Texas hospitals after legislation on abortion. Am J Obstet Gynecol 2022. https://doi.org/10.1016/j.ajog.2022.06.060. S0002-9378(22)00536-1.

129. Available at: https://www.supremecourt.gov/opinions/21pdf/19-1392_6j37.pdf. Accessed January 2, 2023.

130. Health and Human Services Letter to Health Care Providers. Available at: https://www.hhs.gov/sites/default/files/emergency-medical-care-letter-to-health-care-providers.pdf. Accessed January 2, 2023.

Updates in Genetic Screening for the General Obstetrician

Taylor M. Dunn, MS, CGC[a],*, Akila Subramaniam, MD, MPH[b]

KEYWORDS

- Cell-free DNA • Noninvasive prenatal screening • Prenatal genetic screening
- Expanded carrier screening

KEY POINTS

- Noninvasive prenatal screening for common aneuploidies should be offered to all pregnant patients as a first-tier screening option within the first trimester.
- At this time, cell-free DNA screening for rare subchromosomal microdeletions and microduplications, rare autosomal trisomies, single-gene conditions, and genome-wide analysis for copy number variations is not recommended.
- Carrier screening, either targeted or expanded, should be offered with appropriate counseling to all pregnant patients and those considering pregnancy.
- Detailed pretest and posttest counseling reviewing the benefits, limitations, and implications of screening results should be provided to all patients offered prenatal genetic screening.

INTRODUCTION

The purpose of prenatal genetic screening is to identify pregnancies at an increased risk of chromosomal abnormalities and reproductive partners at an increased risk to have a pregnancy with an autosomal recessive or X-linked genetic condition. With this knowledge and appropriate counseling, patients can make well-informed decisions regarding their pregnancy and reproductive options. Historically, prenatal genetic screening was primarily offered to patients considered to be at high risk based on their age, ultrasound findings, family history, or reported ancestry; however, a disadvantage to this screening approach is that many affected pregnancies and at-risk partners may not be identified. For this reason, the American College of Obstetricians and Gynecologists (ACOG) and the American College of Medical Genetics and

[a] Department of Genetics, University of Alabama at Birmingham, 1720 2nd Avenue South, VH1L108B, Birmingham, AL 35294-0019, USA; [b] Division of Maternal Fetal Medicine, Department of Obstetrics and Gynecology, University of Alabama at Birmingham, 1700 6th Avenue South, Women and Infants Center, 10270, Birmingham, AL 35249, USA
* Corresponding author.
E-mail address: taylordunn@uabmc.edu

Obstet Gynecol Clin N Am 50 (2023) 493–507
https://doi.org/10.1016/j.ogc.2023.03.005
0889-8545/23/© 2023 Elsevier Inc. All rights reserved.

obgyn.theclinics.com

Genomics (ACMG) endorse offering aneuploidy screening, including cell-free DNA screening (cfDNA), and carrier screening to all pregnant patients, regardless of age, ancestry, or family history.[1–4] While prenatal genetic screening is not a new concept to obstetric health care providers, due to rapid advancements in screening technologies, the number of screening options has drastically increased, and providers are faced with the challenges of understanding the variety of screening options available, providing appropriate pretest and posttest counseling, integrating broad screening into routine prenatal care, and staying up to date on evolving guidelines and recommendations. In this article, we will summarize current recommendations for the newer cfDNA technology, provide updates for carrier screening, highlight important points to discuss in pretest and posttest counseling, and provide guidance on how to identify patients that should be referred to genetic specialists.

ANEUPLOIDY SCREENING
Background

The purpose of aneuploidy screening is to assess fetal risk of chromosomal abnormalities, historically trisomy 21 (Down syndrome), during pregnancy. While serum analyte screening and ultrasound have been clinically available for decades, cfDNA has transformed our ability to identify fetuses at increased risk of chromosomal abnormalities. cfDNA, also referred to as noninvasive prenatal screening or noninvasive prenatal testing (NIPT), analyzes fragments of DNA originating from the pregnancy, primarily placental trophoblast cells, circulating in the pregnant patients' bloodstream. There are multiple methodologies used for cfDNA, with the most common being massively parallel shotgun sequencing and single nucleotide polymorphisms–based analysis. Each methodology has advantages and limitations in certain clinical situations, and detection rates may vary slightly between laboratories; however, 1 methodology has not been found to be superior in all clinical scenarios.

cfDNA was designed to screen for the three most common aneuploidies seen in pregnancy: trisomy 21 (Down syndrome) (T21), trisomy 18 (T18), and trisomy 13 (T13). When cfDNA became commercially available in 2011, it only screened for these aneuploidies in singletons and was typically only offered to pregnant patients at increased risk of fetal aneuploidy based on age at delivery, family history of chromosomal abnormalities, or ultrasound abnormalities.[5] However, given the higher detection rate and lower screen positive rate when compared to older screening methodologies, cfDNA has rapidly been integrated into routine prenatal care as the most sensitive and specific screening method for pregnancies at increased and average risk of fetal aneuploidy.[1,4,6]

There are many benefits of cfDNA when compared to serum analyte screening including detection of fetal aneuploidies at as early as 9 to 10 weeks' gestation and the ability to be performed any time after. Additionally, ACMG recently published a systematic evidence review reporting that the use of cfDNA screening reduced the number of diagnostic tests performed by at least one-third and up to ~80% depending on the study.[6] However, it is important that obstetric health care providers and patients understand the limitations of cfDNA, most notably that cfDNA is screening and not a diagnostic testing.

Current Recommendations

In 2020, ACOG and the Society for Maternal-Fetal Medicine (SMFM) published updated clinical management guidelines on screening for fetal chromosomal abnormalities during pregnancy.[1] They recommend that all pregnant patients, regardless of age or prior risk of aneuploidy, should be offered fetal aneuploidy screening and diagnostic testing options including serum analyte screening (with or without nuchal translucency ultrasound), cfDNA screening, and prenatal diagnostic testing via chorionic villus sampling (CVS) or amniocentesis in each pregnancy.[1] The most notable update was the endorsement that cfDNA is the most sensitive and specific screening test for common fetal aneuploidies in patients of all ages; however, it is emphasized that cfDNA should not be considered diagnostic testing given the potential for false-positive and false-negative results.[1] Furthermore, ACMG recently published an updated practice guideline that strongly recommends cfDNA screening (T21, T18, T13) over traditional screening approaches for all pregnant patients with singleton and twin gestations.[4] ACMG also strongly recommends that cfDNA screening for sex chromosome aneuploidies (SCAs) be offered to all pregnant patients with singleton gestations.[4] It is important to note that regardless of the type of aneuploidy screening used, all patients should be offered a second-trimester ultrasound to evaluate fetal anatomy for any structural abnormalities.[1]

If aneuploidy screening is accepted, ACOG recommends that a single screening approach should be pursued, and multiple screening tests should not be performed simultaneously.[1] In addition, a screening test with a lower detection rate should not be performed after a successful screening test with a higher detection rate. For example, a quad screen should not be performed after successful cfDNA screening. This most commonly occurs when an obstetric health care provider intends to order serum alpha-fetoprotein (AFP) alone to evaluate for neural tube defects, but a quad screen is ordered unintentionally. Given the higher screen positive rate of serum analyte screening, this can result in conflicting screening results and increase patient anxiety without proper counseling.

Special Circumstances

Multifetal gestations

The ACOG guideline briefly reviewed the finding that cfDNA can be performed in twin gestations, but provided minimal guidance on whether this should be offered.[1] ACMG's updated practice guideline strongly recommends cfDNA screening (T21, T18, T13) over traditional screening approaches in twin gestations.[4] While the rate of cfDNA test failure is slightly increased in twin gestations when compared to singletons, the test performance of cfDNA for common aneuploidies is comparable between twin and singleton gestations.[6,7] However, cfDNA screening for SCAs is generally not available in twin gestations because of limitations of the technology.[4] Of note, it is important to report fetal number to the testing laboratory as this has significant implications for data analysis and reporting. Additionally, ACMG reports there are very limited data on cfDNA screening in triplets.[6]

Other conditions

When cfDNA screening became commercially available in 2011, it initially screened for T21 and quickly expanded to include additional common aneuploidies including T18, T13, and SCAs.[5,8,9] ACMG's systematic evidence review reported that while the sensitivity and specificity of cfDNA for SCAs are comparable to those of common aneuploidies, the positive predictive values (PPVs) are substantially lower ranging from 30% (45,X) to 74% (47, XXY; 47, XYY).[6] More recently, testing laboratories have expanded their screening to include select chromosomal microdeletions (eg, 22q11.2), single-gene conditions, rare autosomal trisomies (RATs), and genome-wide screening for large chromosomal deletions and duplications (typically >7 megabases). RATs are autosomal trisomies outside of the common aneuploidies (T21, T18,

T13) and can be associated with significant fetal anomalies, confined placental mosaicism, maternal chromosomal abnormalities, and maternal malignancy.[10]

While the body of research around cfDNA screening for these conditions is growing, ACOG does not recommend routinely screening for these conditions given the PPVs are notably lower than those for common aneuploidies, and clinical utility has not been well established.[1] However, ACMG's updated practice guideline suggests that cfDNA for 22q11.2 deletion syndrome be offered to all pregnant patients with appropriate counseling discussing the reduced sensitivity and specificity when compared to common aneuploidies and SCAs.[4] At this time, ACMG does not recommend routine cfDNA screening for other microdeletions or RATs because of low clinical utility.[4] However, as ACMG highlights, cfDNA is the only laboratory methodology that can identify these conditions at all.[6] With this is mind, there are instances where using expanded cfDNA is reasonable; however, thorough counseling on the limitations of this testing should be provided, preferably by a genetic counselor, maternal-fetal medicine specialist (MFM), or geneticist.[11]

Facilitating Decision-Making

ACOG recommends that all patients should be counseled on aneuploidy screening and diagnostic testing options in each pregnancy; therefore, obstetric health care providers must be able to discuss each patient's risk and the advantages and disadvantages of available screening and diagnostic testing options.[1] When introducing aneuploidy screening and diagnostic testing options, it is important to discuss the purpose of this testing and inform patients of their a priori risk for fetal aneuploidy. These conditions typically occur by random chance at conception and are not usually inherited. The patient's age at delivery is typically used to predict fetal aneuploidy risk; however, family history of chromosome abnormalities or prior affected pregnancy may affect this risk.

It is important to investigate whether the patient wants to know their risk of having a pregnancy affected with a chromosome abnormality. Whether the patient desires to know this information or not, they should be made aware that screening options exist to assess the risk of these conditions. If patients are interested in pursuing screening, providers should discuss their options, relative advantages and disadvantages of each, possible results, and subsequent implications for the pregnancy. A comparison of commonly used aneuploidy screening options is summarized in **Table 1**. A full review of additional serum analyte screening options can be found in ACOG Practice Bulletin 226.[1]

The advantage of serum analyte screening and cfDNA is that the screening is noninvasive with no risk to the pregnancy. The advantage of cfDNA screening over serum analyte screening is the ability to screen for more conditions, a higher detection rate, and a lower false-positive rate. Additionally, cfDNA can be performed at ~10 weeks' gestation and beyond, while serum analyte screening can only be performed at specific times in the first and second trimesters. However, a disadvantage of cfDNA is the possibility for nonreportable results or incidental findings. The advantage of diagnostic testing via CVS or amniocentesis is the definitive diagnosis provided by the results; however, these invasive procedures associated with a small risk of miscarriage. This discussion should be targeted to the individual patient, their a priori risk, as well as their personal values and goals. For example, in pregnant patients older than 35 years, it is important to inform them that serum analyte screening will likely return screen positive given their age-related a priori risk.

Pretest Counseling for cfDNA

- Conditions being screened for: Patients should be made aware of the conditions included in cfDNA. It is important to note that while cfDNA may report fetal sex, it

Table 1
Features of commonly used aneuploidy screening methodologies

Screening Method	Gestational Age for Screening (Weeks)	Conditions and Anomalies Screened For	Detection Rate for Trisomy 21	Methodology
Cell-free DNA	9–10 to term	T21, T18, T13, SCAs	99%	Sequencing of placental cfDNA
NT alone	10–14	Aneuploidy, structural anomalies	70%	NT measurement
Quad	15–22	T21, T18, NTDs	81%	hCG, AFP, uE3, DIA
Integrated	10–14 15–22	T21, T18, NTDs	96%	NT measurement, PAPP-A, hCG hCG, AFP, uE3, DIA
Anatomy scan	18–22	Structural anomalies, soft markers	50%	Ultrasound

Abbreviations: AFP, alpha-fetoprotein; cfDNA, cell-free DNA screening; DIA, dimeric inhibin A; hCG, human chorionic gonadotropin; NT, nuchal translucency; NTDs, neural tube defects; PAPP-A, pregnancy-associated plasma protein-A; uE3, unconjugated estriol.

Data from American College of Obstetricians and Gynecologists' Committee on Practice Bulletins—Obstetrics; Committee on Genetics; Society for Maternal-Fetal Medicine. Screening for Fetal Chromosomal Abnormalities: ACOG Practice Bulletin, Number 226. Obstet Gynecol. 2020;136(4):e48-e69. https://doi.org/10.1097/AOG.0000000000004084

is intended to provide information on fetal risk of common aneuploidies that may have significant implications for the pregnancy.

- Possible result types: Patients should be made aware of possible result types including positive, negative, and inconclusive or no-call results. They should understand that a positive result is not diagnostic, a negative result does not rule out the possibility of a genetic condition, and that cfDNA results are not always straightforward. Additionally, patients with obesity should be informed that chance of screen failure or no-call result increases with increasing maternal weight. Patients should also be informed that a second sample may be requested.
- Potential for incidental findings: Because cfDNA screening involves analysis of maternally derived cell-free DNA, it is possible to detect maternal chromosome abnormalities or malignancy, although these are rare. This can include mosaic Turner syndrome, trisomy X, microdeletions, and microduplications.
- Potential cost to the patient: While ACOG, SMFM, and ACMG endorse cfDNA screening for all pregnant patients, it is important to consider that this screening may not be covered by a patient's insurance. Obstetric providers should be knowledgeable on the billing procedures practiced by the testing laboratory they use. Additionally, patients can be encouraged to discuss their eligibility for coverage and remaining deductible with their insurance providers to better estimate their potential out-of-pocket cost.[12]
- Procedure for results disclosure: Patients should be made aware of the time frame within which they will be notified about their results.[12] Additionally, it is important to review how patients will be notified. For example, will results be disclosed via a phone call, a message in the patient portal, a notification from the testing laboratory, or at their next visit.

Posttest Counseling

- Results disclosure within a timely manner: Patients should be notified of their results within a reasonable time frame. When needed, this allows patients time to consider their options for further evaluation. In a prenatal setting, delays in communicating results could limit diagnostic testing options and pregnancy management decisions.[12]

Positive cfDNA Results

- Disclose positive screening result: Patients should be informed that there is an increased chance for their fetus to have the specified condition; however, the patient should understand that a positive screening result is not diagnostic for the fetus. Providers should emphasize that no irreversible decisions should be made based solely on cfDNA screening results.
- Review PPV: It important to discuss the PPV or the likelihood that the fetus is truly affected with the specified condition. Typically, testing laboratories will report a patient-specific PPV. Because PPVs incorporate disease prevalence, they are expected to be lower in average-risk populations when compared to those in high-risk populations. Additionally, PPVs may vary between laboratories, as each laboratory may include different factors when calculating patient-specific PPVs. For example, some laboratories use clinical outcome data, while others use analytical data. There are also online tools available to providers to calculate PPVs. One example is the NIPT/Cell Free DNA Screening Performance Calculator created by the Perinatal Quality Foundation and the National Society for Genetic Counselors (https://www.perinatalquality.org/Vendors/NSGC/NIPT/) which

estimates PPVs for many conditions based on estimates of population preva-lence.[13] Another option is the Positive Predictive Value of Cell Free DNA Calcu-lator developed by a group at the University of North Carolina at Chapel Hill (https://www.med.unc.edu/mfm/nips-calc/).[14] This calculator is unique in that the provider can adjust the gestational age in addition to the pregnant patient's age. This calculator uses sensitivity and specificity data from validation studies from four commonly used cfDNA testing platforms. A limitation of this calculator is that PPVs can only be estimated for common autosomal aneuploidies (T21, T18, T13).

- Review specified condition: Providers should summarize common features of the specified condition and associated prognosis.
- Potential for false-positive results: With any screening test, there is a potential for false-positive results. False-positive results can be related to the limitations of cfDNA or may be caused by many fetoplacental or maternal abnormalities including confined placental mosaicism, co-twin demise, or maternal chromo-somal abnormalities.
- Refer for genetic counseling and MFM consult: All patients who receive a positive cfDNA result should undergo genetic counseling and be offered diagnostic testing.
- Briefly review diagnostic testing options: Depending on gestational age, patients should be informed of diagnostic testing options including CVS, amniocentesis, or postnatal genetic testing.
- Provide the patient a copy of their results.

Negative cfDNA Results

- Review negative predictive value: Patients who receive a negative or low-risk screening result should be informed that while a negative result significantly re-duces the risk of the conditions evaluated, it does not guarantee that the fetus is unaffected. It is important to communicate the residual risk, or the chance that the fetus is affected despite a negative screening result. Patients receiving a negative result should be made aware that false negatives are rare, but possible.
- Review limitations of cfDNA: It is important to remind the patient that there are many genetic conditions that are not evaluated for by cfDNA. Additionally, cfDNA does not screen for open neural tube defects (ONTDs); therefore, serum AFP to screen for ONTDs should be offered at 15 to 20 weeks' gestation. Furthermore, cfDNA does not replace routine anatomy ultrasound screening.
- Provide the patient a copy of their results.

No-Call and Nonreportable cfDNA Results

An important quality metric used in cfDNA is fetal fraction, the percentage of placental cfDNA fragments over the total amount, which includes maternal and placental cfDNA fragments. Fetal fraction increases with gestational age and decreases with increasing maternal weight.[15] The fetal fraction is commonly found to be 10% by 10 weeks' gestation in the general population.[16] Because cfDNA performance improves- with higher fetal fraction, the likelihood of a no-call result is increased for samples with a fetal fraction below 3% to 4%.[16] There are many potential causes of low fetal fraction, which are outlined below.

- Review result: Notify the patient that the testing laboratory was unable to provide a fetal risk for the specified conditions. If the testing report includes further details on why testing was unable to be performed, or why the laboratory could not make a high-confidence call, this should be shared with the patient.

- Discuss potential causes of no-call results: Some no-call results are due to specimen quality issues where testing cannot be performed. Other times, testing can be performed, but a high-confidence call cannot be made after analysis. cfDNA can be influenced by many fetoplacental and maternal factors including gestational age, maternal weight, medications (eg, low-molecular-weight heparin), underlying medical conditions (eg, autoimmune conditions, malignancy), and fetoplacental aneuploidy.[16–18] When a pregnant patient receives a no-call result, they should be made aware of common causes including early gestational age and increased maternal weight. It is also important to inform the patient that there is an increased risk of fetal aneuploidy, especially trisomy 18, trisomy 13, and triploidy.[1,19,20] One testing laboratory has developed a fetal fraction-based risk model that adjusts for prior risk, maternal weight, gestational age, and the fetal fraction to better predict the likelihood of chromosomal abnormality (T13, T18, triploidy) for pregnancies with low fetal fraction.[21]
- Refer for genetic counseling: Given the information above, patients with no-call results should be referred for genetic counseling and comprehensive ultrasound and offered diagnostic testing.
- Consider offering cfDNA redraw: The testing laboratory may provide additional guidance on the likelihood of receiving a result with a second sample. For example, fetal fraction is expected to increase with gestational age; therefore, the likelihood of receiving a result may increase with greater gestational age. However, patients should be aware that a second no-call result is possible, further delaying diagnostic testing.

Incidental Findings on cfDNA

- Review result: Notify the patient that the testing laboratory reported an incidental or atypical finding. Similar to a positive screening result, patients should be informed that cfDNA is not diagnostic. Potential incidental findings can include concern for maternal chromosome abnormality, an atypical finding outside the scope of the test, or concern for maternal malignancy.
- Refer for genetic counseling and MFM consult: Any patient receiving an atypical cfDNA result (eg, positive, no-call, incidental finding) should be referred to an MFM for further evaluation and genetic counseling. It can be helpful to inform that patient that prenatal diagnostic testing or maternal testing may be offered.
- Discordant fetal sex: It is important to compare the reported fetal sex with that observed on ultrasound. If external genitalia observed on ultrasound are discrepant with cfDNA results, patients should be referred for genetic counseling and MFM consult. While the cfDNA result may be negative, the fetus may be at risk of a disorder of sex development or a genetic condition associated with sex reversal or ambiguous genitalia. Other possible explanations include laboratory error or vanishing twin.

While there are many aneuploidy screening options, cfDNA has emerged as a primary screening tool. As described above, there are many benefits of cfDNA; however, the pretest and posttest counseling discussions around cfDNA and subsequent results are much more nuanced than traditional serum analyte screening. A summary algorithm for aneuploidy screening including follow-up steps for each result type is provided in **Fig. 1**. Because cfDNA is now recommended for all pregnant patients, it is imperative obstetric health care providers understand the benefits and limitations

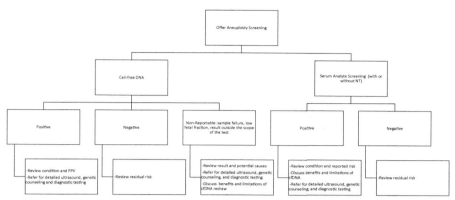

Fig. 1. A summary algorithm for aneuploidy screening including follow-up steps for each result type.

of this testing, and are equipped to provide appropriate pretest and posttest counseling.

CARRIER SCREENING
Background

The goal of carrier screening is to identify patients who are at increased risk to have a child with an inherited autosomal recessive or X-linked genetic condition. Typically, carriers of these conditions are asymptomatic and have a negative family history. Ideally, carrier screening is performed before pregnancy to allow reproductive partners to consider the full range of reproductive options available.[2] Partners at increased risk should be informed of their reproductive options including refraining from having biological children together, adoption, use of donor gamete/embryo, preimplantation genetic testing for monogenic disorders, diagnostic testing during pregnancy, or postnatal diagnostic testing.

In the past, carrier screening was offered based on a patient's reported ancestry or family history. However, we continue to learn that this screening approach is flawed and limits many patients' access to information that may have significant impacts on reproductive decision-making.[22] For this reason, professional organizations are endorsing pan-ethnic screening to ensure equitable care for patients of all ethnicities.[22] Furthermore, the decreasing cost of next-generation sequencing has allowed for simultaneous evaluation of more genes and disease-causing variants within these genes at a more affordable cost, increasing patients' access to broad screening.[22] However, the rapid expansion and implementation of carrier screening has introduced many complexities that have only begun to be addressed by ACOG and ACMG.

Current Recommendations

In 2017, ACOG stated that ethnic-specific, pan-ethnic, and expanded carrier screening (ECS) are all acceptable screening strategies for patients.[2] As seen in **Table 2**, ACOG specifically recommends that all pregnant patients and those considering pregnancy should be offered carrier screening for cystic fibrosis (CF), spinal muscular atrophy (SMA), and hemoglobinopathies.[2] In addition, those with a family history of intellectual disabilities or personal history of ovarian insufficiency should

Table 2
ACOG and ACMG carrier screening recommendations

Conditions	ACOG[2,3]	ACMG[22]
CF + SMA + hemoglobinopathies + risk-based screening (eg, fragile X, Ashkenazi Jewish ancestry)	Recommend offering to all patients	Tier 1, not recommended
Conditions with carrier frequency ≥1 in 100	Recommendation for ECS	Tier 2, not recommended
Conditions with carrier frequency ≥ 1 in 200 (including X-linked conditions)	Not addressed	Tier 3, recommend offering to all patients
Conditions with carrier frequency <1 in 200	Not addressed	Tier 4, not recommended for all patients. Should be considered for consanguineous partners, those with relevant personal or family history, and partners who desire maximum information.

Abbreviations: ACMG, American College of Medical Genetics and Genomics; ACOG, American College of Obstetricians and Gynecologists; CF, cystic fibrosis; ECS, expanded carrier screening; SMA, spinal muscular atrophy.

Data from Committee Opinion No. 690: Carrier Screening in the Age of Genomic Medicine. Obstet Gynecol. 2017;129(3):e35-e40; and Gregg AR, Aarabi M, Klugman S, et al. Screening for autosomal recessive and X-linked conditions during pregnancy and preconception: a practice resource of the American College of Medical Genetics and Genomics (ACMG). Genet Med. Oct 2021;23(10):1793-1806

be offered carrier screening for fragile X syndrome.[2] While ACOG recognizes that ethnicity-based screening has limitations, they still recommend specific screening for patients based on ethnicity (eg, Ashkenazi Jewish), personal medical history, or family history.[3] ACOG addresses that pan-ethnic or ECS can be offered depending on patients' interest. If ECS is offered, only conditions meeting the following criteria should be included: carrier frequency ≥1 in 100, well-defined phenotype, onset early in life, detrimental effect on quality of life, or cognitive or physical impairment requiring medical intervention.[2]

In contrast, in 2021, ACMG recommended that all pregnant patients or those planning a pregnancy should be offered ECS, stating that screening based on self-identified ancestry or socially defined groups is inequitable.[22] To provide additional guidance on what carrier screening options should be offered to patients, ACMG proposed a tiered approach (see **Table 2**) and recommended that all patients should be offered tier 3 carrier screening which includes autosomal recessive and X-linked conditions with a carrier frequency greater than 1 in 200.[22] Furthermore, if pregnant patients and their reproductive partner elect to proceed with simultaneous carrier screening because of time constraints, ACMG recommends that the reproductive partner be offered tier 3 carrier screening for autosomal recessive conditions only.[22]

Special Circumstances and Future Direction

As many obstetric care providers are aware, there are many barriers to carrier screening uptake in partners of pregnant patients who are known carriers. These barriers can include insurance coverage/cost, logistical challenges, and lack of understanding of the potential implication of the results.[23] One screening methodology that can overcome this challenge is single-gene NIPT (sgNIPT), which can provide fetal risk assessment for certain conditions without a paternal blood sample. Carrier screening with reflex to sgNIPT for CF, SMA, sickle cell disease, and alpha and beta thalassemias first became commercially available in 2019, with a reported analytical sensitivity of >98% and specificity of >99.9%.[24] While this methodology is still considered screening and should not replace diagnostic testing, it can provide an accurate fetal risk assessment to help guide counseling discussions around diagnostic testing.

Pretest Counseling

- Purpose of screening: Patients should be informed that carrier screening is intended to identify healthy reproductive partners that are at risk of having a pregnancy or child affected by certain inherited genetic conditions. In most cases, carriers are not expected to have symptoms of these conditions.
- Follow-up for positive results: Patients should be informed that subsequent testing for their partner may be recommended depending on their results. Furthermore, the option of prenatal diagnostic testing should be introduced.
- Potential health implications of carrier status: Pregnant patients should be informed that carriers for certain conditions may be at increased risk to develop associated clinical features. For example, Duchenne muscular dystrophy carriers are atincreased risk of cardiac disease, and fragile-X premutation carriers are at increased risk of primary ovarian insufficiency.[22]
- Review benefits and limitations of targeted versus expanded screening: While it is unrealistic to review all conditions that are being screened for on ECS, patients should be provided with general information about the groups of conditions being screened for (eg, inheritance, severity, carrier frequency). Additionally, patients should be informed that when more genes are analyzed, it is more likely to be found as a carrier.
- Limitations of screening: Patients should be informed that a negative carrier screening result greatly reduces, but does not completely eliminate, their risk to be a carrier or have an affected child.

Common Misconceptions

- "I don't have any personal or family history of genetic conditions": Patients should be informed that carrier screening is intended to identify healthy reproductive partners at risk of having an affected pregnancy or child. In most cases, carriers are not expected to have symptoms of these conditions. Furthermore, most biological parents of a child with a genetic condition have no related family history. One study of 12,000 individuals who underwent carrier screening reported that around 88% of individuals found to be carriers for CF, SMA, or fragile X syndrome had no family history.[25]
- "I am not from a high-risk ethnic group": It is important for patients to understand that while people of specific ethnic groups may have a higher chance to be a carrier for certain conditions, any person of any ethnicity can be a carrier. Furthermore, many people may not know their full ancestry.
- "If I find out I am a carrier, it won't change anything for this pregnancy": Patients should be made aware that there are more options than invasive diagnostic testing or termination of affected pregnancies. Even if partners decline these

options, they can learn more about the genetic condition, available treatments, interventions, and identify support groups and medical specialists.

Posttest Counseling

Positive result

- Review the conditions the patient was found to be a carrier for: It is important to provide general information on the natural history of the specified condition(s) and their inheritance. Review that this result is not diagnostic for the fetus. Additionally, it is important to notify patients if their carrier status is associated with health implications.
- Discuss next steps: For patients found to be a carrier for autosomal recessive conditions, their reproductive partner should be offered screening either for the specific condition or expanded screening. For patients found to be carriers for an X-linked condition, male reproductive partners do not need to be screened.
- Referral for genetic counseling or MFM consultation: Patients or reproductive partners found to be carriers can be referred for genetic counseling to provide in-depth counseling on the variant identified, the associated genetic condition, inheritance pattern, risk for the current or potential pregnancy, and prenatal and postnatal testing options.
- Provide the patient a copy of their results.

Negative result

- Review residual risk: Patients should be informed that a negative carrier screening result greatly reduces the risk of being a carrier, but does not completely eliminate the chance.[22] After a negative carrier screening result, each individual still has a residual risk to be a carrier, which is typically provided by the testing laboratory. This residual risk is still present given all causative genes may not be known, all genes associated with a condition may not be evaluated, all causative variants may not be detected because of technical limitations, and variants may be misclassified.[22]
- Review limitations of carrier screening: It is important to remind the patient that there are many genetic conditions that are not evaluated by carrier screening (eg, de novo variants). A negative carrier screening does not eliminate the risk to have a child with a genetic condition.
- Provide the patient a copy of their results.

SUMMARY

Prenatal genetic screening, including aneuploidy screening and carrier screening, has expanded drastically with rapid advancements in DNA sequencing technologies. This expansion has challenged obstetric health care providers as they are expected to integrate broad screening into routine prenatal care, understand these complex technologies, and appropriately counsel on the results. As our understanding of genetic variants and conditions continue to evolve, it is imperative that obstetric health care providers are well informed on current guidelines and recommendations to provide consistent and equitable care to all patients. Furthermore, obstetric providers that do not feel equipped to appropriately counsel their patients on screening options or results should consider a referral to a genetic counselor, MFM specialist, or other genetics specialist to help facilitate this process.[12]

CLINICS CARE POINTS

- Multiple studies have illustrated that cfDNA is the most sensitive and specific screening test for common fetal aneuploidies in patients of all ages, and should be offered to all pregnant patients with singleton and twin gestations as a first-tier screening option. However, false-positive and false-negative results are possible, and cfDNA should not be considered diagnostic testing.
- The body of research around cfDNA screening for rare microdeletions, rare autosomal trisomies, single-gene conditions, and genome-wide analysis is growing; however, routine cfDNA screening for these conditions is generally not recommended given the low positive predictive values (PPVs) and limited clinical utility.
- Important points to review in pretest counseling for cfDNA include what conditions are being screened for, possible result types and their implications for the pregnancy, potential cost to the patient, and procedure for results disclosure.
- When disclosing a positive cfDNA result, it is important to review that screening results are not diagnostic, provide the positive predictive value, discuss the natural history of the specified condition, and offer a referral for genetic counseling and MFM consultation to further discuss the results and diagnostic testing options.
- When disclosing a no-call result, it is helpful to review common causes including sample failure, early gestational age, increased maternal weight, and fetal aneuploidy. A discussion around the benefits and limitations of cell-free DNA redraw should occur, and patients should be offered a referral for genetic counseling and MFM consultation for further evaluation.
- Research suggests that ethnicity and family history based carrier screening approaches are flawed and inequitable. To promote more equitable care, pan-ethnic carrier screening, either targeted or expanded, should be offered with appropriate counseling to all pregnant patients and those considering pregnancy.
- When disclosing a positive carrier screening result, it is important to review the natural history of the condition(s), the inheritance patterns, and whether their carrier status is associated with health implications. Reproductive partner screening should be offered if a patient is found to be a carrier for an autosomal recessive condition. If a patient is found to be a carrier only for an X-linked condition, male reproductive partners do not need to be screened.
- When disclosing a negative cfDNA or carrier screening result, it is important to review residual risks and limitations of the screening.

DISCLOSURE

The authors have nothing to disclose.

REFERENCES

1. American College of Obstetricians and Gynecologists' Committee on Practice Bulletins-Obstetrics. Committee on Genetics SfM-FM. Screening for Fetal Chromosomal Abnormalities: ACOG Practice Bulletin, Number 226. Obstet Gynecol 2020;136(4):e48–69.
2. Committee Opinion No. 690: Carrier Screening in the Age of Genomic Medicine. Obstet Gynecol 2017;129(3):e35–40.
3. Committee Opinion No. 691: Carrier Screening for Genetic Conditions. Obstet Gynecol 2017;129(3):e41–55.

4. Dungan JS, Klugman S, Darilek S, et al. Noninvasive prenatal screening (NIPS) for fetal chromosome abnormalities in a general-risk population: An evidence-based clinical guideline of the American College of Medical Genetics and Genomics (ACMG). Genet Med 2022. https://doi.org/10.1016/j.gim.2022.11.004.

5. Palomaki GE, Kloza EM, Lambert-Messerlian GM, et al. DNA sequencing of maternal plasma to detect Down syndrome: an international clinical validation study. Genet Med 2011;13(11):913–20.

6. Rose NC, Barrie ES, Malinowski J, et al. Systematic evidence-based review: The application of noninvasive prenatal screening using cell-free DNA in general-risk pregnancies. Genet Med 2022;24(9):1992.

7. Dyr B, Boomer T, Almasri EA, et al. A new era in aneuploidy screening: cfDNA testing in >30,000 multifetal gestations: Experience at one clinical laboratory. PLoS One 2019;14(8):e0220979.

8. Palomaki GE, Deciu C, Kloza EM, et al. DNA sequencing of maternal plasma reliably identifies trisomy 18 and trisomy 13 as well as Down syndrome: an international collaborative study. Genet Med 2012;14(3):296–305.

9. Samango-Sprouse C, Banjevic M, Ryan A, et al. SNP-based non-invasive prenatal testing detects sex chromosome aneuploidies with high accuracy. Prenat Diagn 2013;33(7):643–9.

10. Scott F, Bonifacio M, Sandow R, et al. Rare autosomal trisomies: Important and not so rare. Prenat Diagn. Sep 2018;38(10):765–71.

11. Shaw J, Scotchman E, Chandler N, et al. Preimplantation genetic testing: Noninvasive prenatal testing for aneuploidy, copy-number variants and single-gene disorders. Reproduction 2020;160(5):A1–11.

12. Committee Opinion No. 693: Counseling About Genetic Testing and Communication of Genetic Test Results. Obstet Gynecol 2017;129(4):e96–101.

13. NIPT/Cell Free DNA Screening Performance Calculator. Available at: https://www.perinatalquality.org/Vendors/NSGC/NIPT/. Accessed November 22, 2022.

14. Positive Predictive Value of Cell Free DNA Calculator. Available at: https://www.med.unc.edu/mfm/nips-calc/. Accessed November 22, 2022.

15. Kinnings SL, Geis JA, Almasri E, et al. Factors affecting levels of circulating cell-free fetal DNA in maternal plasma and their implications for noninvasive prenatal testing. Prenat Diagn 2015;35(8):816–22.

16. Canick JA, Palomaki GE, Kloza EM, et al. The impact of maternal plasma DNA fetal fraction on next generation sequencing tests for common fetal aneuploidies. Prenat Diagn 2013;33(7):667–74.

17. Wang E, Batey A, Struble C, et al. Gestational age and maternal weight effects on fetal cell-free DNA in maternal plasma. Prenat Diagn 2013;33(7):662–6.

18. Suzumori N, Ebara T, Yamada T, et al. Fetal cell-free DNA fraction in maternal plasma is affected by fetal trisomy. J Hum Genet 2016;61(7):647–52.

19. Palomaki GE, Kloza EM, Lambert-Messerlian GM, et al. Circulating cell free DNA testing: are some test failures informative? Prenat Diagn 2015;35(3):289–93.

20. Revello R, Sarno L, Ispas A, et al. Screening for trisomies by cell-free DNA testing of maternal blood: consequences of a failed result. Ultrasound Obstet Gynecol 2016;47(6):698–704.

21. McKanna T, Ryan A, Krinshpun S, et al. Fetal fraction-based risk algorithm for non-invasive prenatal testing: screening for trisomies 13 and 18 and triploidy in women with low cell-free fetal DNA. Ultrasound Obstet Gynecol 2019;53(1):73–9.

22. Gregg AR, Aarabi M, Klugman S, et al. Screening for autosomal recessive and X-linked conditions during pregnancy and preconception: a practice resource

of the American College of Medical Genetics and Genomics (ACMG). Genet Med 2021;23(10):1793–806.
23. Carlotti K, Hines K, Weida J, et al. Perceived barriers to paternal expanded carrier screening following a positive maternal result: To screen or not to screen. J Genet Couns 2021;30(2):470–7.
24. Tsao DS, Silas S, Landry BP, et al. A novel high-throughput molecular counting method with single base-pair resolution enables accurate single-gene NIPT. Sci Rep 2019;9(1):14382.
25. Archibald AD, Smith MJ, Burgess T, et al. Reproductive genetic carrier screening for cystic fibrosis, fragile X syndrome, and spinal muscular atrophy in Australia: outcomes of 12,000 tests. Genet Med 2018;20(5):513–23.

Prenatal Contraceptive Counseling

Lauren Thaxton, MD, MBA, MS[a], Lisa G. Hofler, MD, MPH, MBA[b],*

KEYWORDS

- Contraception counseling • Postpartum contraception
- Immediate postpartum LARC • Tubal ligation

KEY POINTS

- Counseling about family planning and desired birth spacing is an essential component of pregnancy care.
- It is a best practice to include contraception conversations at a standard prenatal visit around 32 weeks to permit time for planning inpatient postpartum contraception such as long-acting reversible contraception or tubal surgery, if desired.
- The postpartum hospitalization is a unique window for access to contraception: patients are known to not be pregnant and they have access to health coverage and health-care providers.
- Special considerations for contraception in the postpartum time include venous thromboembolism risk, lactation, and uterine involution.

INTRODUCTION
Birth Spacing and Family Planning

Discussions about patients' desires (or not) for future pregnancies and ideal family size are a vital component of prenatal care. The antenatal window offers a unique opportunity to collaboratively discuss how to reach a patient's reproductive goals: postpartum patients are more likely to have health-care coverage and an established relationship with a care provider, and they do not have the time pressure of an immediate concern for unplanned pregnancy.

Ideal spacing between pregnancies is best determined by the patient. Clinicians can, however, contextualize conversations by providing medical information about the risks and benefits of certain timing. The World Health Organization (WHO) recommends birth spacing of 2 to 3 years[1] while the American College of Obstetricians and

[a] Department of Women's Health, Dell Medical School, University of Texas, 2508 Greenlawn Parkway, Austin, TX 78757, USA; [b] Department of Obstetrics & Gynecology, University of New Mexico Health Sciences Center, 1 University of New Mexico, MSC10 5580, Albuquerque, NM 87131, USA
* Corresponding author. Division of Complex Family Planning, University of New Mexico School of Medicine, 1 University of New Mexico, MSC10 5580, Albuquerque, NM 87131.
E-mail address: lhofler@salud.unm.edu

Obstet Gynecol Clin N Am 50 (2023) 509–523
https://doi.org/10.1016/j.ogc.2023.03.006
0889-8545/23/© 2023 Elsevier Inc. All rights reserved.

Gynecologists (ACOG)[2] recommends at least 6 months with a discussion of risks and benefits between 6 and 18 months. Short interpregnancy intervals (IPIs) are defined as a new pregnancy occurring less than 18 months after giving birth. Observational studies indicate short IPIs are associated with an increase in maternal and fetal adverse outcomes, including uterine rupture in people attempting a trial of labor after an earlier cesarean delivery, low birth weight, preterm birth, and newborns that are small for gestational age.[3] Yet, more than a third of deliveries (35%) in the United States demonstrate a short IPI.[4] Short IPIs are even more common among people of color and are one contributing factor in the disparities in birth outcomes. For all these reasons, the federal government has set a Healthy People 2030 target to reduce the incidence of short IPI birth to 26.9%.

Postpartum Sexual Function

Commonly, clinicians encourage 6 weeks of pelvic rest after birth, yet nearly half of women have resumed intercourse before that time and nearly all have resumed intercourse by 3 months postpartum.[5] Because there is no particular risk of sexual intercourse before 6 weeks (other than short IPI) and many return to sex sooner than that, clinicians could instead focus on preparing patients for intercourse on a timeline of the patient's choosing. This counseling should include information about expected return to fertility and anticipatory guidance about postpartum sexual function.

The postpartum state is associated with bodily changes including weight fluctuation, vaginal atrophy, perineal lacerations and healing, incontinence and pelvic floor disorders, all of which might affect a person's sexual desire and satisfaction. Additionally, postpartum depression, poor sleep, or relational conflict might also affect sexual health. These associations are poorly studied as are interventions,[6] so it is unsurprising that many postpartum care providers feel uncomfortable bringing up the topic of postpartum sexual satisfaction. Using screening tools such as the Female Sexual Function Index[7] universally for pregnant and postpartum patients could help providers identify and respond to dysfunction where it exists.

Patient-Centered Counseling

Once desired birth spacing and a timeline for return to intercourse have been established, contraceptive knowledge and access are necessary to help people achieve these goals. Clinics should implement systems that promote client-centered, shared decision-making around contraception.[8] This model of counseling draws on the reproductive justice framework, acknowledging historical injustices of reproductive coercion that disproportionately affect people of color, recognizing provider biases that can affect counseling and centering the patient's voiced priorities and preferences; **Box 1** contains additional resources. In addition to providing nonbiased counseling, clinicians and health systems must be prepared to deliver on patient-expressed desires for the full range of contraceptive options in a timely manner. This should include the ability to start and stop a chosen method of contraception because contraceptive preferences could also change during the course of one's life span.

Metrics of success around postpartum contraception should reflect the goal of providing quality counseling and timely access to patient-desired contraceptive options, rather than establishing a target for use of any particular method. The Person-Centered Contraceptive Counseling Measure[8] is a 4-item measure that was endorsed by the National Quality Forum and could be used by clinics to quantify the quality of patient experience (see **Box 1**).

Quality prenatal contraception counseling should also include information about unique postpartum considerations such as lactation, increased venous

---

Box 1
Additional resources for contraceptive counseling and provision

Improving Contraceptive Counseling through Shared Decision-Making Curriculum

   Available at https://www.innovating-education.org/2016/03/2743/

Person-Centered Contraceptive Counseling Measure

   Available at https://pcccmeasure.ucsf.edu/

American College of Obstetricians and Gynecologists Postpartum Contraceptive Access
Initiative Resources

   Available at https://pcainitiative.acog.org/

SPIRES Postpartum IUD Insertion Training Demonstration

   Available at https://www.youtube.com/watch?v=uMcTsuf8XxQ

---

thromboembolism (VTE) risk, and comorbidities of pregnancy such as hypertension, diabetes, and cardiac disease. With all these considerations, it is a best practice to include contraception conversations at one or more standard prenatal visits around 32 weeks to permit time for ongoing discussion and planning.

DISCUSSION
Contraceptive Method Overview and Effectiveness

Many contraceptive options are currently available in the United States (**Table 1**). The most commonly used methods include oral contraceptive pills, long-acting reversible contraception (LARC, which includes the contraceptive implant and intrauterine devices [IUDs]), and permanent contraception.[9]

The US Centers for Disease Control and Prevention (CDC) uses a 3-tiered system of contraceptive efficacy, with the most effective methods (contraceptive implants and IUDs, and the permanent methods of vasectomy and tubal sterilization, all with effectiveness >99%) categorized as tier 1 (**Fig. 1**).[10] User-dependent prescription methods, with typical use effectiveness around 90% to 95%, are categorized as tier 2, and less-effective methods are tier 3.

Postpartum patients may safely use the full range of contraceptive options after delivery. There are, however, some considerations unique to the postpartum population and additional contraceptive methods only available in the postpartum period, including lactational amenorrhea and immediate postpartum LARC.

Contraceptive Method Eligibility During the Postpartum Period

The CDC publishes the US Medical Eligibility Criteria for Contraceptive Use[10] (US MEC), which provides recommendations about using contraceptive methods for patients with certain medical conditions and other characteristics. These recommendations are intended to assist health-care practitioners in counseling patients through the contraceptive decision-making process. Each medical condition or characteristic is assigned a category for each contraceptive method, ranging from 1, a condition for which there is no restriction for the use of the contraceptive method, to 4, a condition that represents an unacceptable health risk if the contraceptive method is used (**Table 2**). Many clinicians consider category 1 and 2 methods acceptable for use, and category 3 and 4 methods generally unacceptable. Under some circumstances, a category 3 contraceptive method might be the only acceptable option for some patients, and this choice requires careful shared decision-making and ongoing monitoring.

Table 1
Contraceptive methods commonly used in the United States

	Method	Timing of Use	Typical Use Pregnancy Risk	Example Brand Name(s)
Estrogen and progestin: CHC	COCPs	Daily	Tier 2: 9%	Dozens of COCP brands
	Contraceptive patch	Weekly	Tier 2: 9%	Xulane, Twirla
	Combined vaginal ring	Monthly	Tier 2: 9%	NuvaRing
Progestin-only contraception (POC)	Contraceptive implant	FDA approved: 3 y Evidence-based: 5 y	Tier 1: 0.05%	Nexplanon
	Hormonal IUDs	3–8 y	Tier 1: 0.2%	Kyleena Liletta Mirena Skyla
	POPs	Daily	Tier 2: 9%	Norethindrone: Heather, Nora-Be, Lyleq Drospirenone: Slynd
	Injectable contraception	Every 12 wk	Tier 2: 6%	Depo-Provera, Depo-SQ, DMPA
	Progestin-only ring	Yearly	Tier 2: 9%	Annovera
Nonhormonal contraception	Copper IUD	FDA approved: 10 y Evidence-based: 12+ y	Tier 1: 0.8%	Paragard
	Female permanent contraception	Indefinitely	Tier 1: 0.5%	Tubal ligation, salpingectomy
	Male permanent contraception	Indefinitely	Tier 1: 0.15%	Vasectomy
	Internal and external condoms	With each act of intercourse	Tier 3: 18%–21%	Durex, FC2, Glyde, Lifestyles, Trojan
	Diaphragm	With each act of intercourse	Tier 2: 12%	Caya
	Contraceptive vaginal gel	With each act of intercourse	Not categorized	Phexxi
	Spermicide	With each act of intercourse	Tier 3: 28%	Conceptrol, Encare, VCF
	Contraceptive sponge	With each act of intercourse	Tier 3: 12% if nulliparous; 24% if parous	Today Sponge
Behavioral contraception	Withdrawal	With each act of intercourse	Tier 3: 22%	
	Lactational amenorrhea (LAM)	Up to 6 mo after birth	Not categorized	
	Fertility awareness-based methods (FABM)	Continuously	Tier 3: 24%	Standard Days, Sympto-Thermal, Two-Day

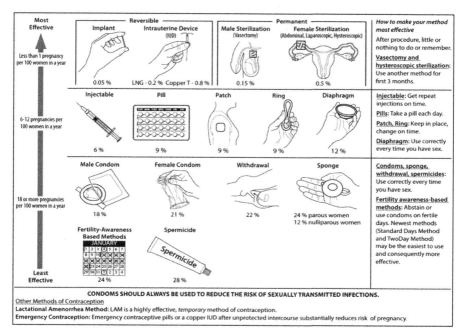

Fig. 1. Effectiveness of contraceptive methods. The percentages indicate the number out of every 100 women who experienced an unintended pregnancy within the first year of typical use of each contraceptive method. (*Adapted from* World Health Organization. (2011). Family planning: a global handbook for providers: 2011 update: evidence-based guidance developed through worldwide collaboration. World Health Organization. Available at https://apps.who.int/iris/handle/10665/44028; and Trussell J. Contraceptive failure in the United States. Contraception. 2011;83(5):397 to 404; with permission)

The US MEC specifically comments on certain postpartum characteristics, in addition to general medical conditions. **Table 3** summarizes medical eligibility for different contraceptive methods at different times during the postpartum period. All methods except estrogen-containing methods, and IUDs in the setting of postpartum sepsis, are generally acceptable to initiate at any time during the postpartum period.

Table 2
Categories of medical eligibility criteria for contraceptive use

Category	Definition
1	A condition for which there is no restriction for the use of the contraceptive method
2	A condition for which the advantages of using the method generally outweigh the theoretic or proven risks
3	A condition for which the theoretic or proven risks usually outweigh the advantages of using a contraceptive method
4	A condition that represents an unacceptable health risk if the contraceptive method is used

From Tepper NK, Curtis KM, Cox S, Whiteman MK. Update to U.S. Medical Eligibility Criteria for Contraceptive Use, 2016: Updated Recommendations for the Use of Contraception Among Women at High Risk for HIV Infection. MMWR Morb Mortal Wkly Rep 2020;69:405 to 410. DOI: https://doi.org/10.15585/mmwr.mm6914a3

Table 3
Medical eligibility for postpartum contraceptive use by timing of method initiation and breastfeeding status

Method	<21 d BF	<21 d NBF	21 d–4 wk[a] / 21 d–30 d BF	21 d–30 d NBF	4 wk[a]–42 d / 30 d–42 d	>42 d
Copper IUD[b]	<10 min: 1 >10 min: 2	<10 min: 1 >10 min: 2	2	2	1	1
Hormonal IUD[b]	2	<10 min: 1 >10 min: 2	2	2	1	1
Implant	2	1	2	1	1	1
DMPA	2	1	2	1	1	1
POC	2	1	2	1	1	1
CHC	4	4	3	With VTE risk factors: 3 No VTE risk factors: 2	With VTE risk factors: 3 No VTE risk factors: 2	BF: 2 NBF: 1

Abbreviations: BF, breastfeeding; CHC, combined hormonal contraception; DMPA, depot medroxyprogesterone acetate; IUD, intrauterine device; NBF, non-breastfeeding; POC, progestin-only contraception; VTE, venous thromboembolism.
[a] This time category boundary is 4 wk for IUDs and 30 d for all other methods.
[b] Postpartum sepsis is a category 4 condition for immediate postpartum IUD placement.
Adapted from Tepper NK, Curtis KM, Cox S, Whiteman MK. Update to U.S. Medical Eligibility Criteria for Contraceptive Use, 2016: Updated Recommendations for the Use of Contraception Among Women at High Risk for HIV Infection. MMWR Morb Mortal Wkly Rep 2020;69:405 to 410. DOI: https://doi.org/10.15585/mmwr.mm6914a3

Special Consideration: Venous Thromboembolism

Pregnancy and the postpartum period are associated with an increased risk of VTE; this risk seems to decrease gradually after birth (**Fig. 2**).[11] Because estrogen-containing contraceptive methods also increase the risk of VTE, the timing of postpartum contraceptive initiation depends on the method chosen.

The CDC considers nonhormonal and progestin-only methods, such as progestin-only pills (POPs), depot medroxyprogesterone acetate (DMPA), and the contraceptive implant and IUDs, to be safe to use immediately postpartum, assigning these methods category 1 status.

In contrast, because pregnancy increases the risk of VTE, combined hormonal contraception (CHC: estrogen-containing pills, contraceptive patches, and the combined vaginal ring) is not assigned a category 2 status until greater than 21 days postpartum for people without risk factors for VTE. For people with additional risk factors for VTE but conditions that would not otherwise contraindicate combined hormonal methods, including age 35 years or older, immobility, transfusion at delivery, obesity, postpartum hemorrhage, postcesarean delivery, preeclampsia, or smoking, estrogen-containing contraception should not be used until more than 42 days postpartum.

Special Consideration: Breastfeeding

The CDC considers progestin-only and nonhormonal contraceptive methods safe for use with breastfeeding, assigning these methods category 1 or 2 through 30 days postpartum and category 1 thereafter[10] (see **Table 3**). The effect of progestin-only

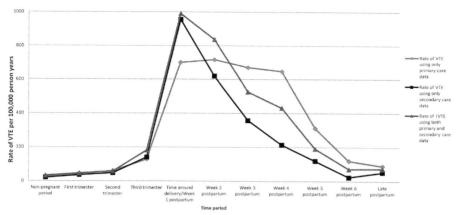

Fig. 2. Risk of venous thromboembolism around pregnancy and the postpartum period. (*From* Abdul Sultan A, Tata LJ, Grainge MJ, West J. The incidence of first venous thromboembolism in and around pregnancy using linked primary and secondary care data: a population based cohort study from England and comparative meta-analysis. PLoS One. 2013;8(7):e70310. Published 2013 Jul 29)

contraception on breastfeeding continues to be extensively studied. Available evidence indicates no impact of progestin-only contraception on lactogenesis, on exclusive breastfeeding, or on any breastfeeding.[12,13] Theoretic concerns about impaired milk production are not borne out by any research to date.[14,15]

Special Consideration: Hypertension in Pregnancy

Because CHC can increase arterial blood pressure among some users, estrogen-containing methods should be avoided in people with hypertensive disease.[16,17] However, patients with a history of high blood pressure during pregnancy, when the current blood pressure is normal, may use any contraceptive method safely because the US MEC considers even estrogen-containing methods to be category 2.

Special Consideration: Peripartum Cardiomyopathy

Just as estrogen can increase cardiovascular complications with hypertensive disease, estrogen-containing contraceptive methods can similarly increase cardiovascular risk for patients with peripartum cardiomyopathy. The US MEC considers all CHC category 4 within the first 6 months of diagnosis and for patients with New York Heart Association (NYHA) Functional Class 3 or 4, and category 3 for all other people with peripartum cardiomyopathy. In contrast, all progestin-only and nonhormonal methods are category 1 or 2 regardless of timing after peripartum cardiomyopathy diagnosis or NYHA functional class.[18]

Immediate Postpartum Long-Acting Reversible Contraception

Contraceptive implants and IUDs, categorized as LARC, are a group of highly effective contraceptive methods that provide similar contraceptive efficacy to permanent contraception, with the benefit of rapid return to fertility after discontinuation.[19] The progestin-only contraceptive implant is placed subcutaneously in the inner upper arm and is effective for up to 5 years.[20] One copper-containing and 4 progestin-only IUDs are available in the United States, with effectiveness lasting from 3 years to 12 or more years, depending on the IUD (see **Table 2**).

The immediate postpartum period, before hospital discharge after birth, is an ideal time for people to access a contraceptive implant or IUD if this is their desired post-partum contraceptive method. These LARC methods typically require an office pro-cedure for placement and health systems often require more than one visit to obtain the device; immediate postpartum placement relieves the need for one or more sepa-rate postpartum contraceptive appointments. Hospitals and health systems should work to offer immediate postpartum LARC methods to all people who desire them; ACOG considers this a best practice.[21,22]

Because LARC devices have historically been placed only at outpatient office visits, many states have implemented policies to create payment mechanisms for these de-vices during the inpatient stay for birth.[23] States that have implemented such efforts have improved access to immediate postpartum LARC.[24] Several resources exist to help hospitals and health systems implement immediate postpartum LARC.[25] In particular, ACOG's Postpartum Contraceptive Access Initiative program includes billing, finance, and implementation trainings for clinical and nonclinical personnel.[26]

IMMEDIATE POSTPARTUM IMPLANTS

The contraceptive implant may be placed at any time during the postpartum period. For patients who desire a contraceptive implant before hospital discharge, informed consent should include the same risks and benefits as for office placement. The pro-cedure for immediate postpartum implant placement is also identical to office place-ment. Clinicians who wish to offer contraceptive implants must undergo US Food and Drug Administration (FDA)-required training in implant placement and removal.

IMMEDIATE POSTPARTUM INTRAUTERINE DEVICES

For those patients whose chosen contraceptive method is an IUD, the discussion around timing of placement includes additional considerations in the immediate post-partum period. Immediate postpartum IUD placement can be very convenient for pa-tients, particularly those undergoing cesarean delivery or for those who choose epidural anesthesia for birth; even unmedicated patients note the IUD placement is generally convenient and the baby distracts them from the procedure.[27] In addition, the risk of uterine perforation is extremely low in the immediate postpartum period; of-fice IUD placement carries a low, but increased, risk of uterine perforation, particularly among people who are postpartum and breastfeeding.[28]

Immediate postpartum IUD placement may come with other risks. Patients should be aware that birth circumstances such as ongoing postpartum hemorrhage or atony, or intra-amniotic inflammation and/or infection, might preclude IUD placement. In these circumstances, often patients who desire immediate postpartum IUD can plan later office placement as a backup. Risk of IUD expulsion is higher after immedi-ate postpartum placement (overall 10.2% expulsion rate); IUDs placed immediately af-ter cesarean birth have lower expulsion rates than those placed after vaginal birth (3.5% vs 14.8%).[29] When placed immediately after vaginal birth, copper IUDs have lower expulsion rates than hormonal IUDs (12.4% vs 27.4%); after cesarean birth, expulsion rates are not statistically different between IUD types. IUD expulsion risk is higher for IUDs placed in the first few days after birth (13.2% expulsion rate), compared with immediately after the delivery of the placenta. Expulsion risk de-creases in the early postpartum (2–3 weeks after birth) period and beyond.[30,31] People generally recognize an expulsion in the postpartum period and can have another IUD placed without delay. Finally, the incidence of missing IUD strings, or strings that do not extrude from the uterine cervix, is higher after immediate postpartum IUD placement.

IMMEDIATE POSTPARTUM INTRAUTERINE DEVICE INSERTION TECHNIQUE

Research suggests that placing an IUD immediately after delivery of the placenta reduces expulsion risk, as does fundal placement of the device. The procedure for placing an IUD at the time of cesarean delivery is straightforward; the manufacturer's inserter may be used to deploy the IUD at the uterine fundus, or the device may be removed from its inserter and placed at the fundus using a sterile ring forceps or the surgeon's hand. Before placement, it is recommended to trim the strings of a hormonal IUD to approximately 10 to 12 cm, inclusive of the IUD; copper IUD strings do not require trimming. Following IUD placement, the hysterotomy is closed in the usual manner.

For immediate postplacental IUD placement after vaginal birth, the manufacturer's inserter is not sufficiently lengthy to reach the uterine fundus. The IUD must be sterilely removed from the manufacturer's inserter and placed at the uterine fundus, most often using a long ring or Kelly forceps. Similar to placement at cesarean delivery, hormonal IUD strings should be trimmed to approximately 10 to 12 cm before placement, and copper IUD strings do not require trimming. Ultrasound guidance is not necessary for placement but might be helpful as clinicians gain experience in the procedure.

Lactational Amenorrhea

Breastfeeding confers many maternal and neonatal benefits, including reduced risk of obesity in both the newborn and the mother, reduced infections and hospitalizations of the newborn, and reduced maternal risks of breast and ovarian cancer. Exclusive breastfeeding can also be used as a temporary method of contraception.

When a newborn is put to the breast to feed, prolactin is released, providing a negative feedback to the hypothalamus and ceasing the pulsatile release of gonadotropin releasing hormone. Downstream, this results in cessation of the release of luteinizing hormone (LH) from the pituitary; the lack of LH surge results in suppression of ovulation. This hypothalamic hypogonadism is the mechanism for lactation as a contraception method as well as a method of maintaining amenorrhea after birth.

People relying on lactational amenorrhea as a method of contraception should be counseled that 3 criteria must be met for this method to be effective:

1. It must be less than 6 months from the birth,
2. They must be exclusively breastfeeding, and
3. They must be amenorrheic.

In the absence of any one of these criteria, the efficacy of lactation as a contraceptive method declines.[32]

Exclusive breastfeeding also results in lower circulating estrogen, which affects vulvovaginal health; breastfeeding women should be counseled about vaginal atrophy. Topical estrogens can be used to treat symptoms such as vulvovaginal itching or pain with vaginal intercourse if they occur.

Combined Hormonal Contraception

The combined oral contraceptive pill (COCP, "the pill") is the most common reversible method of contraception used by US women, representing 14% of the method mix in 2017 to 2019.[9] COCPs include both estrogen and progestin components and function by inhibiting the HPO axis and thereby preventing ovulation. The pill is taken daily to be effective; missed pills are the most common reason for contraceptive failure.

However, there are nondaily, nonoral CHC formulations including the vaginal ring and the patch. The ring is placed into the vagina every month, and the patch is placed on the skin every week.

CHCs offer noncontraceptive benefits that patients might desire including lighter, more regular, and less painful periods. Additionally, they offer nongynecologic benefits including reduction of acne and hair growth as well as cancer risk reduction.[33] Some patients might also prefer CHCs as contraceptive options that they can easily start and stop on their own.

CHCs contain estrogen, which increases the VTE risk. For this reason, they should be deferred until 21 days postpartum for low-risk patients, and through at least 42 days for patients with additional VTE risk factors. All patients who experience peripartum cardiomyopathy should not use CHCs in the first 6 months after birth. Thereafter CHCs are not a preferred method (category 3) but can be considered in patients with normal or mildly impaired cardiac function.

Other absolute contraindications for CHCs include tobacco smoking over age 35, uncontrolled hypertension, current VTE or past VTE with a high risk of recurrence, ischemic heart disease, history of cerebrovascular accident, complicated valvular heart disease, migraine headache with aura, current breast cancer, diabetes with end-organ damage (eg, retinopathy, nephropathy, or neuropathy), severe cirrhosis or liver tumors (adenomas or hepatomas), complicated solid organ transplants, and lupus with positive or unknown antiphospholipid antibody status. Health histories should be reviewed for these contraindications before prescribing CHCs.

Progestin-Only Contraception

Progestin-only contraceptives include the injectable contraceptive DMPA, POPs, the progestin-only vaginal ring, and hormonal IUDs and the contraceptive implant. All these methods can be started immediately after delivery with no effect on breastfeeding or VTE risk. Progestin-only methods do have the side effect of an irregular bleeding pattern. This might not be bothersome in the first few weeks after birth where irregular bleeding is to be expected but some patients find this side effect to be bothersome thereafter.

DMPA is an injection administered intramuscularly or subcutaneously once every 3 months (12–15 weeks) that functions by suppressing ovulation and thickening cervical mucus. Primary side effects of DMPA include irregular bleeding and modest weight gain.[34] Other considerations with DMPA include that once administered, the effects of the shot cannot be reversed, and therefore, people must wait for the DMPA to clear if they experience bothersome side effects. Additionally, the FDA has placed a black-box warning on DMPA that it should not be used for greater than 2 years due to concerns about bone mineral density.[35] Pregnancy and lactation also confer a lower bone mineral density.[36] However, bone mineral density measurement using dual-energy X-ray absorptiometry is studied as an indicator of fracture risk in postmenopausal women, a different population from recently pregnant people or people using contraception to prevent pregnancy. There is no evidence to suggest that low bone mineral density in a reproductively aged population confers the same risk. Additionally, changes in bone mineral density that occur both with DMPA and pregnancy and lactation have been found to be reversible. For these reasons, ACOG[37] and the WHO[37] both agree that usage beyond 2 years is acceptable after weighing risks and benefits.

POPs are taken orally once daily and function primarily by thickening cervical mucus. POPs have a shorter half-life than COCPs and therefore efficacy decreases quickly with missed doses. A new POP approved by the FDA in 2019 utilizes drospirenone as the active progestin and therefore has a longer half-life than norethindrone POPs. This might be a more efficacious and realistic option for postpartum parents.

Nonhormonal Contraception

Barrier methods of contraception create physical barriers preventing sperm and egg from meeting, or methods that inactivate sperm. These include condoms (both external and internal), diaphragms, the sponge and cervical caps, spermicides, or nonhormonal vaginal gels that lower vaginal pH. These methods must be used with every episode of intercourse, which might be difficult to plan when parenting. Additionally, the diaphragm, sponge, and cervical cap are designed for the nonpostpartum anatomy; initiation of these methods is recommended to be delayed until 6 weeks after delivery for this reason. Condoms are also effective at preventing sexually transmitted infections and can be purchased over the counter, which might make them more accessible to busy postpartum patients. All the methods within this category are nonhormonal, which might be a priority for some people.

Postpartum Tubal Permanent Contraception

Tubal permanent contraception is among the most popular contraceptive methods.[9] In this form of permanent contraception, the fallopian tube is interrupted via a clip or ring device, or is partially or completely removed, preventing ovum transport after ovulation so that sperm and egg cannot meet. The immediate postpartum period is a convenient time for tubal surgery: the patient is known to not be pregnant, insurance coverage is known, and no additional health-care visits are needed. For a few days after term vaginal birth, the uterine fundus and fallopian tubes can be accessed through a small infraumbilical minilaparotomy incision, and for most people the fallopian tubes are easily accessible at the time of cesarean delivery. Several techniques have been described for postpartum tubal surgery, most commonly variations of partial salpingectomy.[38] Complete salpingectomy is becoming an increasingly prevalent method for postpartum tubals; in 2013, the Society of Gynecologic Oncology recommended discussion of salpingectomy at the time of sterilization for ovarian cancer prevention and in 2015 ACOG followed suit although large studies of complication rates have not yet been published.[39]

It is imperative that health systems offer postpartum permanent contraception. People who do not obtain their desired postpartum tubal surgeries are significantly more likely to experience unintended short interval pregnancy.[40] Hospitals, labor and delivery units, and operating rooms should devise systems to prioritize access to postpartum sterilization.[41]

For people covered through federal health insurance programs, most commonly Medicaid, informed consent for tubal sterilization must be obtained at minimum 30 days before the anticipated surgery. This requirement was enacted after pervasive reports of patients undergoing sterilization without full informed consent. Because the federal consent must be completed ahead of time, and because immediate postpartum LARC also requires preplanning, it is a best practice to include postpartum contraception conversations at a standard prenatal visit around 32 weeks.

Vasectomy

Vasectomy is a form of permanent contraception in which the vas deferens is interrupted, preventing sperm from entering semen. Three months following the procedure, the patient should have a confirmatory semen analysis to confirm the absence of sperm; a second form of contraception should be used until azoospermia is confirmed. Vasectomy can be performed at any point during a pregnancy, thereby leveraging the pregnancy status as a second form of contraception. Compared with salpingectomy, vasectomy is less expensive, safer, and more effective—yet this method of contraception is much less common.[9] Some pregnant people will still prefer their own permanent contraception in the event they have another sexual partner (change of partners, multiple partners, or rape).

Timing of Postpartum Visits

As noted, many postpartum patients resume intercourse before the standard 6-week postpartum visit. Studies indicate that the earliest return to fertility in a nonbreastfeeding woman is about 3 weeks and many will ovulate before resumption of first menses. Additionally, problems with breastfeeding such as inadequate latch or concerns for poor milk production and resultant supplementation tend to occur early in the postpartum period. Postpartum mood disorders including depression tend to occur early (in the first few weeks) after delivery. For all these reasons, it has been suggested that we reconsider the timing of the postpartum visits.[42] ACOG recommends a first postpartum visit within 2 to 3 weeks, which will give clinicians the opportunity to address contraception, mood, and breastfeeding in a timely manner.[43] A second visit at 4 to 6 weeks postpartum can be used to transition chronic health conditions such as hypertension and diabetes to primary care and to place intrauterine contraception for those that did not have an IUD placed before then.

SUMMARY

Clinicians can leverage the long-term relationships forged with their patients over the antenatal period to discuss complex issues including desired family size and spacing. Clinicians can review contraceptive tools to meet these goals while weighing patient priorities as well as medical risks and contraindications. If a patient desires a postpartum contraceptive method, health systems should mobilize to provide these methods as soon as medically possible, including providing all nonestrogen containing methods before hospital discharge.

CLINICS CARE POINTS

- Approach conversations about birth spacing, family size, and desired contraception from a model of shared decision-making.
- Utilize the US CDC Medical Eligibility Criteria as a reference when addressing contraception in the context of medical comorbidities.
- Special postpartum considerations include elevated VTE risk, hypertensive disorders, lactation, and cardiomyopathy.
- Placement of LARC devices and fulfillment of sterilization requests during postpartum hospitalization increases access to devices and surgeries that might otherwise be out of reach for patients with inadequate health-care coverage.

DISCLOSURE

Dr Hofler reports no financial disclosures relevant to the content of this article. Dr Thaxton reports no financial disclosures relevant to the content of this article.

REFERENCES

1. RHR_policybrief_birthspacing_eng.pdf. Available at: https://apps.who.int/iris/bitstream/handle/10665/73710/RHR_policybrief_birthspacing_eng.pdf. Accessed January 2, 2023.

2. Interpregnancy Care. Obstetric Care Consensus No. 8. American College of Obstetricians and Gynecologists. Obstet Gynecol 2019;133(1):e51–72.

3. Conde-Agudelo A, Rosas-Bermúdez A, Kafury-Goeta AC. Birth spacing and risk of adverse perinatal outcomes: a meta-analysis. JAMA 2006;295(15):1809–23.

4. Gemmill A, Lindberg LD. Short Interpregnancy Intervals in the United States. Obstet Gynecol 2013;122(1):64–71.

5. Sok C, Sanders JN, Saltzman HM, et al. Sexual Behavior, Satisfaction, and Contraceptive Use Among Postpartum Women. J Midwifery Wom Health 2016;61(2): 158–65.

6. Leeman LM, Rogers RG. Sex after childbirth: postpartum sexual function. Obstet Gynecol 2012;119(3):647–55.

7. Rosen R, Brown C, Heiman J, et al. The Female Sexual Function Index (FSFI): a multidimensional self-report instrument for the assessment of female sexual function. J Sex Marital Ther 2000;26(2):191–208.

8. Patient-Centered Contraceptive Counseling. Committee Statement No. 1. American College of Obstetricians and Gynecologists. Obstet Gynecol 2022;139: 349–53.

9. Daniels K, Abma JC. Current contraceptive status among women aged 15–49: United States, 2017–2019. NCHS data brief, no 388. Hyattsville, MD: National Center for Health Statistics; 2020.

10. Curtis KM, Tepper NK, Jatlaoui TC, et al. U.S. Medical Eligibility Criteria for Contraceptive Use, 2016. MMWR Recomm Rep (Morb Mortal Wkly Rep) 2016;65(No. RR-3):1–104.

11. Jackson E, Curtis KM, Gaffield ME. Risk of venous thromboembolism during the postpartum period: a systematic review. Obstet Gynecol 2011;117(3):691–703.

12. Turok DK, Leeman L, Sanders JN, et al. Immediate postpartum levonorgestrel intrauterine device insertion and breast-feeding outcomes: a noninferiority randomized controlled trial. Am J Obstet Gynecol 2017;217(6):665.e1–8.

13. Truitt ST, Fraser AB, Grimes DA, et al. Combined hormonal versus nonhormonal versus progestin-only contraception in lactation. Cochrane Database Syst Rev 2003;2:CD003988.

14. Levi E, Avila K, Wu H. O17Immediate postpartum contraceptive implant placement and breastfeeding success in women at risk for low milk supply: A randomized non-inferiority trial. Contraception 2022;116:73.

15. Phillips SJ, Tepper NK, Kapp N, et al. Progestogen-only contraceptive use among breastfeeding women: a systematic review. Contraception 2016;94(3): 226–52.

16. Cardoso F, Polónia J, Santos A, et al. Low-dose oral contraceptives and 24-hour ambulatory blood pressure. Int J Gynaecol Obstet Off Organ Int Fed Gynaecol Obstet 1997;59(3):237–43.

17. Chasan-Taber L, Willett WC, Manson JE, et al. Prospective study of oral contraceptives and hypertension among women in the United States. Circulation 1996;94(3):483–9.

18. Pregnancy and Heart Disease. ACOG Practice Bulletin No. 212. American College of Obstetricians and Gynecologists. Obstet Gynecol 2019;133:e320–56.

19. Averbach S, Hofler L. Long-Acting Reversible Contraception With Contraceptive Implants and Intrauterine Devices. JAMA 2022;327(20):2013–4.

20. McNicholas C, Swor E, Wan L, et al. Prolonged use of the etonogestrel implant and levonorgestrel intrauterine device: 2 years beyond Food and Drug Administration–approved duration. Am J Obstet Gynecol 2017;216(6):586.e1–6.

21. Immediate Postpartum Long-Acting Reversible Contraception. Committee Opinion No. 670. American College of Obstetricians and Gynecologists. Obstet Gynecol 2016;128:e32–7.

22. Increasing Access to Contraceptive Implants and Intrauterine Devices to Reduce Unintended Pregnancy. Committee Opinion No. 642.American College of Obstetricians and Gynecologists. Obstet Gynecol 2015;126:e44–8.

23. Medicaid Reimbursement for Postpartum LARC. Available at: https://www.acog.org/programs/long-acting-reversible-contraception-larc/activities-initiatives/medicaid-reimbursement-for-postpartum-larc. Accessed January 2, 2023.

24. Steenland MW, Vatsa R, Pace LE, et al. Immediate Postpartum Long-Acting Reversible Contraceptive Use Following State-Specific Changes in Hospital Medicaid Reimbursement. JAMA Netw Open 2022;5(10):e2237918.

25. Palm HC, Degnan JH, Biefeld SD, et al. An initiative to implement immediate postpartum long-acting reversible contraception in rural New Mexico. Am J Obstet Gynecol 2020;222(4S):S911.e1–7.

26. U.S. Postpartum Contraceptive Access Initiative. Published July 22, 2015. Available at: https://pcainitiative.acog.org/. Accessed January 2, 2023.

27. Carr S, Singh R, Espey E, et al. Post-Placental IUD Insertion: A Mixed Methods Assessment of Women's Experiences [22N]. Obstet Gynecol 2016;127:120S.

28. Reed SD, Zhou X, Ichikawa L, et al. Intrauterine device-related uterine perforation incidence and risk (APEX-IUD): a large multisite cohort study. Lancet Lond Engl 2022;399(10341):2103–12.

29. Jatlaoui TC, Whiteman MK, Jeng G, et al. Intrauterine device expulsion after postpartum placement. Obstet Gynecol 2018;132(4):895–905.

30. Averbach SH, Ermias Y, Jeng G, et al. Expulsion of intrauterine devices after postpartum placement by timing of placement, delivery type, and intrauterine device type: a systematic review and meta-analysis. Am J Obstet Gynecol 2020;223(2):177–88.

31. Averbach S, Kully G, Hinz E, et al. Early vs Interval Postpartum Intrauterine Device Placement: A Randomized Clinical Trial. JAMA 2023;329(11):910–7.

32. Curtis KM, Jatlaoui TC, Tepper NK, et al. U.S. Selected Practice Recommendations for Contraceptive Use, 2016. MMWR Recomm Rep (Morb Mortal Wkly Rep) 2016;65(No. RR-4):1–66.

33. Bahamondes L, Valeria Bahamondes M, Shulman LP. Non-contraceptive benefits of hormonal and intrauterine reversible contraceptive methods. Hum Reprod Update 2015;21(5):640–51.

34. Dianat S, Fox E, Ahrens KA, et al. Side Effects and Health Benefits of Depot Medroxyprogesterone Acetate: A Systematic Review. Obstet Gynecol 2019;133(2):332–41.

35. DEPO-PROVERA® CI Boxed Warning medroxyprogesterone acetate injectable suspension, for intramuscular use | Pfizer Medical Information - US. https://www.pfizermedicalinformation.com/en-us/depo-provera/boxed-warning. Accessed January 2, 2023.

36. Karlsson C, Obrant KJ, Karlsson M. Pregnancy and lactation confer reversible bone loss in humans. Osteoporos Int J Establ Result Coop Eur Found Osteoporos Natl Osteoporos Found USA 2001;12(10):828–34.

37. Depot Medroxyprogesterone Acetate and Bone Effects. Committee Opinion No. 602. American College of Obstetricians and Gynecologists. Obstet Gynecol 2014;123:1398–402.

38. Lawrie TA, Kulier R, Nardin JM. Techniques for the interruption of tubal patency for female sterilisation. Cochrane Database Syst Rev 2016;8. https://doi.org/10.1002/14651858.CD003034.pub4.

39. Zamorano AS, Mutch DG. Postpartum salpingectomy: a procedure whose time has come. Am J Obstet Gynecol 2019;220(1):8–9.

40. Thurman AR, Janecek T. One-year follow-up of women with unfulfilled postpartum sterilization requests. Obstet Gynecol 2010;116(5):1071–7.

41. Access to Postpartum Sterilization. ACOG Committee Opinion No. 827. American College of Obstetricians and Gynecologists. Obstet Gynecol 2021;137:e169–76.

42. Speroff L, Mishell DR. The postpartum visit: it's time for a change in order to optimally initiate contraception. Contraception 2008;78(2):90–8.

43. Optimizing Postpartum Care. ACOG Committee Opinion No. 736. American College of Obstetricians and Gynecologists. Obstet Gynecol 2018;131:e140–50.

Prenatal Care for the Obese and Severely Obese Pregnant Patient

Dawn Palaszewski, MD*

KEYWORDS

- Prenatal care • Pregnancy • Antepartum • Obese • Obesity

KEY POINTS

- Obesity is an increasingly common health problem in the United States.
- When a woman is obese, there are increased risks of antepartum, intrapartum, and post-partum complications.
- As the severity of a complication seems to be "dose-related," the higher the body mass index the greater the risk for morbidity or mortality.

INTRODUCTION/HISTORY/DEFINITIONS/BACKGROUND

Obesity is an increasingly common health problem in the United States. A body mass index (BMI) of 30.0 or higher falls within the obesity range. Obesity can be subdivided into categories of Class I that is a BMI of 30 to less than 35, Class II that is a BMI of 35 to less than 40, and Class III that is a BMI of 40 or higher and sometimes classified as "severe" obesity. The National Health and Nutrition Examination Survey (NHANES) is used to collect data on the prevalence of chronic conditions such as obesity in the population. Results from 1999–2000 to 2017–March 2020 showed that among US adults aged 20 years and over the prevalence of obesity increased from 30.5% to 41.9% and the prevalence of severe obesity increased from 4.7% to 9.2%. The prevalence of obesity has likewise increased substantially among women of reproductive age. The prevalence of obesity among women 20 to 39 years of age increased from 29.8% in 2001–2002 to 39.7% in 2017–2018. The NHANES also collects data on the proportion of women who had a healthy weight before pregnancy, and this number is decreasing. The percentage of females delivering a live birth who had a healthy weight before pregnancy was 42.1% in 2018, 41.0% in 2019, and 40.0% in 2020.[1] The prevalence of obesity before pregnancy varies by race or ethnic group. For American Indian and Alaska Native, the prevalence is 40%, for non-Hispanic Black 39%, for Hispanic 32%, for non-Hispanic White 26%, and for non-Hispanic Asian 10%.[2]

University of South Florida Morsani College of Medicine
* 4033 Medicci Lane, Wesley Chapel, FL 33543.
E-mail address: dawnpalaszewski@gmail.com

Obstet Gynecol Clin N Am 50 (2023) 525–534
https://doi.org/10.1016/j.ogc.2023.03.013
0889-8545/23/© 2023 Elsevier Inc. All rights reserved.

obgyn.theclinics.com

Definition of Obesity

The term obesity refers to the amount of adipose tissue a person is carrying. As this is a complex item to accurately measure, a screening test was needed to determine which individuals might be at higher or lower risk for certain medical complications. The concept of BMI was to stratify patients into risk groups for having a weight that negatively impacts their health. It took into consideration both height and weight as BMI is calculated as weight in kilograms divided by the square of the height in meters. The cutoff of 30 in a nonpregnant patient represents a reasonable cutoff in balancing sensitivity and specificity for identifying those at risk for disease from excess body fat. It does not account for individual differences in frame size, lean body mass, and fat distribution patterns.[3] For example, a professional athlete may have a BMI of 35+ but it is due to increased lean body mass. As this is a screening test and the term obesity projects the idea of fat shaming, it may be best to use the terms healthy weight and unhealthy weight when counseling a patient.

Implications of Higher Maternal BMI During Pregnancy

Obesity can have many effects on pregnancy. When a woman is obese, there are increased risks of antepartum, intrapartum, and postpartum complications (**Box 1**). This article specifically addresses the issues of fetal abnormalities, cardiac dysfunction, obstructive sleep apnea (OSA), gestational diabetes mellitus, preeclampsia, stillbirth, cesarean delivery, failed trial of labor, venous thrombosis, and difficulty breastfeeding. The fetuses of obese pregnant women are at risk of both macrosomia and impaired growth. The infants born to these women tend to have more body fat and long term are at an increased risk of childhood obesity, metabolic syndrome, autism spectrum disorders, childhood developmental delay, and attention-deficit/ hyperactivity disorder.[4] However, if the mother has comorbidities often associated with pregnancy such as hypertensive disorders of pregnancy the fetus may actually be growth restricted. It is for these reasons that prenatal care needs to be individualized for these patients. As the severity of a complication seems to be "dose-related," the higher the BMI the greater the risk for morbidity or mortality.

Prepregnancy obesity contributes to the racial and ethnic disparities observed in maternal morbidity rates. One study found that 3% to 15% of the associated disparities between racial/ethnic groups and severe maternal morbidity are mediated by prepregnancy obesity.[5]

MANAGEMENT STRATEGIES: PRECONCEPTION WEIGHT LOSS

Care to achieve a healthy pregnancy outcome in an obese woman should ideally start in the preconception period. Weight loss before pregnancy should be encouraged as even small weight reductions may have improved pregnancy outcomes. Women should be informed by their provider of the risks of obesity and the benefits of weight loss before pregnancy. Diet and exercise should be discussed. Medications for weight loss are not recommended during pregnancy or preconception due to safety concerns. Increasing numbers of women of reproductive age are having bariatric surgery. It is strongly recommended that they wait 12 to 24 months before conceiving. Bariatric surgery-related weight loss is associated with reduced risks of gestational diabetes, hypertensive disorders, large for gestational age (LGA) infants, cesarean delivery, and postpartum hemorrhage compared with controls that did not undergo bariatric surgery and had a BMI similar to the treated women's presurgery BMI. However, bariatric surgery is associated with micronutrient deficiencies, surgical complications, as well as small for gestational age (SGA) infants, preterm birth, congenital abnormalities,

---

Box 1
Obesity complications related to pregnancy

- Spontaneous abortion
- Fetal congenital abnormalities
- Cardiac dysfunction
- Proteinuria
- Obstructive sleep apnea
- Nonalcoholic fatty liver disease
- Gestational diabetes mellitus
- Preeclampsia
- Stillbirth
- Indicated preterm birth
- Spontaneous preterm birth
- Cesarean delivery
- Failed trial of labor
- Endometritis
- Wound rupture or dehiscence
- Venous thrombosis
- Difficulty breastfeeding
- Postpartum anemia
- Postpartum depression
- Fetal macrosomia or impaired growth
- Infants at an increased risk of childhood obesity, metabolic syndrome, autism spectrum disorders, childhood developmental delay, and attention-deficit/hyperactivity disorder.

---

and perinatal mortality, which are increased if the pregnancy occurs too soon after surgery.[3] Multidisciplinary collaboration of the obstetrician, nutritionist, primary care provider, and bariatric surgeon is recommended during pregnancy. Guidelines for nutrition management after bariatric surgery do not exist for pregnancy, but they are adapted from the bariatric surgery guidelines. Postsurgical complications include anastomotic leaks, bowel obstruction or ischemia, internal or ventral hernias, and band erosion or migration. During pregnancy, it is important to evaluate for postsurgical complications when gastrointestinal symptoms occur. Fewer and less severe pregnancy complications are observed with restrictive procedures such as sleeve gastrectomy compared with Roux-en-Y gastric bypass surgery; for this reason, restrictive procedures may be favored in those who have not yet completed childbearing.[6]

Management: modification of standard prenatal care routines

Despite attempts at weight loss before conceiving, many women will still begin pregnancy in an obese BMI category. Obstetric care providers will need to modify prenatal care in the setting of obesity for safety and effectiveness. Modifications of care will be needed in expected weight gain, nutritional recommendations, screening tests, thromboprophylaxis, ultrasound, antenatal testing, and timing and mode of delivery.

MANAGEMENT: RECOMMENDED WEIGHT GAIN AND NUTRITIONAL INTERVENTIONS

Counseling regarding weight gain during pregnancy is based on the Institute of Medicine (IOM) recommendations. These are total weight gain of 25 to 35 lbs for women with a normal BMI, 15 to 25 lbs for overweight women, and 11 to 20 lbs for obese women. Prepregnancy BMI is typically used for this counseling, and as mentioned above, it may be helpful to refer to healthy and unhealthy weight. The recommended weight gain is the same for patients in all classes of obesity. These recommendations were made after it was found by gaining the suggested weight that there were few SGA infants. There are limited data regarding short-term and long-term maternal and newborn outcomes so the IOM did not recommend lower targets for weight gain for pregnant women with more severe degrees of obesity.[4,7,8]

Inadequate weight gain and gestational weight loss should not be encouraged for obese pregnant women. Studies have looked at consequences in these situations. There are some perceived benefits such as decreased cesarean section rate, decreased risk of a LGA infant, and decreased postpartum weight retention but an increased risk of a SGA infant. A systematic review focused on outcomes in obese women with gestational weight loss and identified an increased risk of SGA below the 10th percentile (adjusted odds ratio [OR], 1.76; 95% CI, 1.45–2.14) and 3rd percentile (adjusted OR, 1.62; 95% CI, 1.19–2.20).[4]

Women who are obese can actually be malnourished in the context of overnutrition due to the consumption of energy-dense but nutrient-poor diets. They also have diminished energy reserves and may have suboptimal status of one or more key micronutrients needed to support healthy fetal development. Obesity has been shown to be negatively associated with maternal iron, vitamin B12, and folate status. Circulating vitamin D may be low due to it being a fat-soluble vitamin sequestered by adipose tissue. Women who are undernourished during pregnancy have an increased risk of delivering an SGA infant. Maternal obesity is a risk factor for neural tube defects and as obese women may have lower folate levels during pregnancy, they may need greater folic acid supplementation.[9] Several clinical practice guidelines have recommended 5 mg of folic acid supplementation daily for women with a BMI of 30 or greater at least 1 month before conception and continued during the first trimester.[10] Owing to the folate and vitamin B12 deficiencies, obese women can also have megaloblastic anemia. Maternal nutrition should be assessed in all pregnant women and interventions such as dietary modifications or vitamin supplementation initiated as necessary.[9] A dietician referral should be considered for obese women, especially those who have had bariatric surgery.

MANAGEMENT: SCREENING FOR CONGENITAL FETAL COMPLICATIONS

Obese women are at an increased risk of fetal structural congenital anomalies, especially congenital heart defects and neural tube defects as mentioned above. There is evidence of a dose–response relationship with BMI.[3] Unfortunately, detection of congenital anomalies by ultrasonography is reduced with increasing BMI. One retrospective cohort study examined ultrasound images for pregnant women at 18 to 24 weeks of gestation who underwent either standard or targeted ultrasonography and detection of anomalous fetuses decreased with increasing maternal BMI by at least 20% in obese women compared with normal weight women. A transvaginal approach in the first trimester, using the maternal umbilicus as an acoustic window, tissue harmonic imaging, or fetal MRI could be used to try to improve imaging.[4] Cell-free DNA test failures are also more common in patients with obesity. Increasing

BMI is associated with decreased fetal fraction. Obese women should be counseled about the limitations of ultrasound in identifying structural anomalies. They should receive further genetic counseling and testing in the case of cell-free DNA screening test results that are not reported by the laboratory or are uninterpretable.[3]

MANAGEMENT: SCREENING FOR OBESITY-RELATED COMORBIDITIES

Early in pregnancy, obese women should be screened for pregestational type 2 diabetes mellitus (DM) such as with a glycated hemoglobin test (Hgba1c), as obesity is a risk for this comorbidity likely due to a relative insulin resistance. With the addition of the insulin resistance due to pregnancy, prediabetic women may become diabetic during the pregnancy (**Box 2**). If the screen is abnormal a formal glucose tolerance test may be needed to confirm. If the early testing is normal then a glucose challenge test at 24 to 28 weeks to screen for gestational diabetes should be performed.[11]

Obesity is a risk factor for OSA. Screening by history can be done and if it is suspected then the patient referred to a sleep medicine specialist. Obesity can have a synergistic effect with OSA, thereby increasing morbidity and severity of complications such as chronic hypertension and type 2 DM. The impact of sleep apnea on enhanced stress responses, endothelial damage, and metabolic alterations are the same changes that are associated with adverse pregnancy outcomes including preterm birth and fetal growth restrictions.[12] The specific effects of OSA versus the other comorbidities associated with OSA (obesity, DM, hypertension) make it difficult to determine the precise impact of just OSA. Women with OSA compared with women without OSA had a fivefold higher risk of dying before discharge from the hospital.[13]

Screening for high blood pressure and proteinuria should occur as for all women. However, obese women are more likely to have underlying disorders such as chronic hypertension before pregnancy.[4] Also, the estimated risk of preeclampsia doubles for every increase of 5 to 7 in the BMI. A relationship between obesity class and preeclampsia has also been documented with the risk three to four times as high for obesity Class II or III as for Class I.[3] Low-dose aspirin (81 mg/day) is used during pregnancy to prevent or delay the onset of preeclampsia. Many obese women will have risk

---

Box
2 Risk factors for pregestational type 2 diabetes mellitus

- Have prediabetes
- Are overweight
- Are 45 years or older
- Have a parent, brother, or sister with type 2 diabetes
- Are physically active less than three times a week
- Have ever had gestational diabetes (diabetes during pregnancy) or given birth to a baby who weighed over 9 pounds
- Are an African American, Hispanic or Latino, American Indian, or Alaska Native person. Some Pacific Islanders and Asian American people are also at higher risk.

From Diabetes risk factors (2022) Centers for Disease Control and Prevention. Centers for Disease Control and Prevention. Available at: https://www.cdc.gov/diabetes/basics/risk-factors.html.

factors for developing preeclampsia, and therefore, aspirin will be recommended from 12 weeks until birth of the baby.[14]

It has been proposed that pregnant women at risk for cardiac disease be screened with transthoracic echocardiography. For example, guidelines from the California Maternal Quality Care Collaborative recommend echocardiography for pregnant women with a history of cardiac disease or four or more risk factors. Risk factors included age 40 years or older, BMI 35 or greater, black race, chronic hypertension, prepregnancy diabetes, and substance use.[15]

Pregnancy is a well-established risk factor for venous thromboembolism (VTE). The risk is fourfold to fivefold increased during pregnancy and the puerperium. There is also an increased risk in obese gravidas with odds ratios ranging from 1.7 to 5.3 greater than normal weight gravidas.[16] Owing to this increased risk of VTE, thromboprophylaxis can be considered when obese pregnant women are hospitalized before delivery, on bed rest, or having surgery during the antenatal period.[10]

MANAGEMENT: ROLE OF ULTRASOUNDS

It has been suggested that ultrasounds be performed early for dating and to assess for twins, at 14 to 16 weeks for early anatomy, at 20 to 22 weeks for routine morphologic assessment, at 28 to 32 weeks to aid in detection of late-onset fetal growth restriction, and anytime in the third trimester for excessive fetal growth.[10] As fundal height measurements do not adequately assess fundal growth as a proxy for fetal growth and clinical palpation of fetal parts in markedly compromised, serial ultrasound for fetal growth may be indicated more frequently in the Class 3 obese patients. Additional ultrasounds may be obtained for antepartum fetal surveillance.

MANAGEMENT: FETAL SURVEILLANCE

The goal of antepartum fetal surveillance is to reduce the risk of stillbirth. Maternal obesity has been identified as a risk factor for stillbirth and as BMI increases the risk of stillbirth increases. Compared to individuals with BMI less than 30, the hazard ratio for stillbirth is 1.71 for prepregnancy BMI 30.0 to 34.9; 2.00 for BMI 35.0 to 39.9; 2.48 for BMI greater than 40; and 3.16 for BMI at 50 or higher. An interaction has also been shown between obesity and gestational age where compared with individuals of normal BMI 18.5 to 25. If BMI is 30 or greater than there is an adjusted hazard ratio of 3.5 (95% CI, 1.9–6.4) at 37 to 40 weeks and 4.6 (95% CI, 1.6–13.4) at greater than 40 weeks. Antepartum fetal surveillance should be considered. One suggested strategy is for a patient with prepregnancy BMI of 35.0 to 39.9 to have weekly testing starting at 37/0 weeks and for a patient with prepregnancy BMI of 40 or higher to have weekly testing starting at 34/0 weeks.[17]

MANAGEMENT: ANTENATAL PREPARATIONS FOR DELIVERY

Labor and delivery care should be considered prenatally. Accommodations in the outpatient and inpatient settings will be necessary for obese patients, and this may influence the facility for delivery. Larger beds, wheelchairs, blood pressure cuffs, and so forth will need to be available. Consultation with an anesthesiologist should be obtained ideally before labor to allow time to develop an anesthetic plan. There are challenges with management of anesthesia and an increased risk of cesarean deliveries for obese women. Obese women have increased risks of anesthesia-related complications, particularly related to general anesthesia. Studies have shown that obesity increases the risk of epidural analgesic failure, failed tracheal intubation, and fatal airway obstruction and hypoventilation during emergence and recovery from general anesthesia. Neuraxial anesthesia should be used whenever possible for obese patients. Preparations such as ensuring the availability of additional airway equipment can be made in advance.[3]

Controversy exists regarding the optimal timing of delivery of obese women. As noted above increasing BMI is an independent risk factor for stillbirth and there is a higher risk of stillbirth at term in women with each increase in BMI class. One study showed that compared with women at 41 weeks with a normal BMI, there was a higher risk of stillbirth in women of obesity Class I at 39 weeks (OR 1.15 95% CI 1.00–1.31), at 38 weeks for obesity Class II (OR 1.21 95% CI 1.04–1.41), and at 37 weeks for obesity Class III (OR 1.30 95% CI 1.11–1.52).[18] The early induction of labor should be considered to reduce the risk of stillbirth, but currently there is no consensus on the timing. Some studies have shown that expectant management in obese women is associated with decreased rates of cesarean delivery without increased incidence of adverse outcomes compared with elective induction of labor (after 37 weeks).[19] In other studies, induction of labor at 38 weeks appeared to lower the risk of cesarean delivery without compromising maternal outcomes[20] or labor induction at 39 weeks was associated with reduced risk of cesarean delivery among women with obesity regardless of parity, age, or comorbidity status.[21] Many obese women will have other medical indications for induction of labor such as preeclampsia or gestational diabetes, but it may be reasonable to consider a 39 week induction of labor for those who do not.

There is an increased risk of cesarean delivery among overweight and obese women compared with normal weight women. One meta-analysis showed that the unadjusted odds ratios for cesarean delivery are 1.46 (95% CI, 1.34–1.60), 2.05 (95% CI, 1.86–2.27), and 2.89 (95% CI, 2.28–3.79) among overweight, obese, and severely obese women, respectively, compared to normal weight women.[4] Obesity alone is not an indication for elective cesarean section; however, as emergency cesarean section operative and anesthetic risks are higher, an informed discussion should be held with women regarding the mode of delivery during prenatal care rather than waiting until labor.[10] The data on a trial of labor after cesarean (TOLAC) section are mixed and again a decision on attempting TOLAC versus a scheduled repeat cesarean section should involve shared medical decision-making.[4]

Breastfeeding is affected by maternal obesity. Obese women are less likely than normal weight women to initiate breastfeeding or exclusively breastfeed. They also breastfeed for shorter durations. An elevated progesterone level which prevents the progesterone decline that leads to lactogenesis, latching difficulties due to large breasts, increased cesarean delivery, and depression are all factors that can cause issues. Early breastfeeding support should be offered[3] (see Article 8 in this monograph for more information on breastfeeding counseling and education)

SUMMARY

Obesity is an increasingly common health problem in the United States, including among reproductive age women. There are increased risks of antepartum, intrapartum, and postpartum complications among obese women. Prenatal care will need to be modified for this population (see Clinics care points). Obese women are recommended to lose weight before pregnancy and gain less weight during pregnancy, 11 to 20 lbs weight gain for all obesity classes. Women who are obese may actually be malnourished and have deficiencies in micronutrients. Women should have appropriate culturally sensitive diet and exercise counseling. Obese women should be screened early in pregnancy for pregestational diabetes mellitus, OSA, depression, elevated blood pressure, and proteinuria. Thromboprophylaxis can be considered when these women are hospitalized before delivery, on bed rest, or having surgery during the antenatal period. There are limitations of ultrasound in detecting fetal structural abnormalities at increasing BMIs. One of the main screening tests for fetal aneuploidy, cell-free DNA, also has a higher failure rate in patients with obesity. Patients should be counseled about these limitations. It has been suggested that ultrasounds are performed early for dating and potentially more often depending on the degree of obesity to monitor for anomalies and growth. Maternal obesity is a risk factor for stillbirth which increases as BMI increases. Consultations with other specialists may be necessary during prenatal care based on a woman's medical complications—for example, a sleep medicine specialist. An anesthesiology consult should be obtained before labor to be prepared for delivery. Early breastfeeding support is also recommended if a woman plans to breastfeed. The early induction of labor could help avoid complications such as stillbirth without increasing the risk of cesarean section and a 39-week induction may be reasonable. Even though obese women are at an increased risk of cesarean section, an elective cesarean section is not indicated by obesity alone. The mode of delivery should be discussed with all obese patients considering risks versus benefits and implementing shared medical decision-making.

CLINICS CARE POINTS

- Inform women of the risks of obesity and the benefits of weight loss before pregnancy.
- After bariatric surgery, one should wait 12 to 24 months before conceiving.
- Recommended weight gain is 11 to 20 lbs for obese women. Less is not encouraged.
- Assess maternal nutrition and recommend dietary supplementation as necessary.
- A dietician referral is optimal, especially those post-bariatric surgery.
- Counsel about the limitations of ultrasound in identifying structural anomalies.
- Provide further genetic counseling and testing in the case of cell-free DNA screening test results that are not reported by the laboratory or are uninterpretable.
- Screen early in pregnancy for pregestational type 2 diabetes mellitus and follow up a normal screen with screen for gestational diabetes.
- Screen for obstructive sleep apnea and if suspected, refer to a sleep medicine specialist.
- Obese pregnant women like all women should be screened for depression.
- Screen for development of hypertensive diseases of pregnancy.
- Recommend aspirin 81 mg/day starting at 12 weeks gestation to minimize risk of preeclampsia.
- Consider screening echocardiography for pregnant women with a BMI of 35 or greater with multiple risk factors for underlying cardiac disease.
- Consider thromboprophylaxis when hospitalized before delivery, on bed rest, or having antenatal surgery.
- Consider ultrasounds early for dating and to assess for twins, $\sim$ 15 weeks for early anatomy, at 20 to 22 weeks for routine morphologic assessment, at 28 to 32 weeks for fetal growth, and anytime in the third trimester for fetal growth or antepartum fetal surveillance as indicated.
- Given the increased risk of stillbirth antepartum surveillance is suggested:
  ○ If a prepregnancy BMI of 35.0 to 39.9: weekly testing starting at 37/0 weeks.
  ○ If a prepregnancy BMI of 40+: weekly testing starting at 34/0 weeks.

- Determine accommodations needed for inpatient settings due to obesity; this may influence the chosen facility for delivery.
- Anesthesiology consult before labor to develop an anesthetic plan.
- If no other medical indications for induction of labor it seems reasonable to induce at 39 week to improve outcomes.
- Obesity alone is not an indication for elective cesarean section; however, since operative and anesthetic risks are higher have an informed discussion regarding the mode of delivery.
- The data on a trial of labor after cesarean (TOLAC) section are mixed and a decision to attempt TOLAC should involve shared medical decision-making.
- Offer prenatal breastfeeding support to obese women who desire to breastfeed.

DISCLOSURE

The author has no commercial or financial conflicts of interest.

REFERENCES

1. Division of Health and Nutrition Examination Surveys. NHANES interactive data visualizations. Washington, DC: National Center for Health Statistics; 2021. Available at: http://www.cdc.gov/nchs/nhanes/visualization/. Available at: Accessed March 1 2023.
2. Centers for Disease Control and Prevention. CDC WONDER. About natality, 2016-2020 expanded). Available at: https://wonder.cdc.gov/natality-expanded-current.html. Accessed March 1, 2023.
3. Creanga AA, Catalano PM, Bateman BT. Obesity in pregnancy. N Engl J Med 2022;387:248–59.
4. American College of Obstetricians and Gynecologists' Committee on Practice Bulletins – Obstetrics. Obesity in pregnancy; ACOG Practice Bulletin, Number 230. Obstet Gynecol 2021;137(6):e128–44.
5. Siddiqui A, Azei W, Egorova N, et al. Contribution of prepregnancy obesity to racial and ethnic disparities in severe maternal morbidity. Obstet Gynecol 2021;137:864–72.
6. Fisher S, Stetson B, Kominiarek M. Pregnancy after bariatric surgery. JAMA 2023; 329(9):758–9.
7. Institute of Medicine. Weight gain during pregnancy: re-examining the guidelines. Washington, DC: National Academies Press; 2009. Available at: https://pubmed.ncbi.nlm.nih.gov/20669500/. Accessed March 1, 2023.
8. Weight gain during pregnancy. ACOG Committee Opinion No. 548. American College of Obstetricians and Gynecologists. Obstet Gynecol 2013;121:210–2.
9. Killeen SL, O'Brien EC, McAuliffe FM. Maternal and fetal normal and abnormal nutrition. In: Hod M, et al, editors. New Technologies and perinatal medicine. 1st edition. Boca Raton: CRC Press; 2019. p. 7–10.
10. Simon A, Pratt M, Hutton B, et al. Guidelines for the management of pregnant women with obesity: a systematic review. Obes Rev 2020;21(3):e12972.
11. US Preventive Service Task Force. Screening for Gestational Diabetes – USPSTF recommendation Statement. JAMA 2021;326(6):531–8. Available at: https://www.uspreventiveservicestaskforce.org/uspstf/recommendation/gestational-diabetes-screening. Accessed March 1, 2023.

12. Romero R. Badr A role for sleep disorders in pregnancy complications: challenges and opportunities. Am J Obstet Gynecol 2014;210:3–11.
13. Facco FL, Chan M, Patel SR. Common sleep disorders in pregnancy. Ostet Gynecol 2022;140:321–39.
14. American College of obstetricians and Gynecologists and the Society for maternal-fetal medicine practice Advisory "Low-dose aspirin use for the prevention of preeclampsia and related morbidity and mortallity. 2021. Available at: https://www.acog.org/clinical/clinical-guidance/practice-advisory/articles/2021/ 12/low-dose-aspirin-use-for-the-prevention-of-preeclampsia-and-related-morbidity-and-mortality. Accessed March 1, 2023.
15. Abelman S, Burd J, Muir M, et al. Implementation of guideline for transthoracic echocardiography screening for pregnant women with risk for cardiac disease. Obstet Gynecol 2022;139(1). 64-64S.
16. Mission J, Marshall N, Caughey A. Pregnancy risks associated with obesity. Obstet Gynecol Clin North Am 2015;42:335–53.
17. Outpatient Antenatal Fetal Surveillance. ACOG Committee Opinion No. 828. American College of Obstetricians and Gynecologists. Obstet Gynecol 2021; 137:e177–97.
18. Eberle A, Czuzoj-Shulman N, Abenhaim H. The risk of stillbirth at term and timing of delivery in obese women. Obstet Gynecol 2020;135:48S–9S.
19. Staudenmaier E, Chatterton C, Montanez M, et al. Induction of labor compared with expectant management and risk of cesarean delivery in obese women. Obstet Gynecol 2019;133:63S–4S.
20. Eberle A, Czuzoj-Shulman N, Abenhaim H. Induction of labor at 38 weeks and risk of cesarean delivery among obese women: a retrospective propensity match study. Obstet Gynecol 2020;135:44S.
21. Glazer K, Danilack V, Field A, et al. Term labor induction and cesarean delivery risk among obese women with and without comorbidities. Am J Perinatol 2022; 39(2):154–64.

Updates on Evaluation and Treatment of Common Complaints in Pregnancy

Brenna McGuire, MD

KEYWORDS

- Pregnancy • Common complaints • Fatigue • Nausea • Vomiting • Headaches
- Skin changes

KEY POINTS

- Pregnancy can affect many organ systems in the body that lead to new and concerning symptoms for patients.
- Obstetric clinicians should be familiar with the causes, diagnosis, and management of pregnancy-associated symptoms.
- Many conditions during pregnancy are benign and will resolve in the postpartum period.
- Clinicians should be aware of "red flag" symptoms during pregnancy that warrant further workup.
- Management of common conditions during pregnancy should include both pharmacologic and non-pharmacologic approaches.

INTRODUCTION

During pregnancy, many hormonal and physiologic changes occur, which lead to symptoms that are new and concerning to the patient. Almost every organ system in the body is altered by pregnancy. It is essential that obstetric clinicians provide guidance, reassurance after ruling out any significant pathology, and adequately treat common pregnancy-associated complaints. The following is a brief review with updates on the evaluation and treatment of some common symptoms that women may experience during pregnancy. This article is organized based on common presenting complaints. Each section reviews the changes in maternal physiology that may be the sole etiology of the patient's concern as well as other diagnoses that need to be considered during the evaluation.

Department of Obstetrics and Gynecology, University of New Mexico Hospital, UNM Obstetrics & Gynecology, MSC10 5580, 1 University of New Mexico, Albuquerque, NM 87131, USA
E-mail address: blmcguire@salud.unm.edu

Obstet Gynecol Clin N Am 50 (2023) 535–547
https://doi.org/10.1016/j.ogc.2023.03.016
0889-8545/23/© 2023 Elsevier Inc. All rights reserved.

obgyn.theclinics.com

COMPLAINTS OF FATIGUE
Physiologic Fatigue and Management

More than 90% of women experience some level of fatigue during pregnancy and the postpartum period. During the first trimester, rising levels of beta-human chorionic gonadotropin (HCG) and shifting levels of estrogen and progesterone lead to increased levels of reported fatigue. During the second and third trimesters, changing physiology and increased caloric demands lead to a sense of exhaustion that can cause a decline in a woman's mental and physical ability to work and complete daily activities. Although it is a common problem due to physiologic changes (constitutional fatigue), it is important to rule out (by history, examination, or testing) some of the more serious etiologies that need to specifically be ruled out or treated. These include anemia, depression, or sleep disturbances.

During pregnancy, women should be counseled that fatigue may be worse during the first trimester when changing levels of hormone are at their highest. Many patients report increasing fatigue during the third trimester due to the rapid increase of fetal growth and resulting caloric demands. Musculoskeletal discomfort with the enlarging uterus also contributes to sleep disturbances. Women should be counseled to rest as much as possible by adjusting sleep schedules for earlier bedtime and addition of daytime naps. Dietary recommendations suggest eating a balanced diet during pregnancy with particular attention to adequate consumption of iron, protein, and total caloric intake ($\sim$1800–2400 calories/day).

Recently, exercise during pregnancy has been determined to be a possible way to decrease symptoms of fatigue. The American College of Obstetricians and Gynecologists currently recommends 20 to 30 minutes of moderate to intense physical activity and regular exercise at least 5 days per week.[1] A recent meta-analysis showed consistent exercise during pregnancy and the postpartum period significantly improved fatigue levels and mental health scores.[2] Women should be encouraged to continue safe exercise routines during pregnancy to help improve levels of fatigue.

Anemia: Anemia during pregnancy is a normal physiologic change due to expanding plasma volume. During pregnancy, women require 27 mg of iron per day to maintain a normal hematocrit during this time of blood volume expansion. This is most often achieved with diet and the addition of prenatal vitamins. However, many women enter pregnancy already having iron deficiency anemia. During pregnancy, all women are evaluated for baseline anemia with the initial prenatal laboratory tests. Those identified with anemia should be evaluated further for decreased iron stores. The standard approaches for iron deficiency anemia is to increase iron intake by either diet (iron-rich foods such as liver) and/or oral iron supplement. These should be offered initially with follow-up in 4 to 6 weeks to evaluate patient's response. In cases of severe anemia or lack of response to oral medication, further testing should be considered to rule out hemoglobinopathies or hemolytic issues.

Over the past decade, intravenous (IV) parenteral iron administration during pregnancy has been shown to be superior in the treatment of iron deficiency anemia. [3] In the past, IV iron was expensive, labor intensive to administer, and carried some risk of medication reactions. The current preparations are more "user-friendly." Therefore, IV iron should be considered early in pregnant women who are not responsive to or do not tolerate oral iron. Three meta-analyses have evaluated the benefits and risks of oral iron versus parenteral iron supplementation. For treatment of iron deficiency, parenteral or IV iron was found to have fewer side effects and fewer medication reactions and had a greater likelihood of achieving a desired hemoglobin level after 4 weeks of administration. In addition, IV iron is safe for administration in the second and third trimester and can be used in individuals who cannot tolerate oral supplementation. Newer guidelines also suggest IV iron administration in patients who have anatomic abnormalities that would change iron absorption including history of bariatric surgery.[3] It is also important to consider using IV iron in anemic patients beyond 30 weeks as it promotes a much more rapid correction of anemia before delivery. The recommended formulation during pregnancy is infusion of ferric carboxymaltose, low molecular weight iron dextran, or ferric derisomaltose. Iron sucrose is a commonly chosen formulation and widely available. However, it requires four to five separate infusions to reach optimal levels, which can be prohibitive for some patients.

Sleep Disturbance: Although much of this is due to the musculoskeletal discomfort, emotional stressors, nausea, gastric esophageal reflux disease, and frequent urination of advancing pregnancy, it is important to evaluate for possible other causes. Restless leg syndrome occurs with increasing frequency as the pregnancy progresses. One can simply ask the patient if her legs bother her at night. Treatment options include iron supplementation (oral or IV) as well as non-pharmacologic therapies or medications.[4] Sleep apnea is becoming a common diagnosis in the general population. In turn, it seems to be even more common among pregnant patients. This may be due to the increase in obesity, which complicates the pregnancy. The presence of sleep apnea in pregnancy has been associated with preeclampsia, gestational diabetes, and cardiac issues.[5] A good history or screening questionnaire can help determine if a referral to a sleep specialist is indicated. A simple screening test is STOP, which inquires about *s*noring, *t*iredness, *o*bserved apnea, and high blood *p*ressure.[6] A positive response on two out of the four questions raise a concern for sleep apnea. This survey has proven an effective screening tool in nonpregnant individuals; it is not proven with pregnant individuals. A positive screen would prompt a referral for a sleep study for evaluation and potential initiation of a continuous positive airway pressure device.

INTEGUMENTARY SYSTEM COMPLAINTS

Skin Changes: Many women notice a change in their skin during pregnancy. These can be categorized as hormonally related or pregnancy-specific. Pregnancy-specific conditions include pruritic urticarial papules and plaques of pregnancy, prurigo of pregnancy, pruritic folliculitis of pregnancy, pemphigoid gestationis, and impetigo herpetiformis. The last two have been associated with some complications of pregnancy. Management of these conditions is beyond the scope of this review. By far, the most common skin conditions that patients report are related to hormonal changes. These include darkening of the breasts and nipples, melasma, linea nigra, striae gravidarum, varicose veins, and acne.[7] Although many of these conditions are temporary and resolve postpartum, they can cause significant distress for patients.

To prevent melasma or darkening of the skin during pregnancy, women should be counseled to limit sun exposure and wear a high-potency, broad-spectrum sunscreen. Severe epidermal melasma can be treated postpartum with a combination of hydroquinone, corticosteroids, and topical tretinoin. It is important to reassure women that this is normal and most often temporary. A second common complaint that women have in pregnancy is development of striae gravidarum or stretch marks. There are many topical treatments that women can safely use including emollients, vitamin E oil, and cocoa butter. There are multiple topical treatments advertised specifically for prevention of stretch marks that include centella asiatica extract, panthenol, hyaluronic acid, and collagen elastin. However, further studies are needed to evaluate the safety and efficacy of these treatments. At this time, they should not be encouraged for widespread use.[8] Women should be counseled that following pregnancy, many stretch marks will fade, although few disappear completely. Some postpartum treatment options include tretinoin therapy and laser treatment options.

Hair Changes: Hormonal changes during pregnancy commonly cause hair follicles to enter a prolonged anagen phase which may be noted by the patient as thickening of the hair or more hair growth, especially on the face. This is primarily due to the increase of androgen levels that occur with pregnancy. The sharp drop in hormonal levels after delivery results in synchronized hair follicles moving into the telogen phase. This often results in a pronounced hair loss — known as Telogen effluvium, typically occurs postpartum and resolved without treatment over 6 to -12 months. In contrast, complains of hair loss during pregnancy may represent a pathologic condition, and a close scalp examination to identify patterns of loss such as in patch, presence of lesions, and associated skin changes is warranted.

Oral Changes: Patients may report bleeding gums or growths on the gums.[9] The high hormonal levels of pregnancy increase angiogenesis within the gums and is seen as worsening gingivitis or gingival hyperplasia[10] Typically, this seems to be a worsening of a preexisting dental problems. In turn, this can lead to a pyogenic granuloma or epulis: a polypoid friable growth from the oral mucosa, lips, and even the tongue. It is estimated that 2% to 5% of pregnant women will develop a pyogenic granuloma during pregnancy.[11] Granuloma can be over a centimeter in diameter and thus interfere with eating. The best treatment of gingivitis is a dental referral for a cleaning and evaluation. It is generally not recommended to remove the granuloma unless they are severely symptomatic.[12,13] Typically, most of the granulomas and the hyperplasia will resolve over the first few months postpartum.[13] It should be noted that many dentist may be uncomfortable or unwilling to provide dental work to pregnant women. The obstetric provider may need to work with the dentist in their community to identify those that are willing to provide dental care during pregnancy.

Ptyalism gravidarum is an excess secretion of saliva with volumes up to 2 L per day.[14,15] Patients will complain that they cannot swallow this excess saliva due to the bad taste. They will commonly carry a cup to spit into. It is unclear as to the cause for this complaint, although it is often associated with nausea and vomiting during pregnancy. There seems to be no effective treatment during pregnancy. The use of lozenges/hard candy or gum will help temporarily, but generally the condition does not resolve until postpartum.

GASTROINTESTINAL COMPLAINTS

Nausea and Vomiting of Pregnancy: It is a common symptom during the first trimester. Approximately 80% of pregnancies are affected by some level of daily nausea or vomiting due to the rising levels of ßhCG that peak at approximately 10 weeks.[16] Women with a multiple gestation pregnancy or gestational trophoblastic disease often have worse symptoms due to the higher levels of ßhCG. Many women have symptoms that persist until the mid-second trimester with typical resolution by 20 weeks. Despite being common, it is one of the most undertreated conditions during pregnancy. It is commonly minimized by clinicians as a normal part of pregnancy and many women are hesitant to seek treatment due to safety concerns about medications in the first trimester.

Pathologic nausea and vomiting or hyperemesis gravidarum only affects 0.3% to 1% of pregnancies and is associated with dehydration, weight loss, and malnutrition and often requires inpatient hospitalization and treatment. There are many conditions which present with nausea and vomiting that are mistaken for normal pregnancy physiologic changes. Some of these include gastroenteritis, chronic *Helicobacter pylori*, molar pregnancy, diabetic ketoacidosis, and thyrotoxicosis. It is important when evaluating patients to consider using a validated measure to assess symptom severity such as the Motherisk-PUQE (pregnancy-unique quantification of emesis and nausea) scoring system.[16] In this way, clinicians can identify patients with severe symptoms that warrant further workup. For women who show signs of severe disease on the PUQE (score $\geq$ 13) consider workups for pathologic causes.

Treatment of nausea and vomiting during pregnancy starts with prevention. Early recognition and treatment are the key to preventing complications and decreasing risk of hospitalization. The most effective approach to prevention is to counsel patients on lifestyle modification in combination with the use of doxylamine and vitamin B6. These can be purchases as over-the-counter medications. There is a prescription version of these components with a time-released formulation that may provide better results for some women. Studies have shown that women who take a prenatal vitamin to optimize nutritional stores of B6 before pregnancy have decreased rates of reported nausea and vomiting during pregnancy.[17] During the first trimester, it is recommended that women are advised to eat small, frequent meals and to avoid spicy and fatty foods, although there is little published evidence that this decreases the severity of vomiting during pregnancy.

Many women desire options for pharmacologic and non-pharmacologic treatment of nausea during pregnancy. The pharmacologic approach begins with prevention efforts using B6 and doxylamine with the addition of either promethazine, prochlorperazine, or diphenhydramine. If symptoms continue, ondansetron or metoclopramide is commonly added to a patient's regimen. (Please note that ondansetron is NOT a first-line medication therapy due to risks of cardiac issues.) For those patients who prefer to decrease pharmacologic intervention, herbal therapies such as ginger, spearmint syrup, *Elettaria cardamomum*, and *Matricaria chamomilla* provide safe and effective alternatives.[18] A systematic review on the efficacy of alternative treatments showed that ginger may be more effective than vitamin B6 at high doses, although less effective with prolonged treatment greater than 60 days.[18] One suggested regime recommends 1000 mg of ginger daily.[19] During pregnancy, clinicians must accurately assess the severity of nausea and vomiting to identify possible pathologic causes and recommend appropriate regimens. Women are offered both pharmacologic options and non-pharmacologic alternatives so that they may make informed choices about their treatment plans. If nausea and vomiting continue past 20 weeks gestation, other causes, such as gastric disorders (*H pylori* or reflux), eating disorders (bulimia), and pancreatitis/liver disorders, should be explored.

Cholestasis: During pregnancy, high levels of estrogen will cause a change in bile composition, which in turn can result in cholestasis. The most common symptom is that of generalized pruritus (that may present on hand and feet) without a clear associated rash (other than excoriations from scratching).[20] This presents in the third trimester, with the diagnosis being confirmed with elevated total bile salts concentrations. The incidence varies greatly worldwide from less than 1% to 27%.[21] The etiology is complex but seems to have three components: genetic susceptibility, hormonal factors, and environmental factors.[22] The diagnosis is primarily clinical with confirmation by total bile salt elevation and not an elevated bile acid ratio.[23] The presence of jaundice is uncommon with intrahepatic cholestasis of pregnancy (ICP) and should prompt a further evaluation for other liver etiologies.

Severe cholestasis is defined as bile acids over 40 μmol/L and occurs in about 20% of case.[24] It should be noted that pruritus may appear before the elevations in bile salts.[25] For this reason in the situation with pruritus with concerns for cholestasis but normal bile acids, weekly testing of bile acids is recommended. It is important to identify this condition early and begin treatment it as cholestasis is associated with sudden fetal death—likely due to sudden development of a fetal arrhythmia or vasospasm.[26,27] The bile acids readily cross the placenta and accumulate in the fetus. The risk of fetal demise increases with higher serum bile acid levels. Levels of 40–99 μmol/L have a twofold increased risk of death, whereas levels greater than 100 μmol/L may have up to a 30-fold increased risk. The recommended management of this condition includes a planned delivery typically by 37 weeks or sooner depending on maternal obstetric history and level of total bile salts.[28] Ursodeoxycholic should be offered to all patients with cholestasis. Although optimal dosing has not been determined, a suggested course is 300 mg two or three times a day until delivery. The pruritus typically improves within 1 to 2 weeks, whereas a reduction in bile acids may take 3 to 4 weeks. Ongoing weekly monitoring of bile acids can be useful to rule out increasing levels that would modify delivery plans. Despite the improvement in maternal status, studies have not been able to demonstrate an improvement of fetal outcomes.[29] For this reason, it is recommended that the delivery plans are based on the highest levels of total bile acids rather than current levels.[30] Antepartum fetal assessment is routinely done with twice weekly with nonstress tests or biophysical profile. However, the value of this assessment has not been proven as fetal death is due to an acute arrhythmia or/and vasospasm.[31] The approach to management has been modified over the past 10 years, so providers need to reference authoritative sources for the most current recommendations.[28]

NEUROLOGICAL SYMPTOMS
Migraine Headaches

Headache is one of the most common ailments affecting women of reproductive age. Many conditions such as migraines, menstrual headaches, and tension headaches can be affected by fluctuating hormonal levels, which are often exacerbated during pregnancy.[32] Many women who suffer from a primary headache syndrome may have worsening symptoms that require attention during their pregnancies. Although headaches in pregnancy are commonly attributed to primary causes, clinicians must identify "red flag" symptoms that indicate a more serious secondary cause such as idiopathic intracranial hypertension, cerebral venous thrombosis, subarachnoid hemorrhage, or preeclampsia. Acute "thunderclap" headaches in pregnancy without a prior primary headache disorder diagnosis, including focal neurological deficits, papilledema, or a postural headache should prompt immediate evaluation with head MRI or CT with limited use of gadolinium.[33]

The most common primary headache syndrome that women present with during pregnancy is migraine without aura. Interestingly, studies have shown that migraines without aura typically improve or remit altogether during pregnancy, whereas migraines with aura are much less likely to improve and often worsen. Migraines without aura typically resolve in nearly 47% of women during the first trimester, 83% of women during the second trimester, and 87% of women during the third trimester.[33] This improvement is likely related to increasing levels of estradiol and a decrease in the hormonal fluctuations that can trigger migraine attacks. Migraines with aura are less likely to improve due to a significantly lower threshold for the onset due to the high estrogen to progesterone ratio during pregnancy.

Management of primary headache symptoms during pregnancy involves diagnosis of headache type and an evaluation of medication history during the initial prenatal care visit. If a history of headaches is identified, behavioral changes should be discussed with patients to decrease the frequency and severity of headaches during pregnancy. These techniques include good sleep hygiene, proper hydration and nutrition, relaxation, and biofeedback techniques. Women should be offered non-pharmacologic interventions such as oral magnesium sulfate 600 mg/d or riboflavin 400 mg/d daily for prophylaxis. There are limited data on the efficacy of these regimens, but initial studies show that they are safe during pregnancy and may lead to a decreased frequency of daily headaches.[34] Beta blockers are commonly used outside of pregnancy for migraine prophylaxis and are an option for prophylaxis in severe cases but may be associated with fetal growth restriction. Many common prophylactic medications for severe migraines such as topiramate and valproic acid are contraindicated due to teratogenic effects and are not recommended during pregnancy.[34]

Acute management of migraine and severe headaches in pregnancy should begin with 1,000 mg oral acetaminophen up to four times a day. Acetaminophen can safely be combined with caffeine which may improve results. However, the maximum dose of caffeine should not exceed 200 mg per day. Products containing butalbital are not recommended during pregnancy due to the risks of rebound headache and the potential for overuse and addiction. Another option for the treatment of refractory migraine headaches is metoclopramide 10 mg (IV or enteral) in combination with diphenhydramine 25 mg (IV or enteral).[35] In general, ergot alkaloids are not recommended during pregnancy as they are classified as category C medications. Opiate-containing medications should be used sparingly for refractory headaches. A recent meta-analysis that evaluated triptan exposure and pregnancy outcomes found there was no significant increase in rates of malformation, prematurity, or spontaneous abortions in those women with migraines with exposure to triptan compared with those patients with migraines and no exposure. A prospective observational study showed that women exposed to triptans during pregnancy demonstrated no increased risk of major birth defects.[35] Overall, triptans should be used as second-line therapy and only in extreme refractory cases. More data are needed to show superiority of treatment compared with the first-line approach. In recent years, the use of noninvasive neurostimulation devices and injectable therapies such as botulinum toxin and peripheral nerve blocks has become a popular way to control severe migraines. Although these therapies have excellent safety profiles, there are currently only limited data related to possible adverse pregnancy outcomes.

Bell's Palsy: It is an acute (evolving over a few hours) peripheral palsy of cranial nerve VII typically involving all three branches. Bell's palsy is characterized by involvement of *both* the upper and lower face. This will present as an asymmetry of the face with smile or grimace and difficulty closing the affected eye. Etiology is unclear but seems to be related to viral infections with herpes simplex activation being the most common theory.[36] Despite this, testing for a viral etiology is not useful. The only testing that may be useful is serology for Lyme disease in areas where it is endemic. There is a twofold to fourfold increased prevalence of Bell's palsy during pregnancy.[37,38] Risk factors include women in the third trimester and those with preeclampsia or obesity.[39] Patients will present fearing that they have had a stroke. If the paralysis was sudden and involves only the lower part of the face, other etiologies such as a stroke should be entertained. Given no other evidence of a stroke, the patient can be reassured that this is a temporary issue and generally will resolve within 6 months. However, patients with complete facial paralysis are less likely to have full resolution.[38,40]

Treatment is primarily to minimize symptoms including analgesics for pain and eye lubrication to prevent corneal dryness. A simple eye patch is not adequate because there is a tendency for the eye to open under the patch with resulting corneal injury.

Waterproof transparent tape can be used to hold the eyelid closed.[41] More recent literature has demonstrated that the use of oral steroids within the first 72 hours improves the speed and completeness of recovery.[38,40] A commonly suggested regimen is prednisone 60 to 80 mg/day for 1 week.[42] If the patient is in the first trimester the use of glucocorticoids may be associated with an increased risk of a fetal cleft palate. Although it is thought that there is a viral etiology, there is no clear benefit of antiviral agents alone. In severe cases, some clinicians will add an antiviral with oral steroids.[42,43] A suggested antiviral regimen for severe Bell's palsy is valacyclovir 1000 mg three times a day for 1 week.

Carpal Tunnel Syndrome: It is a common complaint in pregnancy with pain or numbness in thumb, index finger, and middle finger (median nerve distribution). The incidence is reported between 2% and 35%.[44,45] It is most common in the third trimester likely due to increased fluid retention causing compression rather than the viral etiology seen in nonpregnant women. The symptoms are relatively classic. The diagnosis is based on history and examination demonstrating median nerve distribution. Maneuvers designed to further compress the nerve may improve the diagnosis. The Phalen maneuver is hyperflexion of the wrists. The Tinel maneuver is eliciting pain with percussion over medial nerve. A positive Phalen test is a more sensitive test for indicating a carpal tunnel syndrome (CTS) than the Tinel test.[46]

Treatment is still primarily symptomatic using a splint to keep the wrist in a neutral position, ice pack, and analgesics. The use of NSAIDs has been reported to have no significant benefit compared with placebo in general for CTS.[47] However, as the etiology of CTS in pregnancy may be due to increased fluid, a trial of NSAIDs is reasonable. A splint can be used initially when sleeping. If symptoms continue or worsen, using the splint throughout the day may be beneficial. However, if symptoms do not improve with these interventions or weakness develops in the affected hand, a referral for evaluation for steroid injection, physical therapy, or even surgery is warranted. The problem will typically resolve within a few weeks postpartum, although full resolution may take months.[48] Carpal tunnel complaints will commonly occur in subsequent pregnancies.

CARDIOPULMONARY COMPLAINTS

Shortness of Breath: There are many changes to both respiratory and cardiac functions during pregnancy that are essential for providing adequate oxygenation and metabolic requirements for both the mother and fetus. These major changes include increased tidal volume, increased vital capacity, and decreased overall residual volume. As the uterus grows, women may experience the sensation of hypoventilation and shortness of breath, particularly with activity. As with any major symptoms during pregnancy, it is important to identify pathologic and serious causes of shortness of breath including pulmonary embolism, asthma exacerbation, and peripartum cardiomyopathy.

Physiologic dyspnea of pregnancy occurs in approximately 60% to 75% of women.[49] Most of the time, these symptoms start in the first and second trimester due to progesterone-induced hyperventilation which is required to meet the rising metabolic demands of the pregnancy. The rising level of progesterone can induce edema in the upper airways as well as thickening of nasal pharyngeal mucus. Many women report worsening symptoms of congestion and rhinitis which can impact the sensation of shortness of breath.[49] Workup and management of shortness of breath during pregnancy involves evaluating for signs and symptoms of severe pathologic disease including a full cardiopulmonary examination and vital sign assessment.

Some of the warning signs that should prompt a more in depth workup include:[50]

- Vital signs with tachycardia greater than 120 beats per minute, respiratory rate greater than 24 breaths per minute, and low oxygen saturation less than 95%
- Pulmonary examination findings of severe wheezing, rales, and rhonchi
- Reports of significant lower extremity swelling
- Chest pain with respirations

Once severe pathologic causes have been excluded, management should consist of reassurances that symptoms are normal during pregnancy and use of over-the-counter medications for symptoms management including cetirizine, loratadine, nasal saline sprays, nasal patches, and humidifier use should be encouraged for symptom relief.

Palpitations

Arrhythmias that are perceived as palpitations are the most common cardiac symptom during pregnancy.[51] Hospitalizations for pregnancy-related arrhythmias have increase between 2000 and 2012. Because maternal mortalities due to cardiac complications have also increased markedly, it is important to differentiate the typical palpitations associated with changing maternal physiology from those that may represent a developing cardiac complication. A good history, including prior pre-pregnant events and pre-existing cardiac issues, along with a cardiac examination should be done. An electrocardiogram may help to clarify the type of arrhythmia.[52] There should be a low threshold for doing a transthoracic echocardiogram in the presence of palpitations along with other risk factors for cardiac concerns (obesity, diabetes, strong family history, and so forth). A supraventricular tachycardia that does not cause syncope, dyspnea, or chest pain and quickly resolves with Valsalva maneuvers is not too concerning. However, a paroxysmal supraventricular tachycardia (PSVT) is often caused by an accessory pathway or by reentry within the atrioventricular node.[52] A pregnancy-related arrhythmia may be the first evidence of such a pathway. With a good history, one may determine that the pregnancy is exacerbating a preexisting problem.[53] If the patient describes a rapid tachycardia with an abrupt onset (and perhaps abrupt resolution) along with the symptoms noted above, PSVT should be considered.[53]

Treatment in a stable patient is the Valsalva maneuver or carotid sinus massage. These may block the AV nodal conduction and terminate the tachycardia.[54] If these fail, adenosine (6–18 mg IV) will terminate approximately 90% of PSVT. If the patient is experiencing hemodynamic compromise, direct current cardioversion should be performed.[55,56] There are a number of prophylactic pharmacologic therapies that can be initiated. The choice depends on cardiac structure, presence of WPW syndrome, or evidence of ischemic injury. A cardiologist consult is often helpful in determining ongoing care.

SUMMARY

Women may present during prenatal care with a variety of common and evolving symptoms. In general, levels of fatigue increase in the first and third trimester, and women should be counseled on behavioral modifications, encouraged to optimize nutrition, and continue safe exercise practices to improve levels of fatigue. Evaluation and management of anemia is also vital in ensuring optimal energy levels and preventing intrauterine growth restriction and preterm delivery. Women often present with concerns for skin changes during their pregnancy. Although most are benign and do not cause adverse pregnancy outcomes, they can cause significant distress. Nausea and vomiting, migraine headaches, and other neurologic complaints are common during pregnancy, and attention must be paid to assessment of symptom severity and evaluation of a possible pathologic cause rather than only due to maternal physiology. Palpitations or shortness of breath complaints are commonly normal changes in pregnancy physiology but may also represent the onset of a concerning pathology. Management of any of these conditions depends on the underlying etiology along with the persistence and severity of symptoms. In situations where the etiology of the complaint requires more evaluation or interventions, further in-depth discussions are needed regarding the diagnosis. When appropriate, patients should be offered both pharmacologic and non-pharmacologic treatment options. Counseling regarding proposed treatment should be patient centered with discussion about the risks, benefits, and efficacy so that patients may make informed decisions regarding care during their pregnancy.

CLINICS CARE POINTS

- Every system in the body is affected by hormonal and physiologic changes during pregnancy. Most are benign and will resolve in the postpartum period, but clinicians must be able to recognize "red flag" symptoms that should prompt further workup.
- Women who present with severe fatigue during pregnancy should be evaluated for baseline anemia and supplemented with intravenous iron when appropriate.
- Untreated sleep apnea can cause medical complications during pregnancy and through life.
- Encouraging women to maintain a regular exercise routine in pregnancy can improve feelings of fatigue and improve overall mental health scores for pregnant patients.
- Assessment of nausea and vomiting during pregnancy begins with quantification of severity of symptoms to guide management and assess response to care. The initial treatment involves behavioral changes and over the counter (OTC) medications. If this is not successful pharmaceutical interventions are available.
- Severe nausea and vomiting during pregnancy (PUQE score ≥ 13) should prompt workup for other pathologic causes such as gastroenteritis, chronic H pylori, molar pregnancy, diabetic ketoacidosis, and thyrotoxicosis.
- Cholestasis of pregnancy can be deadly for the fetus. Diagnosis, with close follow-up, medical intervention, and timing of the delivery can minimize fetal compromise.
- Management of migraine headaches during pregnancy initially includes acetaminophen and caffeine with the addition of metoclopramide and diphenhydramine as the initial treatment options. With refractory migraines, medications such as butalbital, opiates, and triptans should be used with caution during pregnancy.
- New onset severe headaches during pregnancy that are associated with focal neurological deficits, papilledema, or a postural changes should prompt further workup with intracranial imaging and neurology consult.
- Bell's palsy treatment, once more serious etiologies are eliminated, consists of reassurance, symptom relief, and oral steroids. Antiviral medications are rarely indicated.
- Carpal tunnel complaints are common with treatment focused on symptom relief.
- Although cardiopulmonary complaints are common, they need to be evaluated carefully to rule out significant cardiac pathology given the increasing incidence of maternal morbidity and mortality from cardiac events.

DISCLOSURE

All authors declare that they have no conflict of interest.

REFERENCES

1. ACOG committee opinion no. 804: physical activity and exercise during pregnancy and the postpartum period: Correction. Obstet Gynecol 2021;138(4):683.
2. Liu N, Wang J, Chen D-dan, et al. Effects of exercise on pregnancy and postpartum fatigue: a systematic review and meta-analysis. Eur J Obstet Gynecol Reprod Biol 2020;253:285–95.
3. Hansen R, Sommer VM, Pinborg A, et al. Intravenous ferric derisomaltose versus oral iron for persistent iron deficient pregnant women: a randomized controlled trial. Arch Gynecol Obstet 2022. https://doi.org/10.1007/s00404-022-06768-x.
4. Picchietti, DL. Restless legs syndrome during pregnancy and lactation. Up To Date. Available at https://www-uptodate-com.libproxy.unm.edu/contents/restless-legs-syndrome-during-pregnancy-and-lactation?search=restless%20legs%20syndrome%20in%20pregnancy&source=search_result&selectedTitle=1~150&usage_type=default&display_rank=1 Accessed March 17, 2023.
5. Dominquez JE, Street L, Louis J. Management of obstructive sleep apnea in pregnancy. Obstet Gynecol Clin North Am 2018;45(2):233–47.
6. Chung F, Yegneswaran B, Liao P, et al. STOP Questionnaire: a tool to screen patients for obstructive sleep apnea. Anesthesiology 2008;108:812–21.
7. Vora RV, Gupta R, Mehta MJ, et al. Pregnancy and skin. J Fam Med Prim Care 2014;3(4):318.
8. Tunzi, M., & Gray, G. R. (2007, January 15). Common skin conditions during pregnancy. American Family Physician. Accessed 28 December, 2022, Available at: https://www.aafp.org/pubs/afp/issues/2007/0115/p211.html.
9. Aldulaimi S, Saenz A. A bleeding oral mass in a pregnant woman. JAMA 2017; 318:293.
10. Jafarzadeh H, Sanatkhani M, Mohtasham N. Oral pyogenic granuloma: a review. J Oral Sci 2006;48:167.
11. Kroumpouzos G, Cohen LM. Dermatoses of pregnancy. J Am Acad Dermatol 2001;45:1.
12. Committee on Health Care for Underserved Women. Oral Health Care During Pregnancy and through the lifespan. ACOG Comm Opin 2013;569:2–3. ACOG.
13. Sills ES, Zegarelli DJ, Hoschander MM, et al. Clinical diagnosis and management of hormonally responsive oral pregnancy tumor (pyogenic granuloma). J Reprod Med 1996;41:467.
14. Thaxter Nesbeth KA, Samuels LA, Nicholson Daley C, et al. Ptyalism in pregnancy - a review of epidemiology and practices. Eur J Obstet Gynecol Reprod Biol 2016;198:47.
15. Bronshtein M, Gover A, Beloosesky R, et al. Characteristics and outcomes of ptyalism gravidarum. Isr Med Assoc J 2018;20:573.
16. Lacasse A, Rey E, Ferreira E, et al. Validity of a modified pregnancy–unique quantification of emesis and nausea (PUQE) scoring index to assess severity of nausea and vomiting of pregnancy. Obstet Anesth Digest 2008;28(3):162–3.
17. Lowe SA, Steinweg KE. Review article: Management of hyperemesis gravidarum and nausea and vomiting in pregnancy. Emerg Med Australasia (EMA) 2021; 34(1):9–15.
18. Khorasani F, Aryan H, Sobhi A, et al. A systematic review of the efficacy of alternative medicine in the treatment of nausea and vomiting of pregnancy. J Obstet Gynaecol 2019;40(1):10–9.
19. Ozgoli G, Goli M, Simbar M. Effects of ginger capsules on pregnancy, nausea and vomiting. J Altern Complement Med 2009;15(3):243–6.

20. Kondrackiene J, Kupcinskas L. Intrahepatic cholestasis of pregnancy-current achievements and unsolved problems. World J Gastroenterol 2008;14:5781.
21. Geenes V, Williamson C. Intrahepatic cholestasis of pregnancy. World J Gastroenterol 2009;15:2049.
22. Pataia V, Dixon PH, Williamson C. Pregnancy and bile acid disorders. Am J Physiol Gastrointest Liver Physiol 2017;313:G1.
23. Huang WM, Gowda M, Donnelly JG. Bile acid ratio in diagnosis of intrahepatic cholestasis of pregnancy. Am J Perinatol 2009;26:291.
24. Lindor KD. Lee RH. Intrahepatic Cholestasis of Pregnancy. Available at https://www-uptodate-com.libproxy.unm.edu/contents/intrahepatic-cholestasis-of-pregnancy?search=Cholestasis%20in%20pregnancy&source=search_result&selectedTitle=1~64&usage_type=default&display_rank=1 Accessed 17 March, 2023.
25. Kenyon AP, Piercy CN, Girling J, et al. Obstetric cholestasis, outcome with active management: a series of 70 cases. BJOG 2002;109:282.
26. Williamson C, Miragoli M, Sheikh Abdul Kadir S, et al. Bile acid signaling in fetal tissues: implications for intrahepatic cholestasis of pregnancy. Dig Dis 2011; 29:58.
27. Sepúlveda WH, González C, Cruz MA, et al. Vasoconstrictive effect of bile acids on isolated human placental chorionic veins. Eur J Obstet Gynecol Reprod Biol 1991;42:211.
28. Lee, RH. Greenberg M. Metz T. et al. Society for Maternal-Fetal Medicine consult series #53 intrahepatic cholestasis of pregnancy published February 2021. Available at https://www.smfm.org/publications/374-smfm-consult-series-53-intrahepatic-cholestasis-of-pregnancy Accessed 17 March, 2023.
29. Walker KF, Chappell LC, Hague WM, et al. Pharmacological interventions for treating intrahepatic cholestasis of pregnancy. Cochrane Database Syst Rev 2020;7:CD000493.
30. Ovadia C, Seed PT, Sklavounos A, et al. Association of adverse perinatal outcomes of intrahepatic cholestasis of pregnancy with biochemical markers: results of aggregate and individual patient data meta-analyses. Lancet 2019;393:899.
31. Lee RH, Incerpi MH, Miller DA, et al. Sudden fetal death in intrahepatic cholestasis of pregnancy. Obstet Gynecol 2009;113:528.
32. Robbins MS. Headache in pregnancy. CONTINUUM: Lifelong Learning in Neurology 2018;24(4):1092–107.
33. Negro A, Delaruelle Z, Ivanova TA, et al. Headache and pregnancy: a systematic review. J Headache Pain 2017;18(1). https://doi.org/10.1186/s10194-017-0816-0.
34. American College of Obstetricians and Gynecologist Clinical Practice Guidleine #3 Headaches in pregnancy and postpartum. Obstet Gynecol 2022;139(5): 944–72.
35. Onorato, K. Dougherty, C. & Ailani, J. (n.d.). Migraine during pregnancy. Practical Neurology. Available at https://practicalneurology.com/articles/2019-may/migraine-during-pregnancy Accessed 17 March, 2023.
36. Jackson CG, von Doersten PG. The facial nerve. Current trends in diagnosis, treatment, and rehabilitation. Med Clin North Am 1999;83:179.
37. Berić A. Peripheral nerve disorders in pregnancy. Adv Neurol 1994;64:179.
38. Vrabec JT, Isaacson B, Van Hook JW. Bell's palsy and pregnancy. Otolaryngol Head Neck Surg 2007;137:858.
39. Shmorgun D, Chan WS, Ray JG. Association between Bell's palsy in pregnancy and pre-eclampsia. QJM 2002;95:359.
40. Cohen Y, Lavie O, Granovsky-Grisaru S, et al. Bell palsy complicating pregnancy: a review. Obstet Gynecol Surv 2000;55:184.

41. MacIntosh PW, Fay AM. Update on the ophthalmic management of facial paralysis. Surv Ophthalmol 2019;64:79.

42. Engström M, Berg T, Stjernquist-Desatnik A, et al. Prednisolone and valaciclovir in Bell's palsy: a randomised, double-blind, placebo-controlled, multicentre trial. Lancet Neurol 2008;7:993.

43. Sax TW, Rosenbaum RB. Neuromuscular disorders in pregnancy. Muscle Nerve 2006;34:559.

44. Mabie WC. Peripheral neuropathies during pregnancy. Clin Obstet Gynecol 2005;48:57.

45. Meems M, Truijens S, Spek V, et al. Prevalence, course and determinants of carpal tunnel syndrome symptoms during pregnancy: a prospective study. BJOG 2015;122:1112.

46. MacDermid JC, Wessel J. Clinical diagnosis of carpal tunnel syndrome: a systematic review. J Hand Ther 2004;17:309.

47. Connor D, Marshall S, Massy-Westropp N. Non-surgical treatment (other than steroid injection) for carpal tunnel syndrome. Cochrane Database Syst Rev 2003;(1):CD003219.

48. McLennan HG, Oats JN, Walstab JE. Survey of hand symptoms in pregnancy. Med J Aust 1987;147:542.

49. Weinberger SE. Maternal adaptations to pregnancy: dyspnea and other physiologic changes of pregnancy. UpToDate. (n.d.). Available at https://www.uptodate.com/contents/maternal-adaptations-to-pregnancy-dyspnea-and-other-physiologic-respiratory-changes?search=respiratory+changes+pregnancy+&source=search_result&selectedTitle=1~150&usage_type=default&display_rank=1 Accessed 14 March, 2023.

50. Patterson KC. Approach to common respiratory problems in pregnancy. In: Lapinsky SE, Plante L, editors. Respiratory disease in pregnancy. Cambridge University Press; 2020. p. 13–24.

51. Vaidya VR, Arora S, Patel N, et al. Burden of Arrhythmia in Pregnancy. Circulation 2017;135:619.

52. Silversides c, Harris L, Yao SC. Supraventricular arrhythmia during pregnancy. UTD Available at: https://www-uptodate-com.libproxy.unm.edu/contents/supraventricular-arrhythmias-during-pregnancy?search=palpitations%20in%20pregnancy&topicRef=443&source=see_link Accessed 17 March, 2023.

53. Lee SH, Chen SA, Wu TJ, et al. Effects of pregnancy on first onset and symptoms of paroxysmal supraventricular tachycardia. Am J Cardiol 1995;76:675.

54. Brugada J, Katritsis DG, Arbelo E, et al. 2019 ESC Guidelines for the management of patients with supraventricular tachycardiaThe Task Force for the management of patients with supraventricular tachycardia of the European Society of Cardiology (ESC). Eur Heart J 2020;41:655.

55. Regitz-Zagrosek V, Roos-Hesselink JW, Bauersachs J, et al. 2018 ESC Guidelines for the management of cardiovascular diseases during pregnancy. Eur Heart J 2018;39:3165.

56. Page RL, Joglar JA, Caldwell MA, et al. 2015 ACC/AHA/HRS Guideline for the management of adult patients with supraventricular tachycardia: a report of the American College of Cardiology/American Heart Association Task Force on Clinical Practice Guidelines and the Heart Rhythm Society. J Am Coll Cardiol 2016; 67:e27.

Prenatal Counseling and Preparation for Breastfeeding

Margarita Berwick, MD*, Adetola F. Louis-Jacques, MD

KEYWORDS

- Breastfeeding • Support • Prenatal care • Infant feeding • Breastfeeding education

KEY POINTS

- Patient education, peer counseling, lactation specialist care, and encouragement are effective strategies for promoting breastfeeding in the prenatal period.
- Patients with anticipated challenges may benefit from additional support including education about signs of adequate milk intake by the newborn, antenatal consultation with a lactation professional focused on identified challenges, antenatal colostrum harvesting, and emotional support.
- Most patients with medical comorbidities, history of breast surgery, and substance use disorders can breastfeed with education and support.

INTRODUCTION

Breastfeeding is the gold standard of infant nutrition, providing well-established dose-dependent benefits to both the breastfeeding individual and the child (**Table 1**). Most recent American Academy of Pediatrics (AAP) guidelines for optimal duration of breastfeeding recommend exclusive breastfeeding for the first 6 months, and continued, along with complementary foods, for 24 months and beyond as mutually desired by parents and their children.[10]

Obstetric care professionals are uniquely poised to make an impact on patients' feeding choices as most women make this decision before conception or early in their pregnancy.[11] Research shows that support delivered in primary care settings is effective in positively influencing breastfeeding rates.[12,13] Strategies for breastfeeding support may include any of the following: education and anticipatory guidance, psychological support, assistance in management of breastfeeding difficulties and obtaining supplies, and referral to community and professional services.

Department of Obstetrics and Gynecology, University of Florida College of Medicine, University of Florida, PO Box 100294, 1600 Southwest Archer Road, Gainesville, FL 32610-0294, USA
* Corresponding author.
E-mail address: mberwick@ufl.edu

Obstet Gynecol Clin N Am 50 (2023) 549–565
https://doi.org/10.1016/j.ogc.2023.03.007
0889-8545/23/© 2023 Elsevier Inc. All rights reserved.
obgyn.theclinics.com

Table 1
Breastfeeding benefits for children and their breastfeeding parents

Maternal Benefits of Breastfeeding	Child Benefits of Breastfeeding
Reduced risk of • Type 2 diabetes mellitus[1] • Ovarian cancer[2] • Breast cancer[3] • Obesity[4] • Cardiovascular disease including stroke, myocardial infarction, and coronary vascular disease[5,6]	Reduced risk of • Respiratory tract infections, otitis media, and gastroenteritis[7–9] • Sudden infant death syndrome (SIDS) (Hauck et al, 2011) • Asthma, food allergies (Ip et al, 2007) • Childhood obesity (Wang et al, 2016) • Childhood leukemia (Su Q et al, 2021) • Inflammatory bowel disease (Xu et al, 2017)

This section explores the current landscape of prenatal interventions to support breastfeeding in the Unites States, including strategies for special circumstances such as support for patients with anticipated challenges and those desiring to breastfeed without antecedent pregnancy.

DISCUSSION
What Are Patient and Provider Perspectives on Prenatal Breastfeeding Support?

Patient perspectives
Factors underlying patients' decisions to breastfeed or formula feed are complex and include age, marital status, income level, race, ethnicity, educational background, family influences, and prior personal feeding experiences of an individual.[14–16] Although many of these factors are non-modifiable, some, including patient perception of provider attitude toward breastfeeding, knowledge about health benefits of breastfeeding, prenatal breastfeeding intention, may be amenable to intervention.

Despite existence of potential opportunities for intervention, only 15% to 29% of patients reported discussing breastfeeding with their clinician.[17,18] In addition, many report feeling unprepared for the challenges of breastfeeding,[19,20] receiving inadequate support, or even being misled or misinformed.[21]

Provider perspectives
Breastfeeding has been consistently designated as one of the top public health priorities in the United States. This view is shared by physicians[22]; however, analyses of physician behaviors showed that breastfeeding discussions are infrequent, inconsistent, and often do not fulfill the recommendations from national guidelines.[17,18] A summary of breastfeeding support guidelines from Unites States Preventive Services Taskforce (USPSTF), AAP, and American College of Obstetricians and Gynecologists (ACOG) applicable to prenatal care is included in **Box 1**.

Among the reasons cited for this deficiency are lack of time, inadequate knowledge, and lack of confidence or skills to address common problems.[27] Surveys of physicians conducted over time also demonstrate that little progress in this area has been made over the past 20 years,[28] and a national survey of US pediatricians even demonstrated decreased belief that benefits of breastfeeding outweigh the difficulties.[29]

Although interventions to increase breastfeeding rates have largely focused on patients, research demonstrated that providing training to health care staff including physicians improves clinical outcomes related to breastfeeding and thus represents an important target for future studies.[30,31]

Box 1

National organization recommendations for breastfeeding support applicable to prenatal care

USPSTF[23]
- Provide 1-on-1 counseling
- Provide supplies
- Provide information about breastfeeding
- Provide psychological support
- Provide hands-on assistance with positioning, latching
- Promote formal educational programs for patients and family members

ACOG[24]
- Develop and maintain knowledge about lactation physiology, management of common problems
- Support each woman's right to breastfeed and decision regarding breastfeeding
- Ask about breastfeeding history
- Work with hospital staff to provide early frequent milk expression

AAP[25]
- Train clinic staff in skills to support breastfeeding, including via telephone
- If possible, use the International Board-Certified Lactation Consultant or another staff with training in breastfeeding
- Engage both parents and other family members
- Initiate conversations about breastfeeding early in prenatal care/ postpartum
- Schedule initial newborn visit by 24 to 48 hours post-discharge
- Refer parents to appropriate educational resources

Surgeon General's Call to Support Breastfeeding[26]
- Educate mothers on benefits of breastfeeding for babies and themselves
- Teach mothers to breastfeed
- Encourage mothers to ask for help with breastfeeding
- Develop systems that guarantee continuity of lactation care at discharge from the hospital
- Include support for lactation as an essential medical service

---

What Types of Prenatal Support for Breastfeeding Have Been Studied?

Emotional support and encouragement

Pooled analyses of US-based trials showed that individual-level interventions such as support and education increase breastfeeding rates.[12] Several studies from diverse patient populations have demonstrated positive effect of provider encouragement on breastfeeding rates; however, these studies are often limited by their retrospective nature and reliance on patient recall.[32–34]

Education and counseling

Educating patients about breastfeeding is one of the key strategies for increasing breastfeeding rates.[26] Three large recent cohort studies demonstrated the efficacy of breastfeeding education in increasing patient knowledge, breastfeeding intention, and in two of the three trials, breastfeeding initiation.[35–38] An older systematic review of 19 US-based studies showed a significant increase in breastfeeding initiation with prenatal education.[37] Timing of education delivery, educational content, and mode of education delivery vary significantly between studies, making it difficult to recommend one approach over another.

Knowledge about health benefits of breastfeeding also has a positive effect on breastfeeding practices.[16,33,39–42] Last, simply educating patients about the recommendations for breastfeeding may also affect patients' breastfeeding practices.[43]

Educational videos

The use of prerecorded breastfeeding education videos has become a popular choice for patient education. Theoretical benefits of video-based education include no demand on provider time, patient ability to access videos at their convenience, and low cost. Data regarding the effect of this type of intervention on breastfeeding are limited.[44,45] The largest study conducted to date found no difference in breastfeeding initiation, exclusivity, or duration either during delivery hospitalization or in the first 6 months postpartum.[45] A study of prenatal video education on antenatal milk expression is currently underway.[46]

Peer support

Peer counselors are typically individuals with successful breastfeeding experience and cultural and socioeconomic background similar to individuals in the community in which they provide the service. Peer counseling interventions have been consistently associated with increased rates of breastfeeding initiation, duration, and exclusivity.[41,47,48] Given their demonstrated efficacy, peer counseling programs have been implemented by Special Supplemental Nutrition Program for Women, Infants and Children programs in many states and are endorsed by the Centers for Disease Control as one of the core strategies to increase breastfeeding rates.

Lactation specialist services

Lactation care may be delivered by practitioners with a range of titles, training, and scope of practice. The most rigorous designation is the International Board-Certified Lactation Consultant (IBCLC). These professionals provide a full scope of lactation care including management of complex cases with exception of prescribing medications except in cases where IBCLC also holds a degree granting them such privileges (eg, MD or APRN). Interventions delivered by lactation specialists have demonstrated efficacy in different patient populations, including those with traditionally low rates of breastfeeding.[49] Team approaches combining the care from a lactation specialist and physician perform better than interventions delivered by a physician alone, and such approaches are highly satisfactory to patients.[20,50]

Hospital policies

The Ten Steps to Successful Breastfeeding are maternity care practices endorsed by the World Health Organization and United Nations Children's Fund for promotion of breastfeeding (**Box 2**). Studies consistently demonstrate that breastfeeding outcomes improve with exposure to increased number of steps.[20,51–54]

Lactation Physiology and Implications for Clinical Management

Knowledge of basic physiology of lactation is important to be able to provide patients with evidence-based counseling, dispel myths, and inform management of some breastfeeding challenges. **Table 2** provides an overview of lactogenesis phases and suggested anticipatory guidance.

SUPPORT FOR BREASTFEEDING IN SPECIAL CIRCUMSTANCES
Breast Anatomy-Related Challenges

Adult breast shape and size vary significantly among individuals and have virtually no impact on ability to breastfeed. Breast examination at initiation of prenatal care and again in late second or third trimester provides an opportunity for identification of potential challenges related to anatomy and identification of other concerns such as lack of breast change over the course of gestation.

Congenital Breast and Nipple Anatomy and Related Challenges

Table 3 provides a description and suggested anticipatory management strategies for most common congenital breast anatomy variations.

Box 2
Ten steps to support breastfeeding (World Health Organization)

1 A. Comply fully with the International Code of Marketing of Breast-milk Substitutes and relevant World Health Assembly resolutions.

1 B. Have a written infant feeding policy that is routinely communicated to staff and parents.

1 C. Establish ongoing monitoring and data management systems.

2. Ensure that staff have sufficient knowledge, competence, and skills to support breastfeeding.

3. Discuss the importance and management of breastfeeding with pregnant women and their families.

4. Facilitate immediate and uninterrupted skin-to-skin contact and support mothers to initiate breastfeeding as soon as possible after birth.

5. Support mothers to initiate and maintain breastfeeding and manage common difficulties.

6. Do not provide breastfed newborns any food or fluids other than breastmilk, unless medically indicated.

7. Enable mothers and their infants to remain together and to practice rooming-in 24 hours a day.

8. Support mothers to recognize and respond to their infants' cues for feeding.

9. Counsel mothers on the use and risks of feeding bottles, artificial nipples (teats), and pacifiers.

10. Coordinate discharge so that parents and their infants have timely access to ongoing support and care.

Acquired Breast Anatomy Alterations and Breast Surgery

Acquired alterations of breast anatomy include breast surgery (augmentation, reduction, lumpectomy, and mastectomy), biopsies, piercings, and tattooing. Any of these alterations have the potential to interfere with breastfeeding through damage to glandular tissue, nerves, and ductal system of the breast. With the exception of complete mastectomy, none of these are indicative of inability to breastfeed.[58,59] However, women with prior breast surgery may have lower rates of breastfeeding initiation, duration, and exclusivity,[60] and in one study of patients with prior breast augmentation, up to 3.7% cited their implant as the reason for not breastfeeding.[60]

Supporting Lactation Without Antecedent Pregnancy

In some cases, such as with surrogacy or adoption, parents may desire to provide their breast milk to the infant without being pregnant. The induction of lactation in these circumstances is possible with a combination of pharmacologic treatment with hormones (usually with combined oral contraceptives containing estrogen and progesterone) and galactagogues (usually dopamine antagonists such as metoclopramide) as well as regular frequent breast stimulation. The detailed descriptions of available regimens, indications, and contraindications for their use are described in ABM Clinical Protocols #9 and #33. Lactation induction is best supervised by professionals with expertise in lactation and experience in use of the medications listed above.

Table 2
Phases of lactogenesis

Lactogenesis Stage and Timing	Physiologic Events	Clinical Findings	Anticipatory Guidance and Management
I (Secretory initiation) From 16–20 wk to 4 d postpartum	Final steps in breast development and maturation are completed during pregnancy under hormonal influence of estrogen, progesterone, and prolactin	Colostrum is produced and may be expressed manually or leak spontaneously	• Reassure patient that leakage of colostrum during pregnancy is normal; disposable or washable bra pads can be used if desired by patient • Help patients initiate of breastfeeding or pumping as soon as possible after birth and ideally within 1 h
II (Secretory activation) Usually within 48–72 h postpartum; may be delayed for up to 10 d	At the time of placental separation progesterone levels decline, and hormonal inhibition of copious milk product ion is removed.	Onset of production of large amount of milk aocompanied < l by color change from yellow to white.	• Patients may experience engorgement which presents as uncomfortable swelling and distention of the breasts associated with onset of stage II lactogenesis • Feeding infant on cue 8–12 times daily or expressing milk at similar time intervals may aid in prevention or reduction of severity of engorgement • Additional efforts to "empty" the breast should not be undertaken due to the risk of development of hyperlactation and worsening symptoms
III (Maintenance) Duration of breastfeeding	Oxytocin stimulates leading to contraction of myoepithelial cells and milk ejection for immediate feeding episode, and prolactin which acts to maintain lactation	Lactation is mainly maintained on supply and demand basis.	• If separation from infant is necessary, milk should be pumped at approximately the same frequency as feeding would occur (5–12 times per day)
IV (Involution) Cessation of breastfeeding	With reduced frequency of feeding, paracrine signals lead to decreased milk production	Breasts may show loss of volume, striae. Small amount of milk may be able to be expressed with pressure or spontaneously for years after lactation is complete.	Explore patient's reasons and feelings about cessation of breastfeeding

Table 3
Common congenital breast anatomy variations and recommended

Anatomy Description	Incidence	Clinical Findings	Management
Insufficient glandular tissue/breast hypoplasia/tuberous breasts	Unknown, likely secondary to absence of a precise/uniform definition[55,56]	Pubertal history of limited breast growth breasts do not increase in size or minimally increase in size during pregnancy. Breasts may be normal in shape or may be described as "tuberous," with narrow base, elongated shape, tissue displacement toward the nipple-areolar complex. Breasts may appear widely spaced and/or significantly asymmetric.	• Optimal management is unknown and breastfeeding outcome cannot be predicted prenatally. • Prenatal consultation with a lactation consultant should be considered. • Optimize conditions for effective lactogenesis • Consider prenatal colostrum harvesting if no contraindications exist (see section below).
Flat or inverted nipples	1%	Inverted nipples are the result of congenital tethering of the nipple to underlying fascia. With gentle pressure to edges of areolae, nipple retracts below the surface. Flat nipples neither retract nor protrude	• No prenatal intervention (breast shells, nipple shapers, exercises) has been shown to permanently alter nipple shape or impact breastfeeding success[57] • Most infants can latch and feed without any intervention • Nipple can be gently drawn out immediately before a breastfeeding session using suction from breast pump.
Polythelia (accessory nipples) with or without polymastia (accessory breast tissue)	1%	Extra nipple with or without breast tissue mound located along the milk like axilla to the inner thigh. Accessory breast tissue shows similar hormonal responses to normally located breast tissue and can develop similar disorders (eg, carcinoma)	• Accessory breast tissue may become enlarged during pregnancy and early postpartum period • Milk production is minimal, and tissue will regress in the absence of stimulation.

Approach to Patients with Anticipated Delay in Lactogenesis Stage II

Up to 44% of postpartum patients in the United States may experience delay in onset of lactogenesis stage II.[61] No uniform definition exists, but several studies defined "delayed" lactogenesis as that taking place more than 72 hours postpartum.[61–64] Risk factors for the delay include a broad range of medical and obstetrical conditions such as obesity, polycystic ovary syndrome (PCOS), pregestational and gestational diabetes, thyroid disease, insufficient glandular tissue, preeclampsia, cesarean delivery, postpartum hemorrhage, and retained placental fragments.[61–66]

Despite the high prevalence of this condition, no uniform approach to management of at-risk patients exists. In addition to receiving maternity care practices that optimize breastfeeding, patients with risk factors for delayed lactogenesis and/or lactation insufficiency may benefit from education about lactation physiology, dose-dependent nature of breastfeeding benefits, and assessment of adequate milk intake by the neonate. *Antenatal* consult with a lactation specialist may be useful to review these subjects as well as strategies for maximizing lactation. Emotional support and encouragement as well as intensive support postpartum are important.

Last, one specific practice that has been shown to be associated with decrease in delayed lactogenesis stage II and improved breastfeeding in the early postpartum period in patients with metabolic and obstetric risk factors is early initiation of breastfeeding or milk expression, ideally within 1 hour of birth.[67]

The Role of Antenatal Milk Expression

Antenatal milk expression refers to collection of breast milk during late pregnancy for storage and use in the early postpartum period. Among benefits of antenatal breast milk expression are reduced rates of formula feeding in the hospital, increased maternal confidence, and increased rate of exclusive breastfeeding in the first week of life.[68] Published regimens of antenatal milk expression vary widely in recommended duration and technique of expression. In most studies, participants started milk expression after 36 weeks of pregnancy; however, protocols initiating expression as early as 32 weeks have been published.[69] Although nipple stimulation has been associated with premature contractions, a scoping review of 20 recent studies demonstrated no increased risk of preterm birth.[69]

BREASTFEEDING AND NEONATAL CONDITIONS
Prematurity

Premature and medically complex infants may have difficulty with coordination of sucking and swallowing and may fatigue easily with attempt at oral feeding. Health benefits of breast milk are particularly advantageous in this group and include lower incidence of necrotizing enterocolitis, sepsis, improved gastrointestinal function, and earlier discharge from the hospital.[70]

Cleft Lip and Palate

Infants with structural abnormalities of the oropharynx such as cleft lip and palate may be able to feed directly from the breast with the use of special techniques and devices.[71] In addition to nutritive benefits of breast milk, breastfeeding promotes optimal growth and development of facial musculature, jaw, and palate, and this benefit extends to infants post-reconstructive surgery of these structures.[72–74] Infants who are unable to feed directly from the breast can be fed expressed breast milk via route most appropriate for their condition, which may involve the use of a regular or specialized bottle, syringe, or medicine cup.

Table 4
Management of select infectious diseases in pregnancy

Breastfeeding Contraindication	Condition	Breastfeeding Management
Breastfeeding or feeding of expressed breast milk contraindicated	Maternal HIV infection	Breastfeeding is contraindicated in settings where breast milk substitutes and sanitary ways of preparing the substitutes are readily available.
Breastfeeding or feeding of expressed milk can occur with appropriate treatment and/or precautions	COVID-19	Ongoing feeding is encouraged. Separation of mother and infant is not necessary. Wash hands thoroughly with soap and water. Cover mouth with cough and sneeze.
	Influenza	Ongoing feeding is encouraged. Separation of mother and infant is not necessary. Wash hands thoroughly with soap and water. Cover mouth with cough and sneeze.
	Active maternal tuberculosis	Expressed breast milk can be fed to the infant by a healthy caregiver. Direct feeding from the breast may resume following 2 wk of appropriate antibiotic treatment when patient is no longer considered contagious.
	Herpetic lesions on the breast	Breastfeed from the unaffected breast. Herpetic lesions must be covered to avoid contact. Milk from the affected breast should be discarded. Hand hygiene and thorough cleaning of pump parts are necessary.
	Shingles	Breastfeed from the unaffected breast lesions must be covered to avoid contact milk from the affected breast should be discarded. Hand hygiene and thorough cleaning of pump parts are necessary.
No restrictions on breastfeeding	Hepatitis B Hepatitis C	Breastfeeding is encouraged. Breastfeeding can continue. If bleeding or severe cracking of the nipple occurs, mothers have traditionally been advised to abstain from directly feeding from or feeding expressed breast milk from the affected side until complete healing occurs.

BREASTFEEDING AND MATERNAL CONDITIONS
Maternal Use of Medications

Individuals taking prescription medications may have concerns regarding medication safety with breastfeeding leading to self-discontinuation or alteration of the dose. Addressing medication concerns early in the course of prenatal care allows time to review safety of a particular medication as well as options for substitution for a medication with more acceptable risk profile when possible. Data regarding breast milk levels and safety of various medications are continually evolving and the most up-to-date information can be found in these resources.

- MotherToBaby
- LactMed
- Dr Thomas Hale's Medications and Mother's Milk
- E-lactancia

Infections

Concerns about transmission of infectious diseases can lead to decision to not breastfeed in patients who do not have a contraindication. **Table 4** summarizes the management guidelines for infections commonly encountered in the United States.

Table 5
Management of select substances and alcohol use in breastfeeding

Substance	Breastfeeding Management
Alcohol	Occasional moderate alcohol consumption defined as consumption of one standard drink per day, may be compatible with breastfeeding, particularly if the parent providing the milk waits at least 2 h before feeding or pumping breast.milk.[76] Heavy alcohol use is not compatible with breastfeeding and should be discouraged in these circumstances.
Tobacco (including e-cigarettes and vaping devices)	Patients who smoke can breastfeed but should never smoke while breastfeeding. Exposure to tobacco smoke prenatally and postnatally is a risk factor for SIDS.[77–80] Data regarding safety of nicotine replacement products (lozenges, gum, and so forth) are limited; however, the use of these products removes infant exposure to other harmful chemicals in smoke and may thus be preferable to ongoing smoking.[81,82]
Marijuana	No uniform guideline exists to guide breastfeeding management due to significant variation of THC content across different products. Accumulating data suggest long-term neurodevelopmental outcomes of THC exposure during pregnancy and lactat.ion.[82] Patient should be discouraged from marijuana use in all forms while breastfeeding.
Opioid use disorder	Accumulating evidence shows that levels of methadone and buprenorphine and their metabolites in breast milk are low, and breastfeeding reduces the severity of neonatal abstinence syndrome.[83,84]
Illicit drugs (amphetamines, PCP, cocaine)	Patients actively using illicit drugs generally should not breastfeed.[10]

Maternal Alcohol and Substance Use

Substance use among pregnant women has increased over the past decade.[75] Providing patients with accurate up-to-date information on risks and benefits of breastfeeding in their specific circumstances is important in helping them make infant feeding decisions and optimizing breastfeeding rates. See **Table 5**.

SUPPORTING LACTATION AT RETURN TO WORK OR SCHOOL

Parents returning to work or school will need to pump and store breast milk to maintain lactation and provide nutrition to the infant during separation. Patients should receive education regarding frequency of pumping which should approximate feeding frequency. Innovations in breast pump technology have led to the development of wearable and hand-free pumps for more convenient pumping. Federal law requires reasonable break time for an employee to express breast milk in the first year of a child's life.

SUMMARY

Exclusive breastfeeding in the first 6 months and continued with introduction of complementary foods for 2 years or longer is the gold standard of infant nutrition, with life-long benefits for children and their breastfeeding parents. Compelling evidence indicates that prenatal care providers can influence patients' infant feeding decisions and increase breastfeeding rates through education, counseling, encouragement, collaboration with lactation professionals, and referral to community resources. Further studies, particularly randomized control trials, are needed to compare prenatal breastfeeding support strategies to each other to identify those that are most effective for widespread implementation.

CLINICS CARE POINTS

- Address infant feeding plans early during prenatal care, ideally starting with the initial prenatal care visit.
- Prenatal care providers should engage the systematic structured learning about breastfeeding from reputable resources. Some recommendations include the breastfeeding curriculum from AAP, ACOG Breastfeeding Toolkit, and the Academy of Breastfeeding Medicine Education page. Links are provided below. If available, shadowing a lactation professional may provide additional insights and skills.
- Educate patients about breastfeeding. Suggested education subjects include breastfeeding as the recommended form of infant feeding, recommended duration of 24 months, health benefits to parent and infant, practical aspects, and realistic description of early breastfeeding.
- Best available evidence indicates that interventions to support breastfeeding are most effective when delivered in a longitudinal manner and incorporating multiple approaches (eg, lactation specialist consultation plus breastfeeding education from MD).
- Work collaboratively with lactation specialists and peer counselors.
- Provide patients with information about community resources for breastfeeding support.
- Inform patients about benefits available through their insurance and federal and state benefits.
- Review patients' medical history and medications and address any concerns regarding breastfeeding.

- Support patients with anticipated challenges by addressing possible problems and creating a proactive plan. When exclusive breastfeeding is not possible, educate patients about health benefits of any breastfeeding or human milk feeding.
- Promote implementation of Ten Steps to Successful breastfeeding.
- Help patients initiate breastfeeding or milk expression as early as possible and ideally in the first hour after birth.

LINKS TO SELECT EDUCATIONAL RESOURCES

AAP Breastfeeding Curriculum: https://www.aap.org/en/learning/breastfeeding-curriculum/.

ACOG Breastfeeding Toolkit: https://www.acog.org/topics/breastfeeding.

Academy of Breastfeeding Medicine Education Center: https://www.bfmed.org/education.

Breastfeeding Handbook for Physicians: https://publications.aap.org/aapbooks/book/428/Breastfeeding-Handbook-for-Physicians.

CONFLICTS OF INTEREST

M. Berwick reports no conflicts of interests. A.F. Louis-Jacques reports no conflicts of interests related to this topic. Current grant support: Robert A. Winn Diversity in Clinical Trials Award Program. National Science Foundation, United States (BCS-2218101). National Institutes of Health, United States NIDA (U01 DA055358-01). Merck for Mothers Safer Childbirth Cities.

REFERENCES

1. Aune D, Norat T, Romundstad P, et al. Breastfeeding and the maternal risk of type 2 diabetes: a systematic review and dose-response meta-analysis of cohort studies. Nutr Metab Cardiovasc Dis 2014;24(2):107–15.
2. Luan NN, Wu QJ, Gong TT, et al. Breastfeeding and ovarian cancer risk: a meta-analysis of epidemiologic studies. Am J Clin Nutr 2013;98(4):1020–31.
3. Unar-Munguía M, Torres-Mejía G, Colchero MA, et al. Breastfeeding mode and risk of breast cancer: a dose-response meta-analysis. J Hum Lact 2017;33(2):422–34.
4. Bobrow KL, Quigley MA, Green J, et al, Million Women Study Collaborators. Persistent effects of women's parity and breastfeeding patterns on their body mass index: results from the Million Women Study. Int J Obes 2013;37(5):712–7.
5. Stuebe AM, Michels KB, Willett WC, et al. Duration of lactation and incidence of myocardial infarction in middle to late adulthood. Am J Obstet Gynecol 2009;200(2):138.e1–1388.
6. Tschiderer L, Seekircher L, Kunutsor SK, et al. Breastfeeding is associated with a reduced maternal cardiovascular risk: systematic review and meta-analysis involving data from 8 studies and 1 192 700 parous women. J Am Heart Assoc 2022;11(2):e022746.
7. Bachrach VR, Schwarz E, Bachrach LR. Breastfeeding and the risk of hospitalization for respiratory disease in infancy: a meta-analysis. Arch Pediatr Adolesc Med 2003;157(3):237–43.
8. Ip S, Chung M, Raman G, et al. Breastfeeding and maternal and infant health outcomes in developed countries. Evid Rep Technol Assess 2007;153:1–186.

9. Wilson K, Gebretsadik T, Adgent MA, et al. The association between duration of breastfeeding and childhood asthma outcomes. Ann Allergy Asthma Immunol 2022;129(2):205–11.

10. Meek JY, Noble L. Section on Breastfeeding. Policy statement: breastfeeding and the use of human milk. Pediatrics 2022;150(1). e2022057988.

11. Declercq ER, Sakala C, Corry MP, et al. Listening to Mothers II: report of the Second National U.S. Survey of women's childbearing experiences: conducted january-february 2006 for childbirth connection by harris interactive(R) in partnership with Lamaze International. J Perinat Educ 2007;16(4):9–14.

12. Patnode CD, Henninger ML, Senger CA, et al. Primary care interventions to support breastfeeding: updated systematic review for the U.S. Preventive services task force. Rockville (MD): Agency for Healthcare Research and Quality (US); 2016. Report No.: 15-05218-EF-1. PMID: 27854403.

13. McFadden A, Gavine A, Renfrew MJ, et al. Support for healthy breastfeeding mothers with healthy term babies. Cochrane Database Syst Rev 2017;2(2): CD001141.

14. Hurley KM, Black MM, Papas MA, et al. Variation in breastfeeding behaviours, perceptions, and experiences by race/ethnicity among a low-income statewide sample of Special Supplemental Nutrition Program for Women, Infants, and Children (WIC) participants in the United States. Matern Child Nutr 2008;4(2):95–105.

15. Beauregard JL, Hamner HC, Chen J, et al. Racial disparities in breastfeeding initiation and duration among U.S. Infants born in 2015. MMWR Morb Mortal Wkly Rep 2019;68(34):745–8.

16. Radzyminski S, Callister LC. Health professionals' attitudes and beliefs about breastfeeding. J Perinat Educ 2015;24(2):102–9.

17. Taveras EM, Li R, Grummer-Strawn L, et al. Mothers' and clinicians' perspectives on breastfeeding counseling during routine preventive visits. Pediatrics 2004; 113(5):e405–11.

18. Demirci JR, Bogen DL, Holland C, et al. Characteristics of breastfeeding discussions at the initial prenatal visit. Obstet Gynecol 2013;122(6):1263–70.

19. Mozingo JN, Davis MW, Droppleman PG, et al. It wasn't working. " Women's experiences with short-term breastfeeding. MCN Am J Matern Child Nurs 2000; 25(3):120–6.

20. Glassman ME, Blanchet K, Andresen J, et al. Impact of breastfeeding support services on mothers' breastfeeding experiences when provided by an MD/IBCLC in the pediatric medical home. Clin Pediatr (Phila). 2022;61(5–6):418–27.

21. Dillaway HE, Douma ME. Are pediatric offices "supportive" of breastfeeding? Discrepancies between mothers' and healthcare professionals' reports. Clin Pediatr (Phila). 2004;43(5):417–30.

22. Meek JY, Nelson JM, Hanley LE, et al. Landscape analysis of breastfeeding-related physician education in the United States. Breastfeed Med 2020;15(6): 401–11.

23. US Preventive Services Task Force, Bibbins-Domingo K, Grossman DC, et al. Primary care interventions to support breastfeeding: US preventive services task force recommendation statement. JAMA 2016;316(16):1688–93.

24. American College of Obstetricians and Gynecologists' Committee on Obstetric Practice; Breastfeeding Expert Work Group. Committee opinion No. 658 summary: optimizing support for breastfeeding as part of obstetric practice. Obstet Gynecol 2016;127(2):420–1.

25. Joan Younger Meek, Amy J. Hatcher, SECTION ON BREASTFEEDING, Margreete Johnston, Mary O'Connor, Lisa Stellwagen, Jennifer Thomas, Julie Ware,

Richard Schanler; The Breastfeeding-Friendly Pediatric Office Practice. Pediatrics 2017;139(5):e20170647.

26. Office of the surgeon general (US); Centers for disease control and prevention (US); office on women's health (US). The surgeon General's Call to action to support breastfeeding. Rockville (MD): Office of the Surgeon General (US); 2011.

27. Sims AM, Long SA, Tender JA, et al. Surveying the knowledge, attitudes, and practices of District of Columbia ACOG members related to breastfeeding. Breastfeed Med 2015;10(1):63–8.

28. Rosen-Carole C, Allen K, Thompson J, et al. Prenatal provider support for breastfeeding: changes in attitudes, practices and recommendations over 22 years. J Hum Lact 2020;36(1):109–18.

29. Feldman-Winter L, Szucs K, Milano A, et al. National trends in pediatricians' practices and attitudes about breastfeeding: 1995 to 2014. Pediatrics 2017;140(4): e20171229.

30. Holmes AV, McLeod AY, Thesing C, et al. Physician breastfeeding education leads to practice changes and improved clinical outcomes. Breastfeed Med 2012;7(6):403–8.

31. Balogun OO, Dagvadorj A, Yourkavitch J, et al. Health facility staff training for improving breastfeeding outcome: a systematic review for step 2 of the baby-friendly hospital initiative. Breastfeed Med 2017;12(9):537–46.

32. Lu MC, Lange L, Slusser W, et al. Provider encouragement of breast-feeding: evidence from a national survey. Obstet Gynecol 2001;97(2):290–5.

33. Kornides M, Kitsantas P. Evaluation of breastfeeding promotion, support, and knowledge of benefits on breastfeeding outcomes. J Child Health Care 2013; 17(3):264–73.

34. Jarlenski M, McManus J, Diener-West M, et al. Association between support from a health professional and breastfeeding knowledge and practices among obese women: evidence from the Infant Practices Study II. Womens Health Issues 2014; 24(6):641–8.

35. Parry KC, Tully KP, Hopper LN, et al. Evaluation of Ready, Set, BABY: a prenatal breastfeeding education and counseling approach. Birth 2019;46(1):113–20.

36. Ahlers-Schmidt CR, Okut H, Dowling J. Impact of prenatal education on breastfeeding initiation among low-income women. Am J Health Promot 2020;34(8): 919–22.

37. Rosen-Carole C, Halterman J, Baldwin CD, et al. Prenatal provider breastfeeding toolkit: results of a pilot to increase women's prenatal breastfeeding support, intentions, and outcomes. J Hum Lact 2022;38(1):64–74.

38. Cohen SS, Alexander DD, Krebs NF, et al. Factors associated with breastfeeding initiation and continuation: a meta-analysis. J Pediatr 2018;203:190–6.e21.

39. Stuebe AM, Bonuck K. What predicts intent to breastfeed exclusively? Breastfeeding knowledge, attitudes, and beliefs in a diverse urban population. Breastfeed Med 2011;6(6):413–20.

40. Ross-Cowdery M, Lewis CA, Papic M, et al. Counseling about the maternal health benefits of breastfeeding and mothers' intentions to breastfeed. Matern Child Health J 2017;21(2):234–41.

41. Houghtaling B, Byker Shanks C, Jenkins M. Likelihood of breastfeeding within the USDA's food and nutrition service special supplemental nutrition program for women, infants, and children population. J Hum Lact 2017;33(1):83–97.

42. Ganju A, Suresh A, Stephens J, et al. Learning, life, and lactation: knowledge of breastfeeding's impact on breast cancer risk reduction and its influence on breastfeeding practices. Breastfeed Med 2018;13(10):651–6.

43. Wallenborn JT, Ihongbe T, Rozario S, et al. Knowledge of breastfeeding recommendations and breastfeeding duration: a survival analysis on infant feeding practices II. Breastfeed Med 2017;12:156–62.

44. Khoury AJ, Mitra AK, Hinton A, et al. An innovative video succeeds in addressing barriers to breastfeeding among low-income women. J Hum Lact 2002;18(2): 125–31.

45. Kellams AL, Gurka KK, Hornsby PP, et al. The impact of a prenatal education video on rates of breastfeeding initiation and exclusivity during the newborn hospital stay in a low-income population. J Hum Lact 2016;32(1):152–9.

46. Demirci J. Prenatal video-based education and postpartum effects. n.d. Available at: https://clinicaltrials.gov/ct2/show/NCT04258709?cond=antenatal+breast+milk+expression&draw=2&rank=1. Accessed 21 Nov, 2022

47. Chapman DJ, Morel K, Anderson AK, et al. Breastfeeding peer counseling: from efficacy through scale-up. J Hum Lact 2010;26(3):314–26.

48. Rhodes EC, Damio G, LaPlant HW, et al. Promoting equity in breastfeeding through peer counseling: the US Breastfeeding Heritage and Pride program. Int J Equity Health 2021;20(1):128.

49. Patel S, Patel S. The effectiveness of lactation consultants and lactation counselors on breastfeeding outcomes. J Hum Lact 2016;32(3):530–41.

50. Bonuck K, Stuebe A, Barnett J, et al. Effect of primary care intervention on breastfeeding duration and intensity. Am J Public Health 2014;104(Suppl 1):S119–27.

51. DiGirolamo AM, Grummer-Strawn LM, Fein SB. Effect of maternity-care practices on breastfeeding. Pediatrics 2008 Oct;122(Suppl 2):S43–9.

52. Beauregard JL, Nelson JM, Li R, et al. Maternity care practices and breastfeeding intentions at one month among low-income women. Pediatrics 2022;149(4). e2021052561.

53. Meyers D, Turner-Maffei C. Improved breastfeeding success through the baby-friendly hospital initiative. Am Fam Physician 2008;78(2):180–2.

54. Alex A, Bhandary E, McGuire KP. Anatomy and physiology of the breast during pregnancy and lactation. Adv Exp Med Biol 2020;1252:3–7.

55. Arbour MW, Kessler JL. Mammary hypoplasia: not every breast can produce sufficient milk. J Midwifery Womens Health 2013;58(4):457–61.

56. Spatz DL. Re: "Is there an association between breast hypoplasia and breastfeeding outcomes? A systematic review" by Kam et al. Breastfeed Med 2022; 17(8):702.

57. Alexander JM, Grant AM, Campbell MJ. Randomised controlled trial of breast shells and Hoffman's exercises for inverted and non-protractile nipples. BMJ 1992;304(6833):1030–2.

58. Bompy L, Gerenton B, Cristofari S, et al. Impact on breastfeeding according to implant features in breast augmentation: a multicentric retrospective study. Ann Plast Surg 2019;82(1):11–4.

59. Kraut RY, Brown E, Korownyk C, et al. The impact of breast reduction surgery on breastfeeding: Systematic review of observational studies. PLoS One 2017; 12(10):e0186591.

60. Jewell ML, Edwards MC, Murphy DK, et al. Lactation outcomes in more than 3500 women following primary augmentation: 5-year data from the breast implant follow-up study. Aesthet Surg J 2019;39(8):875–83.

61. Nommsen-Rivers LA, Dolan LM, Huang B. Timing of stage II lactogenesis is predicted by antenatal metabolic health in a cohort of primiparas. Breastfeed Med 2012;7(1):43–9.

62. Brownell E, Howard CR, Lawrence RA, et al. Delayed onset lactogenesis II predicts the cessation of any or exclusive breastfeeding. J Pediatr 2012;161(4): 608–14.
63. Chapman DJ, Pérez-Escamilla R. Identification of risk factors for delayed onset of lactation. J Am Diet Assoc 1999;99(4):450–6.
64. Mullen AJ, O'Connor DL, Hanley AJ, et al. Associations of metabolic and obstetric risk parameters with timing of lactogenesis II. Nutrients 2022;14(4):876.
65. Lee S, Kelleher SL. Biological underpinnings of breastfeeding challenges: the role of genetics, diet, and environment on lactation physiology. Am J Physiol Endocrinol Metab 2016;311(2):E405–22.
66. Willis CE, Livingstone V. Infant insufficient milk syndrome associated with maternal postpartum hemorrhage. J Hum Lact 1995;11(2):123–6.
67. Parker LA, Sullivan S, Krueger C, et al. Effect of early breast milk expression on milk volume and timing of lactogenesis stage II among mothers of very low birth weight infants: a pilot study. J Perinatol 2012;32(3):205–9.
68. Forster DA, Moorhead AM, Jacobs SE, et al. Advising women with diabetes in pregnancy to express breastmilk in late pregnancy (Diabetes and Antenatal Milk Expressing [DAME]): a multicentre, unblinded, randomised controlled trial. Lancet 2017;389(10085):2204–13.
69. Foudil-Bey I, Murphy MSQ, Dunn S, et al. Evaluating antenatal breastmilk expression outcomes: a scoping review. Int Breastfeed J 2021;16(1):25.
70. Schanler RJ, Shulman RJ, Lau C. Feeding strategies for premature infants: beneficial outcomes of feeding fortified human milk versus preterm formula. Pediatrics 1999;103(6 Pt 1):1150–7.
71. Bessell A, Hooper L, Shaw WC, et al. Feeding interventions for growth and development in infants with cleft lip, cleft palate or cleft lip and palate. Cochrane Database Syst Rev 2011;2011(2):CD003315.
72. Silveira LM, Prade LS, Ruedell AM, et al. Influence of breastfeeding on children's oral skills. Rev Saude Publica 2013;47(1):37–43.
73. Lawrence RM. Transmission of infectious diseases through breast milk and breastfeeding. Breastfeeding 2011;406–73.
74. Mast EE. Mother-to-infant hepatitis C virus transmission and breastfeeding. Adv Exp Med Biol 2004;554:211–6.
75. Salameh TN, Hall LA. Depression, anxiety, and substance use disorders and treatment receipt among pregnant women in the United States: a systematic review of trend and population-based studies. Issues Ment Health Nurs 2020; 41(1):7–23.
76. Anderson PO. Alcohol use during breastfeeding. Breastfeed Med 2018;13(5): 315–7.
77. Hauck FR, Thompson JM, Tanabe KO, et al. Breastfeeding and reduced risk of sudden infant death syndrome: a meta-analysis. Pediatrics 2011;128(1):103–10.
78. Wang L, Collins C, Ratliff M, et al. Breastfeeding reduces childhood obesity risks. Child Obes 2017;13(3):197–204.
79. Su Q, Sun X, Zhu L, et al. Breastfeeding and the risk of childhood cancer: a systematic review and dose-response meta-analysis. BMC Med 2021;19(1):90.
80. Xu L, Lochhead P, Ko Y, et al. Systematic review with meta-analysis: breastfeeding and the risk of Crohn's disease and ulcerative colitis. Aliment Pharmacol Ther 2017;46(9):780–9.
81. Forinash AB, Pitlick JM, Clark K, et al. Nicotine replacement therapy effect on pregnancy outcomes. Ann Pharmacother 2010;44(11):1817–21.

82. Anderson PO. Breastfeeding with smoking cessation products. Breastfeed Med 2021;16(10):766–8.
83. Metz TD, Stickrath EH. Marijuana use in pregnancy and lactation: a review of the evidence. Am J Obstet Gynecol 2015;213(6):761–78.
84. McQueen KA, Murphy-Oikonen J, Gerlach K, et al. The impact of infant feeding method on neonatal abstinence scores of methadone-exposed infants. Adv Neonatal Care 2011;11(4):282–90.

Systemic Oppression, the Impact on Obstetric Care, and Interventions to Achieve Ideal Obstetric Outcomes

Mariam Savabi, MD, MPH*

KEYWORDS

- Oppression • Adverse outcomes • Racism • Maternal morbidity and mortality
- Anti-oppression

KEY POINTS

- Adverse obstetric patient outcomes should not occur because of oppression.
- Many adverse obstetric outcomes are preventable.
- Intentionally interrupting our own participation in the systems of oppression will improve patient outcomes.

INTRODUCTION

As providers of obstetric care, we dedicate our careers to serving patients during some of the most vulnerable times in their life. We take an oath stating we will, "do no harm"[1] to our patients and we strive for ideal patient outcomes. It is estimated that 80% of maternal deaths are preventable.[2] Why, despite our best efforts, are obstetric patients experiencing adverse outcomes? And why are patients who experience adverse outcomes often those who identify with nondominant characteristics such as race, class, sexual orientation, and gender identity, among others?

First, it is *critical* for the medical community to dispel the belief that patients from different backgrounds are genetically predisposed to adverse obstetric outcomes.[2] With that in mind, we must understand how we participate in the system of oppression in order for us to interrupt these adverse outcomes. It is also essential that obstetric providers understand their privilege, power dynamics with patients, and the reality that we are gatekeepers to patient care resources. These factors directly contribute to the adverse outcomes our patients experience.[3]

General Obstetrician and Gynecologist, HealthCare Anti-oppression Institute (Founder), Tacoma, WA, USA
* 1712 6th Avenue, Suite 100, PMB 1238, Tacoma, WA 98405, USA.
E-mail address: msavabi@gmail.com

Obstet Gynecol Clin N Am 50 (2023) 567–578
https://doi.org/10.1016/j.ogc.2023.03.008
0889-8545/23/© 2023 Elsevier Inc. All rights reserved.
obgyn.theclinics.com

This article may deviate from conventional information about prenatal care. However, systemic oppression is the root of the problem when it comes to disparities in adverse patient outcomes. We must understand and explore the root of the issue to achieve better outcomes. This article is written following the guiding human rights principles of reproductive justice.[4]

This article includes:

1. Explore how systemic oppression is upheld in society.
2. Discuss different social identities and outline typical privileged and oppressed groups.
3. Review various "Isms" to discuss adverse outcome patterns and ways to interrupt oppression.

The Ladder of Oppression

Oppression is created by systems and upheld by individuals. To illustrate oppression, a thought exercise is presented by the ladder of oppression[5] ("the Ladder") as shown in **Fig. 1**. We review each rung of the "ladder" and discuss how we participate both consciously and unconsciously in oppression. We can collectively work on dismantling oppression if we have a deep understanding of our position of power, privilege, and targeted identities.

The individual level

Stereotypes are societally enforced thoughts. The bottom of the ladder, or the first rung, is "stereotype." Stereotypes can be a generalization you have seen or experienced regarding a group of people. This can be conscious and unconscious. Medicine teaches obstetric providers to stereotype, or makes assumptions, about patients based on limited information such as appearance, names, primary language, and countless other characteristics. One example of a stereotype is to assume that a patient who is thin is "healthy." Of course we know that this is not true for all thin people, but it is a thought we can have that puts someone "in a box" by observed characteristics. This can become complicated in health care. Stereotypes in health care can be important to glean details about our patients, or a complicated situation, but also require us to consciously question the validity of these stereotypes. Although stereotypes can allow us to quickly assess situations, as the next rung of the ladder shows, stereotypes in patient care can become dangerous for many reasons.

Prejudice is an emotionally connected thought. Prejudice is the next rung on the ladder. Prejudice is a stereotype that has been reinforced with emotion. This can be conscious and unconscious. Prejudice is a feeling or negative attitude toward people from the stereotyped group. Prejudice may be conscious, meaning you know that you

Ladder of Oppression

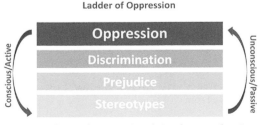

Fig. 1. Ladder of oppression. (*Data from* National Conference for Community and Justice, NCCJ Central Coast Office, based on lesson plan by Jarrod Schwartz 2002.)

have this negative emotion about a group of people. It can also be unconscious, meaning that you may not recognize that you carry those prejudicial thoughts. The goal of implicit bias training[6] is to answer questions regarding stereotypes and prejudice without overthinking your answer. It is supposed to tap into the unconscious parts of yourself that perhaps you do not recognize. It can be disappointing to know that you carry prejudice despite wanting to be a good and kind person but, the truth is, everyone carries prejudice. Society is constantly reinforcing prejudicial thoughts. Prejudicial messages come from the media, our community, politicians, and our places of work. It takes significant introspection, understanding, and desire to interrupt prejudicial thoughts. It is important for us to correct our way of thinking and question what is taught by society because, if we do not, our thoughts can lead to action as shown in the next rung of the ladder.

Discrimination is when stereotypes and prejudice become action. Discrimination is the third rung of the ladder. Discrimination is the implementation of prejudice. Although stereotypes and prejudice are internal, discrimination is an external manifestation, or an action. Discrimination can be conscious and unconscious. Discrimination is present in daily life and is readily identifiable. For example, firing an employee because they become pregnant,[7] harsher sentencing of individuals from targeted groups for the same offense compared with an individual from the privileged group,[8] or paying female-presenting employees less than their equally qualified male-presenting counterparts.[9] There are also instances in which discrimination can be subversive. This is often referred to as a microaggression. Despite calling certain actions "microaggressions," this type of discrimination significantly impacts the targeted individuals.

The systemic level

Oppression is systemic control of society to benefit the privileged and disadvantage the oppressed, which is upheld by institutions of power. Oppression is the top rung of the ladder. Examples of institutions of power include the legal system, education, health care, government, and media, among others. Individuals who create and control these institutions hold positions of power and create protections for the groups to which they belong. In the United States, individuals who created our government and have overseen institutions of power have typically been those that have one or many privileged identities including being white, heterosexual, Christian men. In the United States, we see "those that have, and those that have not." This dynamic has been purposefully created to allow for some to have privilege and resulted in others being oppressed. For those that are privileged to have maximum allocations of resources, they have created a system that consciously oppresses those with targeted identities and diverts resources to the privileged.

Oppression and health care

The ladder of oppression in **Fig. 1** illustrates how oppression is created on a societal overarching level. As individuals, by not questioning or interrupting our participation in the ladder, we unconsciously perpetuate oppression. When we are conscious of the ladder and do nothing to interrupt it, we also perpetuate oppression.

Health care is an institution of oppression. It was created by the privileged to benefit the privileged. As obstetric providers, we have a responsibility to transform this institution from one of oppression to one where patients of all identities have equitable experiences and outcomes. When you read about adverse patient outcomes among individuals with oppressed identities, it is not because of medical predispositions, it is because you, and I, and our colleagues have not done enough to interrupt systems of oppression.

Understanding the ladder, our participation in it, and how it systemically affects patients, is a constant journey of questioning and one that I ask you to join me on. Guidance on how to interrupt these systems in medical contexts is provided more fully below.

The Matrix of Oppression

All social identities fall on the spectrum of privilege and oppression. Some of these identities may be easier to understand as they are visibly obvious or are discussed more frequently in society, such as race. For those who are privileged, the matrix of oppression is a thought exercise. For those who are from targeted or borderline social groups, it is a lived experience. An important distinction to keep in mind is that no oppression is better or worse than another; oppression is always unacceptable.

The sections of the matrix of oppression in **Fig. 2** describe the following.

1. Social identity, which are characteristics defining someone's belonging in a group[10]
2. Privileged social group, which is defined as "access to power enjoyed by a dominant group, giving them economic, political, social and cultural advantages at the expense of members of a marginalized group"[11–13]
3. Border social group, which is a group of people that depending on the circumstances, can pass or have periods of time where they may experience privilege and others when they may experience being targeted

Matrix of Oppression (United States)				
Social Identity	Privileged Social Groups	Border Social groups	Targeted Social Groups	Oppression
Ability	Temporarily Able-Bodied/Able-Minded	Temporary Disabilities and/or Invisible Disabilities	Physical, Mental, Emotional, and/or Learning Disabilities	Ableism
Age	Adult (30–65)	Young Adult (18–29)	Elderly, Young	Ageism
Appearance	Toned, Lean, Euro-centric Features	Average Looking - Not Fit but Not Flabby	Overweight, Underweight, Above/Below Height, Plain	Lookism/Sizeism
Race	White	White Passing or Ambiguous Race	Asian, Black, Latino, Middle Eastern, and Native/Indigenous	Racism
Ethnicity	Anglo-Saxon, Western European	Eastern European	Immigrants or Descendents of Non-European Countries/Do Not Speak English	Ethnocentrism
Immigration Status	American Citizen	Legal/documented Immigrant	Undocumented Immigrant	Xenophobia
Religion	Mainstream Christian	Non-Mainstream Christian	Jews, Muslims, Hindus, Buddhists, Atheists, etc.	Religionism
Sex	Male	Transexual, Intersex (proximity to maleness)	Female	Sexism
Gender/Gender Identitiy	Cisgender	Gender Ambiguous	Transgender, Genderqueer, Non-binary	Genderism
Sexual Orientation	Heterosexual	Bisexual, Pansexual, Asexual	Homosexual	Heterosexism
Class	Rich, Upper-Class	Middle Class (Upper Middle/Lower Middle)	Working/Lower Class	Classism

Fig. 2. Matrix of oppression. (*Modified from* Teaching for Diversity and Social Justice, 3rd Edition, Adams M, Bell LA., Copyright © 2016 Routledge. Reproduced by permission of Taylor & Francis Group.)

4. Targeted social group, which describes the group of individuals that experience systemic oppression and are in direct contrast to the privileged group

The privileged social group has unearned advantages that the social structure has created and is maintained for them to continue to benefit. The targeted, or oppressed, social group has to endure disadvantages based on their identities. "[W]hile unearned advantage can be difficult to see, unearned disadvantage is often highly visible to those who experience it."[3] The lived experience of oppression directly relates to adverse outcomes and statistics in obstetrics.

The matrix of oppression is a complicated exercise to explore. It takes in-depth discussion to dissect where an individual falls on the matrix as well as the relationship that the matrix has with society. It can be difficult to understand each section, and some may argue about whether a certain group should fall into a certain section. The matrix demonstrates generalities that occur in the United States and does not purport to be accurate in every situation. This matrix is also not exhaustive of all social identities.

Intersectional identities

All of us have multiple identities that define our lived experience. Intersectionality is a term that was coined, "...to understand the variety of privileges and/or forms of oppression that one may experience simultaneously..."[14,15] As obstetric providers, it is important for us to consider our own identities when approaching patient care and how this may influence patient outcomes.[16] Our diverse backgrounds and lived experiences can, on the one hand, help us to empathize with individuals from certain backgrounds or who have certain identities that we can relate to or have experience with. On the other hand, our identities can sometimes prevent us from understanding challenges that some individuals experience who have identities and experiences that are different from our own. Indeed, it is equally important to consider how patient experiences and identities may influence their interaction with and outcomes from the health care system.

Although the matrix lists each identity independently, it is important to be mindful of intersectionality and appreciate how several identities make up an individual at all times. Review the matrix and determine where you fall on the spectrum. Then, consider the intersectional and lived experiences of patients to understand how a system created with disadvantages can lead to adverse health outcomes.

"Isms"

This section discusses different 'isms' or oppressions commonly experienced in obstetric care, outcomes that can result from these oppressions, and possible solutions. To thoroughly understand each oppression would require much more time and space than is possible in this article. With this in mind, each section below is meant to provide some information and challenge the reader with respect to how you can be a change agent and anti-oppressive obstetric provider.

Ableism

A person can be privileged in their physical, mental, emotional, or intellectual ability, and it is described as temporary because it can be taken away or lost. A border social group may have a disability that is temporary (eg, a broken foot), and they will return to being able-bodied once healed. There are also invisible disabilities that can allow a person to pass as privileged at some points in their life and be targeted at other points in their life. For example, learning disabilities or autoimmune diseases can sometimes fall under a border social group. The targeted social group is a group that cannot hide their disability. This oppression is referred to as ableism.

Patients with disabilities commonly have adverse obstetric outcomes. In addition, there are unique needs for intellectual, psychiatric, and physical disabilities.[17] There is extensive knowledge regarding the adverse outcomes of patients with disabilities experience in accessing health care, information, and the ability to exercise their reproductive choices safely. Disabled patients have a higher proportion of the following.

1. Preterm births[18,19]
2. Low-birth weight infants[18,19]
3. Stillbirths[19]
4. Cesarean delivery[18]
5. Gestational diabetes
6. Preeclampsia
7. Increased risk for postpartum readmission[18]

Ways to address these outcomes as obstetric providers.

1. Cater prenatal care to the patients' needs[19]
2. Extend times of prenatal visits[19,20]
3. Collaborative interprofessional care team[19]
4. Preconception counseling[17,19]
5. Close and regular postpartum follow-up[19]
6. Make sure that examination tables, access into clinic hallways and rooms, and equipment meet the needs of the patient, or find appropriate accommodations such as going to the operating room to complete care and providing comfort to the patient
7. Explore support systems and create an integrated plan of care
8. Ensure the facility has the appropriate equipment to serve all patients (a legal requirement from the Americans with Disabilities Act).[21]

Lookism/sizeism

Weight stigma also affects patient health outcomes. Weight is regularly used as an inaccurate proxy to health status.[22] Patients may feel judged by the health care system and providers and delay or avoid medical care because of their weight.[23] Patients have sometimes described prenatal care experiences "as negative, humiliating, and stigmatizing" because of the treatment and comments they receive due to their weight.[24] It is well-documented that patients of higher weight often have their medical concerns dismissed, which has led to delay in diagnosis, or even death.[23]

It is important to acknowledge patients do have a higher risk of obstetric complications when they have a higher weight,[25] but nonjudgmental language use and discussions are critical for positive patient care. For obstetrics providers, awareness of bias, listening to patient concerns, and ensuring you are providing evidence-based care for the patient is also essential to achieve as equitable of outcomes as possible.

Patients with a higher weight commonly experience the following obstetric outcomes.

1. Increase in maternal mortality[25]
2. Higher risk of comorbidities such as gestational diabetes, preeclampsia[25]
3. Higher risk of c-section[25,26]
4. Neonatal complications include "higher rates of neonatal meconium aspiration, ventilator support, and neonatal death"[25]
5. Higher risk of depression during and after pregnancy

Ways to address these outcomes as obstetric providers.

1. Have weight scales in each individual room instead of in public places.
2. Ask the patient if they want to know their weight.
3. Outside of obstetric care, collect a weight if it is medically necessary.
4. The Institute of Medicine guidelines for weight gain in pregnancy were developed to minimize occurrence of SGA infant without consideration of impact on maternal short-term and long-term outcomes[27,28]; keep this in mind when discussing weight gain in pregnancy and not relying on these weight gain ranges as definitive recommendations, but rather guidance.
5. Have appropriate equipment and do in-clinic trainings on how to use the equipment correctly and safely (ie, Hoyer lift, weight scales to accommodate higher weight patients, electric examination tables to lower as much as possible)[29] to adequately care for patients in clinic.
6. Discuss possible adverse outcomes that can be experienced by patient and neonate in a nonjudgmental way to facilitate patient collaboration and understanding.

Racism

Race is a social construct and it is inappropriate that there are "biological differences based on physical appearance."[30] The United States has a sinister history related to reproductive care for people of oppressed social identities, especially with respect to race. This has included forced sterilization,[31] experimentation,[32] and exclusion of care,[33] among other cruelties. The historical context of reproductive health care in the United States helps to explain why individuals with certain identities may distrust or approach medicine and obstetrics with more hesitancy.

Despite controlling for other factors such as education and class status, outcomes remain similarly negative for non-white patients. Owing to historical oppression in the United States, Black and Indigenous patients continue to experience the highest rates of adverse outcomes, compared with individuals of other races.[34]

Non-white patients may experience the following obstetric outcomes.

1. Two to three times higher maternal mortality rate[35]
2. Higher risk of preterm birth[36]
3. Non-white infants have higher mortality rates[34]
4. The quality of obstetric care varies for patients that are non-white.[37]

Ways to address these outcomes as obstetric providers.

1. Careful postpartum follow-up for vulnerable patients[38]
2. Restructure medical school curricula to combat racial stereotypes[39]
3. Recruit providers of different racial and ethnic backgrounds as they are more likely to work in communities with patients[40] from similar or racially oppressed backgrounds and have higher patient satisfaction[41]
4. Read and understand information about racial disparities and be cognizant of these outcomes to avoid preventable morbidity and mortality.[42]

A modern example of how oppression is being questioned in health care today is the Maternal Fetal Medicine Units Network Trial of Labor after C-section (TOLAC) calculator. The TOLAC calculator was found to inappropriately lower expected calculated success attempting a TOLAC based on their race and ethnicity. This led to higher rates of repeat c-sections, increased morbidity, and even mortality for non-white patients. It is only when practitioners questioned the validity of including race and ethnicity in the calculator's formula that race and ethnicity were removed.[43] This adjustment will allow for more non-white patients to undergo a TOLAC, thus decreasing their risk of obstetric complications.

Ethnocentrism/xenophobia

The United States is composed of many different cultures, languages, and backgrounds. This can create challenges for non-English speaking patients' access to health care as there are many barriers in understanding a convoluted health care and medical insurance system, which is typically not in their primary language. Patients who come from other countries or speak different languages are noted to commonly have adverse outcomes. These include an increased risk of obstetric trauma and c-sections.[44]

Ways to address these outcomes as obstetric providers.

1. Provide patients with limited English proficiency with a qualified language interpreter as is required for institutions that receive federal funds under Section 1557 of the Affordable Care Act.[45]
2. Create standard operating procedures to ensure that qualified interpreters are available for clinical care.
3. Do not inquire about or report a patient's immigration status to any legal person or institution. In addition, providers may refuse to provide patient immigration-status information unless there is a "warrant or other court order for a specifically identified individual" to any legal entity.[46]
4. Acquaint yourself with the lives of refugee and immigrant patients to better understand their specific needs and risks
5. Provide medical resources in patients' primary language.[47]

Classism

Classism is an important aspect of the Social Determinants of Health (SDoH) and the Healthy People 2030 goals. SDoH is a public health approach to understand what contributes to health disparities and inequities.[48] Examples of SDoH include safe housing and neighborhoods, access to education, income, unpolluted environment, access to healthy foods, and physical activity opportunities. Rural residents also experience "overall higher poverty rates, especially among rural racial and ethnic minority populations."[46] People who have lower socioeconomic status, such as rural communities, have a heavier disease burden and adverse outcomes as they are often exposed to more detrimental SDoH and ultimately suffer the brunt of health disparities.[49] Examples of rural areas with some of the worst health outcomes include the South, Delta Region, the US-Mexico Border, and Tribal Communities.

Adverse outcomes among low-income people include.

1. Increased risk for small for gestational age neonates[50]
2. Increased risk for preeclampsia[50]
3. Increased risk of gestational diabetes[51]
4. Increased risk of preterm birth[52]

Ways to address these outcomes as obstetric providers.

1. Incorporate telemedicine to increase access to patient care[53] for both rural and urban residents.
2. Advocate to expand health insurance coverage.[53]
3. Acknowledge transportation challenges and give leniency when patients are late to appointments.
4. Consider health insurance status before providing procedures and treatments.

5. Learn about and encourage patients to access financial resources that the state or the hospital has to offer.
6. Connect with and learn about local programs that can provide support to your patients during the pregnancy and postpartum. Nurse home visits, postpartum community center groups, group therapy offerings are just a few examples of local programs that can benefit low-income obstetric patients.

SUMMARY

The goal of this article is to invigorate obstetric providers to challenge and transform the institution of medicine to improve patient outcomes and have a more just and equitable health care system. Despite our best efforts, systemic oppression continues to exist in health care and results in adverse outcomes among patients with targeted identities. As the ladder of oppression demonstrates, the system of oppression is upheld by our individual actions. By addressing our stereotypes, prejudice, and discrimination, we can interrupt the actions and thoughts that lead to oppression. This article presents ways to interrupt oppression that are outlined in the "Isms" section that can easily applied and implemented in daily patient care. Recognizing the identities and intersectionality of individuals enables obstetric providers to empathize with patients who share similar or relatable identities and more importantly enables providers to appreciate the diversity of experience and possible challenges patients may encounter with the health care system. The intersectional approach to obstetric patient care and interruption of oppression can lead to ideal patient outcomes.

DISCLOSURES

None.

REFERENCES

1. Hajar R. The physician's oath: historical perspectives. Heart Views 2017;18(4): 154–9.
2. Leimert K, Olson D. Racial disparities in pregnancy outcomes: genetics, epigenetics, and allostatic load. Curr Opin Physiol 2020;13:155–65.
3. Nixon S. The coin model of privilege and critical allyship: implications for health. BMC Public Health 2019;19(1637). https://doi.org/10.1186/s12889-019-7884-9.
4. Reproductive Justice. SisterSong. Available at: https://www.sistersong.net/reproductive-justice. Accessed 1 March, 2023.
5. Schwartz J. Ladder of oppression. National Conference for Community and Justice. Available at: https://www.nccj.org/. Accessed March 1, 2023.
6. Chapman E, Kaatz A, Carnes M. Physicians and implicit bias: how doctors may unwittingly perpetuate health care disparities. J Gen Intern Med 2013;28(11): 1504–10.
7. Byron RA, Roscigno V. Relational power, legitimation, and pregnancy discrimination. Gend Soc 2014;28(3). https://doi.org/10.1177/0891243214523123.
8. Kansal T. Racial disparity in sentencing. Open Society. Published January 2005. Available at: https://www.opensocietyfoundations.org/publications/racial-disparity-sentencing. Accessed 1 March, 2023.
9. Horstman C. Male physicians earn more than women in primary and specialty care. The Commonwealth Fund. Available at: https://www.commonwealthfund.org/blog/2022/male-physicians-earn-more-women-primary-and-specialty-care#:~:text=2022).

&text=Women%20physicians%20make%20less%20than,(%2495%2C000%20compared%20to%20%2457%2C000). Accessed 1 March, 2023.

10. McLeod, S. Social identity theory. simply psychology. Published October 24, 2019. Available at. https://www.simplypsychology.org/social-identity-theory.html. Accessed 1 March, 2023.

11. Anti-Oppression Network. Terminologies of oppression. Available at: https://theantioppressionnetwork.com/resources/terminologies-of-oppression/. Accessed 1 March, 2023.

12. Hill Collins P. Black feminist thought: knowledge, consciousness, and the politics of empowerment. Boston: Unwin Hyman; 1990. p. 221–38. Available at: https://negrasoulblog.files.wordpress.com/2016/04/patricia-hill-collins-black-feminist-thought.pdf. Accessed 1 March, 2023.

13. Adams M, Bell LA, Griffin P. Teaching for diversity and social justice. 2nd ed. Routledge/Taylor & Francis Group; 2007. https://doi.org/10.4324/9780203940822.

14. Cole NL. Definition of intersectionality. ThoughtCo. Available at: thoughtco.com/intersectionality-definition-3026353. Published July 31, 2021. Accessed 1 March 2023.

15. Crenshaw K. Demarginalizing the intersection of race and sex: a black feminist critique of antidiscrimination doctrine, feminist theory and antiracist politics. Univ Chic Leg Forum 1989;(1):138–67.

16. Wilson Y, White A, Jefferson A, et al. Intersectionality in clinical medicine: the need for a conceptual framework. Am J Bioeth 2019;19(2):8–19.

17. D'Angelo A, Ceccanti M, Fiore M, et al. Pregnancy in women with physical and intellectual disability: psychiatric implications. Pensiero Sci 2020;55(6):331–6.

18. Gavin N, Benedict B, Adams K. Health service use and outcomes among disabled Medicaid pregnant women. Wom Health Issues 2006;16(6):313–22.

19. Akobirshoev I, Pariah SP, Mitra M, et al. Birth outcomes among US women with intellectual and developmental disabilities. Disabil Health J 2017;10(3):406–12.

20. Long-Bellil L, Mitra M, Iezzoni LI, et al. The impact of physical disability on pregnancy and childbirth. J Womens Health 2017;26(8):878–85.

21. Americans with Disabilities Act. Available at: https://adata.org/factsheet/ADA-overview. Accessed 1 March, 2023.

22. van Amsterdam N. Big fat inequalities, thin privilege: An intersectional perspective on 'body size.'. Eur J Womens Stud 2013;20(2):155–69.

23. Chrisler J, Barney A. Sizeism is a health hazard. Fat Stud 2017;6(1):38–53.

24. Bombak AE, McPhail D, Ward P. Reproducing stigma: interpreting "overweight" and "obese" women's experiences of weight-based discrimination in reproductive healthcare. Soc Sci Med 2016;166:94–101.

25. Creanga AA, Catalano PM, Bateman BT. Obesity in pregnancy. N Engl J Med 2022;387:248–59.

26. Teefey C, Reforma L, Koelper N, et al. Risk factors associated with cesarean delivery after induction of labor in women with class III obesity. Obstet Gynecol 2020;135(3):542–9.

27. Rasmussen K, Yaktine A. Weight gain during pregnancy: reexamining the guidelines. Inst Med. Published online 2009. Available at: https://www.ncbi.nlm.nih.gov/books/NBK32799/. Accessed 1 March, 2023.

28. Most J, St Amant M, Hsia D, et al. Evidence-based recommendations for energy intake in pregnant women with obesity. J Clin Invest 2019;129(11):4682–90.

29. Maclean L, Edwards N, Garrard M, et al. Obesity, stigma and public health planning. Health Promot Internation 2009;24(1):88–93.

30. Braveman P, Dominguez TP. Abandon "race." Focus on racism. Front Public Health 2021;9(689462):1–8.
31. Gutiérrez E, Fuentes L. Population control by sterilization: the cases of Puerto Rican and Mexican-origin women in the United States. Latinoa Res Rev 2009;7(3): 85–97.
32. Prather C, Fuller T, Jeffries W, et al. Racism, African American women, and their sexual and reproductive health: a review of historical and contemporary evidence and implications for health equity. Health Equity 2018;2(1):249–59.
33. Yearby R, Clark B, Fibueroa J. Structural racism in historical and modern US health care policy. Health Aff 2022;41(2). https://doi.org/10.1377/hlthaff.2021.01466.
34. Infant Mortality. CDC. Available at: https://www.cdc.gov/reproductivehealth/maternalinfanthealth/infantmortality.htm#print. Accessed 1 March, 2023.
35. Hoyert D. Maternal Mortality Rates in the United States, 2020.; National center for Health Statistics. Available at: https://www.cdc.gov/nchs/data/hestat/maternal-mortality/2020/maternal-mortality-rates-2020.htm. Accessed 1 March 2023.
36. Manuck T. Racial and ethnic differences in preterm birth: a complex, multifactorial problem. Semin Perinatol 2017;41(8):511–8.
37. Howell E, Zeitlin J. Quality of care and disparities in obstetrics. Obstet Gynecol Clin North Am 2017;44(1):13–25.
38. Mi T, Hung P, Li X. Racial and ethnic disparities in postpartum care in the greater Boston area during the COVID-19 pandemic. JAMA Netw Open 2022;5(6): e2216355. Available at: https://jamanetwork.com/journals/jamanetworkopen/fullarticle/2793512. Accessed 1 March, 2023.
39. Amutah C, Greenidge K, Mante A, et al. Misrepresenting race — the role of medical schools in propagating physician bias. N Engl J Med 2021;384:872–8.
40. Walker KO, Moreno G, Grumbach K. The association among specialty, race, ethnicity, and practice location among California physicians in diverse specialties. J Natl Med Assoc 2012;104:46–52.
41. LaViest T, Nuru-Jeter A. Is doctor-patient race concordance associated with greater satisfaction with care? J Health Soc Behav 2002;43:296–306.
42. Eliminating Preventable Maternal Mortality and Morbidity. ACOG. Available at: https://www.acog.org/advocacy/policy-priorities/maternal-mortality-prevention. Accessed 1 March, 2023.
43. Buckley A, Sestito S, Ogundipe T, et al. Racial and ethnic disparities among women undergoing a trial of labor after cesarean delivery: performance of the VBAC calculator with and without patients' race/ethnicity. Reprod Sci 2022;29(7):2930–8.
44. Sentell T, Chang A, Ahn HJ, et al. Maternal language and adverse birth outcomes in a statewide analysis. Women Health 2016;56(3):257–80.
45. Section 1557 of the Patient Protection and Affordable Care Act. Available at: https://www.hhs.gov/civil-rights/for-individuals/section-1557/index.html. Accessed 1 March, 2023.
46. HEALTH CARE PROVIDERS AND IMMIGRATION ENFORCEMENT Know Your Rights, Know Your Patients' Rights. Available at: nilc.org/issues/immigration-enforcement/healthcare-provider-and-patients-rights-imm-enf/. Accessed 1 March, 2023.
47. Health Care for Immigrants. ACOG. 2023;Committee Statement No. 4. https://doi.org/10.1097/AOG.0000000000005061
48. Social Determinants of Health. Available at: https://health.gov/healthypeople/priority-areas/social-determinants-health. Accessed 1 March, 2023.
49. McMaughan DJ, Oloruntoba O, Smith ML. Socioeconomic status and access to healthcare: interrelated drivers for healthy aging. Front Public Health 2020;(8): 231. https://doi.org/10.3389/fpubh.2020.00231.

50. Pawar D, Sarker M, Caughey A, et al. A. Influence of socioeconomic status on adverse utcomes in pregnancy. Obstet Gynecol 2020;135:33S.

51. Zhou T, Du S, Sun D, et al. Prevalence and trends in gestational diabetes mellitus among women in the United States, 2006–2017: a population-based study. Front Endocrinol 2022;13. https://doi.org/10.3389/fendo.2022.868094.

52. McHale P, Maudsley G, Pennington A, et al. Mediators of socioeconomic inequalities in preterm birth: a systematic review. BMC Public Health 2022;(22):1134. https://doi.org/10.1186/s12889-022-13438-9.

53. Hostetter M, Klein S. Restoring access to maternity care in rural America. Published September 2021. Available at: https://www.commonwealthfund.org/publications/2021/sep/restoring-access-maternity-care-rural-america. Accessed 1 March, 2023.

Increasing Access: Telehealth and Rural Obstetric Care

Beatriz Tenorio, MD, Capt, USAF, MC[a],
Julie R. Whittington, MD, LCDR, MC, USN[a,b,*]

KEYWORDS

• Telehealth • Telemedicine • Rural obstetrics • Maternity care

KEY POINTS

• There is an increasing need for telemedicine capabilities in rural obstetrics.
• Robust telemedicine programs exist and serve as a valuable model for other health systems.
• Telehealth modalities are well accepted by patients and providers.
• Initiation of telehealth programs may require access to Registered Nurses, Registered Diagnostic Medical Sonographers, and personnel trained in telehealth technology. These professionals can be difficult to find in rural America.

INTRODUCTION

The US Department of Health and Human Resources released their projections regarding supply and demand for women's health service providers for 2018 to 2030 in March 2021.[1] The overarching theme is the mismatch of demand and supply; the need for obstetrician/gynecologists is beyond the providers available. This inadequacy of providers is seen disproportionately throughout the country, specifically in rural America.

Multiple studies have evaluated the disparities in outcomes that stem from socioeconomic factors and geographic access, particularly in rural communities.[2–5] Rural communities are defined as a "county with an urban population of 2.5 to 19.9 K, or 20k + not adjacent to a metropolitan area." The US Maternity Care Deserts Report from March of Dimes in 2022 highlights the difficulties faced in ensuring adequate facilities and providers for safe maternity care.[6] In 2018, there were already issues

[a] Department of Women's Health, Navy Medicine Readiness and Training Command Portsmouth, 620 John Paul Jones Circle, Portsmouth, VA 23708, USA; [b] Department of Obstetrics and Gynecology, Uniformed Services University of the Health Sciences, 4301 Jones Bridge Road, Bethesda, MD 20814, USA
* Corresponding author.
E-mail address: julie.whittington09@gmail.com

Obstet Gynecol Clin N Am 50 (2023) 579–588
https://doi.org/10.1016/j.ogc.2023.03.014
0889-8545/23/Published by Elsevier Inc.

obgyn.theclinics.com

regarding maternity care deserts, with ~34% of counties in the United States being classified as maternity care deserts (lack of maternity care resources, providers, and hospitals/birth centers). This has increased to 36% of counties in the United States being classified as maternity care deserts in the 2022 report, with at least two-thirds of these areas located in rural counties (**Fig. 1**). The report highlights the importance of telehealth in obstetric care to increase access to care in rural areas.[6] Given geographic barriers to care, telehealth has been used and will need to be used further to increase access.

NATURE OF THE PROBLEM

Approximately 18 million women of reproductive age reside in rural communities with nearly half a million deliveries born in rural hospitals each year. Medicare notably covers almost half of all deliveries in the United States, with rural communities tending to have a higher need for Medicaid coverage.[7] In 2020, over 8 million patients of childbearing age lived in counties without an obstetric hospital, with 52.9% of rural counties having no obstetric services. This concerning number is compounded by the fact that there is an increasing closure of maternity wards in rural countries, with 53 (2.7% of rural locations) closing between 2013 and 2018.[6] This trend is projected to continue, decreasing access to obstetric care. This is due to shortages of providers, low volume of births, and low-income communities. Not surprisingly, birthing people in these rural areas are at higher risk for obstetric complications due to the lack of access, such as preterm delivery, maternal mortality, postpartum hemorrhage, and postpartum depression.[3,8] Their infants are also at an increased risk of adverse neonatal outcomes.

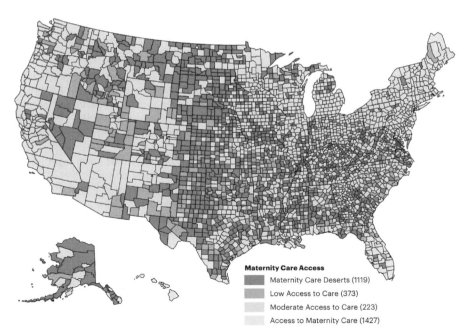

Maternity Care Access

Maternity Care Deserts (1119)
Low Access to Care (373)
Moderate Access to Care (223)
Access to Maternity Care (1427)

Fig. 1. Maternity care deserts. (*From* Brigance, C., Lucas R., Jones, E., Davis, A., Oinuma, M., Mishkin, K. and Henderson, Z. (2022). Nowhere to Go: Maternity Care Deserts Across the U.S. (Report No. 3). March of Dimes. https://www.marchofdimes.org/research/maternity-care-deserts-report.aspx; with permission.)

Decreased access to care has been highlighted by the Centers for Medicare and Medicaid Services (CMS), prompting a brief in 2019 to improve access to maternal health care. Proposal components include further incorporation, utilization, and expansion of telehealth in rural communities.[7] Of note, barriers to obstetric telehealth include challenges with overall telehealth, such as limited access to broadband, cost of equipment/technology, scheduling, and reimbursement for teleconsultation.

TELEHEALTH AND OBSTETRIC CARE

As described in the American College of Obstetricians and Gynecologists (ACOG) Committee Opinion on telehealth, telehealth refers to the "technology-enhanced health care framework that includes services such as virtual visits, remote patient monitoring, and mobile health care." This differs from traditional telemedicine, which refers to "clinical diagnosis and monitoring" delivered by technology.[9] Telemedicine involves real-time patient and provider interaction, whereas other modalities may involve delayed physician involvement or the utilization of technology to assist patients with medical choices. Different telehealth modalities have been evaluated and shown to impact patient outcomes. The modalities include live/real-time virtual visits, store-and-forward "asynchronous telemedicine," teleultrasound, remote patient monitoring, and mobile health (mHealth).

Live/real-time virtual visits have been evaluated as a viable method of increasing access to care, especially in obstetrics. A 2016 quality improvement initiative focused on comparing outcomes between the traditional 14 in-person visits to a 9 to 5 (in-person to virtual visits) framework for low-risk obstetric patients.[10] This study demonstrated noninferiority in obstetric outcomes (no significant differences in C-section, preterm birth, birth weight, or neonatal intensive care unit [NICU]). However, there was a notably higher rate of preeclampsia in the virtual visit cohort. There was also no statistical difference in patient satisfaction between in-person and virtual visits.[11] A limitation of this study was demographics, as the participants were low-risk pregnancies that did not have issues with access to care. Thus, this modality may be more appealing and successful in middle–high-income mothers and is not necessarily generalizable. One qualitative study during coronavirus disease 2019 (COVID-19) looked at the acceptability of virtual visits for the management of diabetes mellitus for patients. It was noted to be satisfactory if it was interspersed with in-person visits.[12]

Virtual visits for high-risk pregnancies were further explored at the University of Pittsburgh Medical Center, where maternal–fetal medicine (MFM) specialists performed telemedicine consultations for higher-risk pregnancies. The patients were treated similarly with in-person prenatal care and five telemedicine visits performed by MFM. Similar results to the low-risk quality improvement project were seen, with similar patient satisfaction and neonatal/maternal outcomes from the in-person versus virtual visit modality. It additionally showed a cost-saving analysis ($90.28/visit) for patients related to travel and work expenses saved with virtual visits.[13]

Robust state networks have emerged as a method to increase access to care. One of the most notable examples is the University of Arkansas for Medical Sciences (UAMS) Institute for Digital Health and Innovation (IDHI) High-Risk Pregnancy Program, which includes:

1. A statewide telemedicine clinic program—where patients are seen virtually in real-time in rural locations
2. Teleultrasound—with remote direction and interpretation, often in real-time with real-time consultation
3. A 24-hour access to MFM consultation for providers

4. A Web site with guidelines for routine and complicated obstetric and neonatal topics for providers
5. A 24-hour nursing call center for both provider and patient support.

This program has an over 95% satisfaction rate for patients, with obstetric (OB) providers noting increased access to care.[14] UAMS IDHI has also established telemedicine, teleultrasound, and teleconsultation for inmates in correctional facilities.[15] This population undoubtedly is at risk for adverse obstetric outcomes due to distance from providers. IDHIs program allows for routine and advanced obstetric services to be continued. A state map of Arkansas with IDHIs sites is helpful to visualize the expansive capabilities (**Fig. 2**). Hawaii is another state with robust telemedicine services. Hawaii is over 90% rural and has limited obstetric resources and significant travel barriers among the islands.[16] Their telehealth services include video consultation, remote patient monitoring, and teleultrasound.[16]

Telemedicine Solutions to Obstetric Care in Rural Counties is a private practice program in Tennessee.[17] It initially started with public and private grant money but is now fully supported by private practice. They use advanced practice nurses and sonographers to visit various sites and evaluate patients. These sites are spaces rented in local

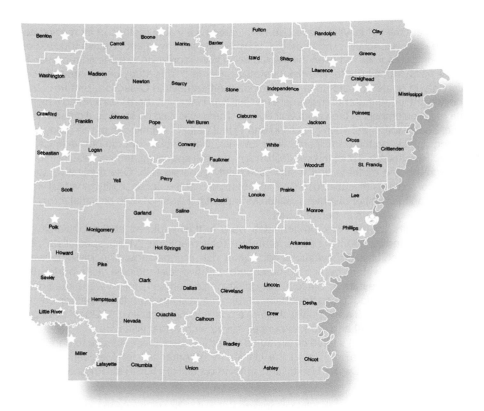

Fig. 2. University of Arkansas for Medical Sciences Institute for Digital Health and Innovation. The University of Arkansas is located centrally in Pulaski County. Note the widespread and thorough Obstetric telehealth network of the rural state. (*Courtesy of* UAMS Institute of Digital Health & Innovation, Little Rock, AR; with permission.)

obstetricians' offices outfitted with telehealth equipment. After completing the ultra-sound or visit, the patient has a teleconference with the MFM specialist. This allows subspecialty obstetric care without the rural patient having to travel.[17]

The Banner Health North Colorado Medical Center uses telehealth to maximize access to obstetricians.[18] They assist family medicine physicians in rural areas with obstetric privileges with inpatient, labor, and delivery management decisions through telemedicine doctor-to-doctor or doctor-to-patient discussions. This is an example of how regionalization of health care may help—allowing women to deliver at their local facilities while still having access to specialists.

"Asynchronous telemedicine"/store-and-forward describes a telehealth modality that involves imaging (eg, ultrasound recordings) to remote specialists for analysis and future consultation. An example is a component of the Arkansas telemedicine network, previously known as ANGELS, where prenatally diagnosed urologic anomalies requiring prenatal urologic consultations were done simultaneously with MFM via teleconsultation. This allowed for consultations in one visit, saving time and effort for both providers and patients.[19]

Real-time ultrasound assessment of the fetus with interpretation and counseling immediately following the sonogram has also been used. To test the accuracy of this modality, a randomized non-inferiority trial was undertaken to compare remotely directed and interpreted ultrasound with in-person ultrasound. It was notable in this study that the detection rates for fetal anomalies were similar between modalities. There was also favorable patient satisfaction with the teleultrasound experience.[20]

Remote patient monitoring has been seen in both prenatal and postpartum care, describing personal health and medical data collected in one location, which is then electronically transmitted to a physician in a different place. Remote monitoring has helped to reduce travel and financial burdens, with patients being given home blood pressure cuffs, handheld fetal Doppler, and education.[21,22] This is often used to aid virtual visits, evaluate otherwise stable patients, and decrease the need for additional visits.[11]

More modalities are included in telehealth. Each modality can contribute to increased access to care. In COVID-19, telehealth coverage specifically expanded virtual visits to include "audio-only" or "phone visits" to improve access. Before COVID-19, virtual visits required live-streaming video with audio to be reimbursable. This was a fundamental change due to the expansion of patients eligible for telehealth visits. During the COVID-19 pandemic and social distancing regulations, telehealth visits increased 63-fold in 2020 alone.[23] A retrospective review of internal medicine visits showed that 26.3% of Medicare patients receiving telehealth lacked digital access in their homes. Although this study population included patients beyond childbearing age, its results suggested that patients located in rural areas, with less broadband access (correlated in rural areas), and required Medicaid were more likely to use phone-only visits versus video–audio visits.

With the laxity in regulation and need for social distancing, there have been debates about whether telehealth coverage should continue to extend to audio-only visits. This study suggested that audio-only telehealth visits allow for increased access to care, as patients who lacked digital access to allow for combined video/virtual audio visits were more likely to be older, African American, require an interpreter, be on Medicaid, and live in areas of low broadband access.[24] The Office of Health Policy notes in their report of Medicare patients and telehealth use that rural patients were less likely to use telehealth services than their urban counterparts, surmised to be due to limitations in broadband access and challenges with Internet availability and affordability.[23]

mHealth is a general term describing patient use of mobile phones or other wireless technology that does not require physician involvement, such as apps. Examples of these programs include Text4baby (smoking cessation in pregnancy text service) and myHealthPregnancy app (prenatal care app).[25]

TELEHEALTH AND RURAL AMERICA

There is an undeniable need for increased access to obstetric care in rural areas. The Government Accountability Office released its report to Congressional Committees in October 2022 regarding maternal health, with one of their strong recommendations including "increasing remote consultations."[21]

Barriers to patients and providers have been observed regarding increasing remote access. For both parties, Internet speeds and connectivity have been limiting factors to the broader implementation of telehealth. In 2020, 20% of US counties had low telehealth access, defined as at least 30% of consumers within the county having low-speed connection needed for adequate broadband access. Of this population, 70% of the counties with the highest proportion of low-speed connections did not have full access to maternity care.[6]

Provider-specific barriers include licensing and payment parity, with licensing involving physicians' ability to provide services outside their state of employment. This comes into play when, in rural counties, half of US counties did not have an OB or a certified nurse midwife. In many cases, the closest provider is across state lines, with the challenges of Medicaid not paying for prenatal care if done out of state. Although the Interstate Medical Licensure Compact (IMLC) attempts to mitigate these state barriers, it is expensive ($700 fee, not including individual state licensure costs), with 14 states not currently participating in IMLC. Payment parity focuses on health insurance reimbursement for telemedicine services, with parity laws varying by state and insurance provider.[13] During COVID-19, many telehealth requirements were waived, and care was reimbursed. However, in November 2022, the CMS released their 2023 Medicare Physician Fee schedule. Its significant telehealth policy included discontinuing reimbursement of audio-only evaluation and management not related to mental/behavioral health care.[26] Regarding this, CMS stated that telehealth services needed to be "analogous to in-person care" so that the service is essentially a substitute for a "face-to-face encounter." Because audio-only visits are not face-to-face, they inherently fail to meet that standard. As discussed previously, phone-only visits may be the only way to ensure access for some patients.

At this time, expansion in telehealth in rural America is predominantly driven by grant-funded programs. The Health Resources and Services Administration currently has the Rural Maternity and Obstetrics Management Strategies program, which provides programs up to a million dollars annually for "innovative, flexible models of care," including telehealth.[27]

FUTURE DIRECTIONS AND LIMITATIONS

There are some limitations to telehealth that should be addressed to maximize its potential fully. One limitation is that while endorsed by multiple government agencies and professional bodies, there needs to be more evidence for non-inferior or improved outcomes.[28] Another limitation of expanding telehealth to rural areas is personnel.[29] There must be nurses to support Labor and Delivery to use telemedicine and teleconsultation on the unit. Using local nursing schools to "feed" rural hospitals would be advisable.[29]

Table 1
Types of telehealth and benefits to rural patients

Telehealth Modality	Description	Benefits for Rural Patients
Virtual visit	Audio and video visit with provider, conducted in real time	Face-to-face encounter with a specialist, no travel required
Asynchronous telemedicine	Imaging is performed and interpreted later by a specialist	Imaging can be performed anywhere if a skilled technician is present and can forward images
Remote patient monitoring	Transmission of data collected by the patient to a provider to use for medical decision-making	Continued interaction with specialists for the management of obstetric complications
mHealth	Patient-managed mobile technology used to deliver information and education	Reinforcement of healthy behaviors and reminders of upcoming visits
Audio only	Real-time telephone visit with a patient and provider	Does not require patient to have Internet access

To introduce telehealth, a health care system must consider the up-front costs associated with establishing a telehealth program. This would include Internet connectivity, cameras, computers, speakers, and microphones; the same equipment would need to be purchased for the other locations.

To expand teleultrasound, Registered Diagnostic Medical Sonographers are needed. Finding-trained sonographers who live in rural locales or are willing to travel to remote locations can be challenging. Teleultrasound is one of the best ways to expand access to MFM for prenatal diagnosis. The CMS suggests creating teleultrasound mentoring programs to expand access to ultrasound images.[20] There is also potential for robotic ultrasound, which a skilled sonographer from another location could control.[16]

The Center for Medicare and Medicaid Services advocates for leveraging cost savings from telehealth to reimburse providers, yet recent policy changes limit some telehealth modalities. With more research on outcomes, the US Government may be more likely to continue supporting various modalities. Military families are often stationed in localities that may have fewer obstetric resources, such as overseas military bases. Some telehealth modalities noted in **Table 1** could be used to help expand obstetric services, including access to MFM specialists in real-time video consultation visits and engaging in remote ultrasound interpretation.

SUMMARY

Telehealth obstetric care has significantly expanded since the COVID-19 pandemic, with both institutions and insurance coverage using telehealth systems to increase access to care. Obstetricians should use this expansion to increase the use of telehealth to benefit the rural obstetric population. Obstetric virtual visits are becoming a more familiar concept to both patients and providers. Telehealth is well accepted by patients and clinicians. Previously established MFM telehealth programs in rural areas can serve as a model for other states or institutions to address the lack of access to care.

CLINICS CARE POINTS

- Audio-only appointments have increased access to care; however, more evidence is needed to show non-inferior versus better outcomes to in-person/video-conference visits.
- Urban hospitals can model telehealth after established programs to extend patient care to rural areas.
- The success of telehealth depends on reliable infrastructure, including broadband Internet.

DISCLOSURE

The authors have no financial disclosures. The views expressed in this article reflect the results of research conducted by the authors and do not necessarily reflect the official policy or position of the Department of the Navy, Department of Defense, or the US Government. B Tenoroio and J.R. Whittington are military service members. This work was prepared as part of their official duties. Title 17 U.S C. 105 provides that "Copyright protection under this title is not available for any work of the US Government." Title 17 U.S C. 101 defines a US Government work as a work prepared by a military service member or employee of the US Government as part of that person's official duties.

REFERENCES

1. Projections of supply and demand for Women's health service providers: 2018-2030. Rockville, Maryland: U.S. Department of Health and Human Services HRaSA, National Center for Health Workforce Analysis; 2021.
2. Mbata O, Garg B, Caughey AB, et al. Differences in perinatal outcomes among rural women by county composition. Am J Perinatol 2022. https://doi.org/10.1055/a-1878-0204.
3. Handley SC, Passarella M, Interrante JD, et al. Perinatal outcomes for rural obstetric patients and neonates in rural-located and metropolitan-located hospitals. J Perinatol 2022;42(12):1600–6.
4. Kozhimannil KB, Interrante JD, Henning-Smith C, et al. Rural-urban differences in severe maternal morbidity and mortality in the US, 2007-15. Health Aff 2019; 38(12):2077–85.
5. Mohamoud YA, Kirby RS, Ehrenthal DB. Poverty, urban-rural classification and term infant mortality: a population-based multilevel analysis. BMC Pregnancy Childbirth 2019;19(1):40.
6. Brigance C., Lucas R., Jones E., et al., Nowhere to Go: maternity care deserts across the U.S. (Report No. 3), 2022, March of Dimes. Available at: https://www.marchofdimes.org/research/maternity-care-deserts-report.aspx.
7. Improving access to maternal health care in rural communities: Issue Brief (2019). Available at: https://www.cms.gov/About-CMS/Agency-Information/OMH/equity-initiatives/rural-health/09032019-Maternal-Health-Care-in-Rural-Communities.pdf.
8. Anglim AJ, Radke SM. Rural maternal health care outcomes, drivers, and patient perspectives. Clin Obstet Gynecol 2022;65(4):788–800.
9. Implementing telehealth in practice. Obstet Gynecol 2020;135(2):e73–9.
10. Pflugeisen BM, McCarren C, Poore S, et al. Virtual visits: managing prenatal care with modern technology. MCN Am J Matern Child Nurs 2016;41(1):24–30.
11. Pflugeisen BM, Mou J. Patient satisfaction with virtual obstetric care. Matern Child Health J 2017;21(7):1544–51.

12. Kozica-Olenski SL, Soldatos G, Marlow L, et al. Exploring the acceptability and experience of receiving diabetes and pregnancy care via telehealth during the COVID-19 pandemic: a qualitative study. BMC Pregnancy Childbirth 2022; 22(1):932.

13. Leighton C, Conroy M, Bilderback A, et al. Implementation and impact of a maternal-fetal medicine telemedicine program. Am J Perinatol 2019;36(7): 751–8.

14. Bhandari NR, Payakachat N, Fletcher DA, et al. Validation of newly developed surveys to evaluate patients' and providers' satisfaction with telehealth obstetric services. Telemed J e Health 2020;26(7):879–88.

15. University of Arkansas for Medical Sciences, Institute for Digital Health and Innovation, Program Guide. University of Arkansas for Medical Sciences, Institute for Digital Health and Innovation. Available at: https://idhi.uams.edu/programs/. Accessed 15 December, 2022.

16. Sullivan C, Cazin M, Higa C, et al. Maternal telehealth: innovations and Hawai'i perspectives. J Perinat Med 2023;51(1):69–82.

17. STORC- telemedicine solutions to obstetric care in rural counties. Available at: https://www.rocob.com/services/telemedicine. Accessed 22 January, 2023.

18. Banner Health launches telehealth for obstetrics. Available at: https://www.bannerhealth.com/newsroom/press-releases/banner-health-launches-telehealth-for-obstetrics. Accessed 22 January, 2023.

19. Rabie NZ, Canon S, Patel A, et al. Prenatal diagnosis and telemedicine consultation of fetal urologic disorders. J Telemed Telecare 2016;22(4):234–7.

20. Whittington JR, Hughes DS, Rabie NZ, et al. Detection of fetal anomalies by remotely directed and interpreted ultrasound (teleultrasound): a randomized non-inferiority trial. Am J Perinatol 2022;39(2):113–9.

21. Thomas NA, Drewry A, Racine Passmore S, et al. Patient perceptions, opinions and satisfaction of telehealth with remote blood pressure monitoring postpartum. BMC Pregnancy Childbirth 2021;21(1):153.

22. Zizzo AR, Hvidman L, Salvig JD, et al. Home management by remote self-monitoring in intermediate- and high-risk pregnancies: A retrospective study of 400 consecutive women. Acta Obstet Gynecol Scand 2022;101(1):135–44.

23. Samson LW TW, Turrini G, Sheingold S. Medicare beneficiaries' use of telehealth in 2020: trends by beneficiary characteristics and location. 2021. Available at: https://aspe.hhs.gov/sites/default/files/documents/a1d5d810fe3433e18b192be4 2dbf2351/medicare-telehealth-report.pdf. Accessed 15 January, 2023.

24. Chen J, Li KY, Andino J, et al. Predictors of audio-only versus video telehealth visits during the COVID-19 pandemic. J Gen Intern Med 2022; 37(5):1138–44.

25. Whittington JR, Ramseyer AM, Taylor CB. Telemedicine in low-risk obstetrics. Obstet Gynecol Clin North Am 2020;47(2):241–7.

26. Telehealth policy changes after the COVID-19 public health emergency. U.S. Department of Health and Human Services. Updated Nov 23, 2022. Available at: https://telehealth.hhs.gov/providers/policy-changes-during-the-covid-19-public-health-emergency/policy-changes-after-the-covid-19-public-health-emergency/. Accessed 15 January, 2023.

27. Rural maternity and obstetrics management strategies (RMOMS) program. 2023, Updated Dec 2022. Available at: https://www.hrsa.gov/rural-health/grants/rural-community/rmoms. Accessed January 15, 2023.

28. DeNicola N, Grossman D, Marko K, et al. Telehealth interventions to improve obstetric and gynecologic health outcomes: a systematic review. Obstet Gynecol 2020;135(2):371–82.

29. Advancing Rural Maternal Health Equity. Centers for Health and Human Services. Available at: https://www.cms.gov/files/document/maternal-health-may-2022.pdf. Accessed January 15, 2023.

Perinatal Depression Treatment Guidelines for Obstetric Providers

Nina E. Higgins, MD[a,b,*], Marquette J. Rose, MD[a],
Tamara J. Gardner, MSN, CNM, PMHNP-BC[c],
Jennifer N. Crawford, PhD[a,b]

KEYWORDS

- Perinatal depression • Reproductive psychiatry • Postpartum depression
- Medication • Psychotherapy

KEY POINTS

- Psychiatric medication for perinatal depression can successfully be managed by front-line providers and should be considered when depression is first identified.
- Risks of medication should be weighed against the risks of untreated mental illness in the perinatal period. Risk versus risk tables provided in this article may facilitate more effective shared decision-making conversations with patients.
- Psychotherapy for depression should also be considered at the time of diagnosis; effective treatments are available.
- Referral to psychiatric and psychological assessment and treatment can be aided by on-site availability of behavioral health providers.

INTRODUCTION

The perinatal period is an especially vulnerable time in which new onset or worsening of previous mood and anxiety symptoms can occur.[1] Collectively, these diagnoses are referred to as perinatal mood and anxiety disorders (PMADs). Although there is a strong association between perinatal anxiety and depression,[2] this article will be focusing specifically on perinatal depression. Perinatal depression is the occurrence

[a] Department of Psychiatry & Behavioral Sciences, University of New Mexico, 2400 Tucker Avenue N.E., 1 University of New Mexico, MSC09-5030, Albuquerque, NM 87131, USA; [b] Department of Obstetrics and Gynecology, University of New Mexico, 2400 Tucker Avenue N. E., 1, MSC09-5030, Albuquerque, NM 87131, USA; [c] Perinatal Associates of New Mexico, 201 Cedar SE, Suite 405 Albuquerque, NM 87106, USA
* Corresponding author. Department of Psychiatry & Behavioral Sciences, University of New Mexico, 2400 Tucker Avenue N.E., 1 University of New Mexico, MSC09-5030, Albuquerque, NM 87131.
E-mail address: negonzales@salud.unm.edu

Obstet Gynecol Clin N Am 50 (2023) 589–607
https://doi.org/10.1016/j.ogc.2023.03.009
0889-8545/23/© 2023 Elsevier Inc. All rights reserved.

of depressive symptoms during the antenatal or postnatal period with an annual incidence of 10% to 20%.[3,4] The consequences of untreated perinatal depression are significant and include negative impacts on maternal health, pregnancy outcomes, and maternal–infant health.[5–7] Postpartum depression increases the risk of suicide, one of the leading causes of pregnancy-related mortality.[8]

Numerous risks associated with untreated depression in pregnancy include, but are not limited to, increased risk of miscarriage,[9,10] increased risk of poor prenatal care,[9] lower use of folic acid or prenatal vitamins,[9,11] lower attendance at regular prenatal appointments,[9] higher risk of cesarean section,[10,12,13] increased risk of preeclampsia,[9,14] risk of preterm birth,[9,10,12,15] risk of low birth weight,[9,10,12,15] increased risk of symptoms worsening postpartum,[9] risk of suicide,[8,9] difficulty bonding with infant,[9] and lower likelihood of breastfeeding.[16] In addition, offspring of mothers who were depressed in pregnancy is at increased risk of difficulty self-soothing,[9] behavioral problems,[9,10] poor neurodevelopmental scores,[9,10] and having a mental health diagnosis later in life.[9]

Given the burden of disease, obstetric providers play a critical role in screening, diagnosis, and treatment of perinatal depression. The American College of Obstetricians and Gynecologists recommend screening patients at least once during the perinatal period with closer monitoring of those with a history of depression.[17] Without access to the initial management of depression during routine prenatal care, treatment can be significantly delayed, as it can take months to establish with a mental health provider, increasing the chances of negative effects on mother and baby.[5–7]

Compounding the importance of bolstering early detection and treatment of perinatal depression is evidence of disparities in mental health access and outcomes generally.[18] Addressing these disparities becomes even more important in the perinatal stage, as Black, Asian, and Native American women, as well as those insured by Medicaid, are less likely to be screened for postpartum depression than White women.[19] Nearly 40% of Black mothers have experienced mental health conditions but are half as likely as White women to receive treatment.[20] These disparities play out in maternal mortality rates, with recent data indicating that mental health conditions are the top contributor to mortality within the postpartum period.[8]

The purpose of this article is to provide pharmacologic and psychological treatment information to help first-line providers more confidently manage perinatal depression. A framework for conducting risk versus risk discussions with patients is provided, and to our knowledge for the first time, risk versus risk tables are provided to encourage and guide such shared decision-making. A brief overview of psychological interventions is provided, along with referral guidance. Finally, a description of our colocated perinatal mental health clinic is provided to illustrate the potential benefits of working closely with behavioral health providers.

PERINATAL PSYCHIATRIC MEDICATION MANAGEMENT
Psychiatric Medication Management Primer

Treatment for perinatal depression is informed by several factors, including severity, past treatment, and minimization of fetal exposures. For patients with mild depression symptoms psychotherapy alone is typically appropriate. For moderate to severe depression symptoms, medication and/or psychotherapy is recommended. Some guiding principles in psychopharmacologic management of depression in pregnancy include (a) use medications that the patient has previously responded to, with the exception of Depakote a known teratogen,[21] (b) use the lowest effective dose that provides symptom relief, and (c) minimize polypharmacy if able.[22] In addition, changes from effective medication once a patient becomes pregnant should not be routine as this increases exposures to the fetus and may result in psychiatric decompensation if the new medication is not effective.

Risk Versus Risk Conversation

Patients often assume that not taking medication in pregnancy means that they have eliminated risk. However, this is not the case considering the risks of untreated perinatal depression listed above. First-line providers should be familiar with the risks of untreated depression in pregnancy and compare them with the risks of proposed medication as part of an informed consent discussion.

In reproductive psychiatry, this is referred to informally as the *risk versus risk* conversation. When provided in a narrative fashion, patients may have difficulty understanding the information to make an informed decision that is right for them and their family. Providers, too, may have difficulty providing all the relevant points in weighing the options. To guide discussion between providers and patients, we have created risk versus risk tables comparing the most common medications' risks with untreated depression (**Table 1**).

A provider may explain:

Both depression and medications have risks in pregnancy, and we will compare these risks to help you make the decision that is right for you. There are three points in pregnancy where we worry about an adverse outcome (left column), first trimester and risk of congenital malformations, all stages of pregnancy and risk for impacts to neurodevelopment, and then risks of complications at or after delivery. The table shows the risks side by side of both depression and a specific medication at each of these time points. Let us review them together for the medications that might be helpful given your symptoms.

We believe this approach has several advantages: improve providers' confidence in discussing options with patients, decrease the risk of providers giving information in a biased way (eg, leaning toward no medication in cases when a patient may benefit from it), and improve patients' ability to compare risks in an easy to reference format. Positive perceptions of treatment and trust in providers contribute to treatment engagement and adherence.[23]

For each class of medication commonly used in the perinatal period, we briefly list known risks in pregnancy and discuss any unique aspects.

Selective Serotonin Reuptake Inhibitors

Selective serotonin reuptake inhibitors (SSRIs) are thought to improve depression, in part, by increasing serotonin availability in the brain. They are often first-line agents for depression and anxiety. The most commonly used SSRIs are sertraline (Zoloft), citalopram (Celexa), escitalopram (Lexapro), fluoxetine (Prozac), and paroxetine (Paxil).

Table 1
Risk versus risk shared decision-making template table

Adverse Outcomes	Untreated Depression	Medication
Risk of congenital malformation		
Risk of negative neurodevelopmental outcome		
Complications at Delivery		

Several recent reviews have covered what is known about the risks of SSRIs in pregnancy.[22,24–26] It is the antidepressant class with the most safety data, being the most studied class of antidepressant in pregnancy.[24]

Most studies that control for maternal depression do not show an increased signal for congenital malformations when used in the first trimester nor increased risk for neurodevelopmental problems in offspring.[27–30] What is more likely, is that maternal depression could be a marker for behaviors (eg, poor prenatal care, substance use) or other genetic or environmental factors, that may increase risk for congenital malformations, complications in pregnancy, or negative neurocognitive consequences in children.[30,31]

There is up to a 30% associated risk of poor neonatal adaptation syndrome (PNAS) at delivery when the neonate is exposed to SSRI in the third trimester.[32] This syndrome usually results in mild symptoms including increased infant fussiness, jitteriness, hypoglycemia, poor muscle tone, and in very rare cases, seizures. Most of the infants do not need additional care other than supportive, and long-term consequences are not seen.[33,34] It is unclear what causes this syndrome, but it may be a mild withdrawal or toxicity.[25] Importantly, stopping antidepressants in the third trimester is not recommended as there is no evidence of decreased PNAS risk, and treatment is removed from the mother in the very vulnerable postpartum period.[22,35]

Another complication associated with third trimester exposure to SSRIs is persistent pulmonary hypertension of the newborn (PPHN); however, it is controversial and unknown if it is a true risk. Studies of the association between PPHN and SSRIs are equivocal and not all studies control for factors known to be independent risks for this condition including prematurity, obesity, smoking, cesarean section, and perinatal depression.[26,36] Women with untreated mental illness also have a higher incidence of those independent risk factors. If a risk exists, it is a low absolute risk.[36] In 2011, the U.S. Food and Drug Administration (FDA) released a statement about PPHN risk, saying "it is premature to reach any conclusion about a possible link between SSRI use in pregnancy and PPHN." They advised health care professionals not alter their current clinical practice of treating depression during pregnancy.[36,37]

Some studies have found a possible small increased rate of postpartum hemorrhage with serotonergic agents; however, it cannot be ruled out that underlying depression or other mental illness is not contributing to this risk.[38] In general, this does not affect our recommendations unless a patient has other risk factors for bleeding.

We recommend using the following table to assist in the risk versus risk conversation when considering an SSRI in pregnancy (**Table 2**).

Selective Serotonin–Norepinephrine Reuptake Inhibitors

Selective serotonin–norepinephrine reuptake inhibitors (SNRIs) act similarly to SSRIs but also affect reuptake of norepinephrine. The most commonly used SNRIs are venlafaxine (Effexor), desvenlafaxine (Pristiq), and duloxetine (Cymbalta). To date, there are less safety data on SNRIs in pregnancy as they are a newer class of antidepressant.

Available data are reassuring that SNRIs are unlikely to be major teratogens.[40,41] Some studies have shown a possible small increase risk of malformations in the first trimester, however, biases by indication could account for these findings.[40] Women who take SNRIs may have a more severe depression that could account for possible increased risk.[42] SNRIs have an independent risk for increasing blood pressure, so monitoring for gestational hypertension is warranted with this class.[43] If the mechanism of PNAS is medication withdrawal or toxicity in the newborn, then the SNRIs likely have a similar risk of this syndrome as the SSRIs. It is unclear if SNRIs have a similar risk of PPHN as the SSRIs.[44] A recent large study looking at antidepressants

Table 2
Selective serotonin reuptake inhibitors versus depression

Adverse Outcome	Untreated Depression	SSRIs
Risk of congenital malformation (3%–5% risk in general population)[39]	• Unknown: May be a marker for behaviors, environmental or behavioral factors that could increase risk for congenital malformations	• Most of the studies controlling for maternal depression have not shown increased risk
Risk of negative neurodevelopmental outcome	• Increased risk of negative impact on intellectual and behavioral functioning in childhood • Increased risk of mental health disorders in offspring	• Studies controlling for underlying maternal mental illness do not show evidence of lower IQ, autism, or behavioral consequences
Complications at delivery	• Risk of miscarriage • Risk of preterm labor • Risk of low birth weight • Risk of preeclampsia • Increase rate of C-section • Risk of worsening mental health symptoms postpartum and difficulty bonding	• Neonatal adaptation syndrome up to 30% risk • Persistent pulmonary hypertension of the new-born controversial risk, if exists low absolute risk • Consider risk of postpartum hemorrhage if patient (pt) has other risk factors for bleeding

and risks of negative neurodevelopmental outcomes in children included the SRNIs and did to find increased risk.[30]

We recommend using the following table to assist in the risk versus risk conversation when considering an SNRI in pregnancy (**Table 3**).

Mirtazapine

Mirtazapine (Remeron) is a noradrenergic and serotonergic antidepressant with similar efficacy to SSRIs in treatment of depression. It not only has indications for insomnia and anxiolysis,[45] but this agent also has unique antiemetic properties which can be helpful in the antenatal period.[46] Literature pertaining to mirtazapine has not demonstrated an increased risk of congenital malformations, spontaneous abortions, or neonatal death.[47] Mirtazapine likely has similar risk of PNAS as the SSRIs.[48] To our knowledge, there are no studies explicitly considering mirtazapine and neurodevelopmental outcomes. However, as mentioned above, studies on other antidepressants that control for maternal mental illness, have not found significant changes in behavior or development in children with in-utero exposure.[30]

We recommend using the following table to assist in the risk versus risk conversation when considering mirtazapine in pregnancy (**Table 4**).

Bupropion

Bupropion (Wellbutrin) is a unique medication that is a norepinephrine and dopamine reuptake inhibitor used to treat depression and for smoking cessation. A small elevated risk of cardiovascular defects has been identified, but these signals are often associated with low absolute risk.[49] Similar to most studies within this population, multiple confounders exist, including confounders of indication given bupropion's use for treatment of smoking cessation. In addition, other studies could not replicate the cardiovascular finding.[29] There is no known increase in risk of miscarriage, prematurity, or low birthweight.[49] To our knowledge, there are no known studies investigating risk of neonatal adaptation syndrome; however, given this risk is usually associated with serotonergic drugs, there is theoretically less risk. A recent large study that looked at antidepressants and risks of neurodevelopmental outcomes in children included bupropion and did not find increased risk.[30]

We recommend using the following table to assist in the risk versus risk conversation when considering bupropion in pregnancy (**Table 5**).

Tricyclic antidepressants

Tricyclic antidepressants (TCAs) block the reuptake of serotonin and norepinephrine in the presynaptic cleft. Their use in general is not first line for depression due to side effect profile and risk of overdose.[50] Available data have not shown an increased rate of congenital malformations when used in the first trimester. TCAs likely have a similar risk of PNAS as SSRIs.[51] Recent studies that included TCAs did not show an increased rate of negative neurodevelopmental outcomes after first trimester exposure.[30] TCAs preferred in pregnancy are nortriptyline or desipramine due to fewer anticholinergic properties and therefore lower likelihood of exacerbating orthostatic hypotension in pregnancy.[26]

We recommend using the following table when considering a TCA in pregnancy (**Table 6**).

Breastfeeding with antidepressants

Most antidepressants have a relative infant dose of less than 10%, which is considered compatible with breastfeeding. All infants should be monitored for excessive sedation, difficulty feeding, difficulty gaining weight, and difficulty meeting

Table 3
Serotonin–norepinephrine reuptake inhibitors versus depression

Adverse Outcome	Untreated Depression	SNRIs
Risk of congenital malformation (3%–5% risk in general population)[39]	• Unknown: May be a marker for behaviors, environmental or behavioral factors that could increase risk for congenital malformations	• Fewer studies compared to the SSRIs • Not likely to increase risk
Risk of negative neurodevelopmental outcome	• Negative impact on intellectual and behavioral functioning in childhood • Increased risk of mental health disorders in offspring	• No evidence of lower IQ or behavioral consequences
Complications at delivery	• Risk of miscarriage • Risk of preterm labor • Risk of low birth weight • Risk of preeclampsia • Increase rate of C-section • Risk of worsening mental health symptoms postpartum and difficulty bonding	• Neonatal adaptation syndrome up to 30% risk • Risk of gestational hypertension • Consider risk of postpartum hemorrhage if pt has other risk factors for bleeding

Table 4
Mirtazapine versus depression

Adverse Outcome	Untreated Depression	Mirtazapine
Risk of congenital malformations (3%–5% risk in general population)[39]	• Unknown: May be a marker for behaviors, environmental or behavioral factors that could increase risk for congenital malformations	• Fewer studies compared to the SSRIs • Available data not showing evidence of increased risk
Risk of poor developmental outcomes	• Increased risk of negative intellectual and behavioral functioning in childhood • Increased risk of mental health disorders in offspring	• No studies explicitly considering mirtazapine and developmental outcomes exist; however, studies on other antidepressants have not found significant increased risk
Complications at delivery	• Risk of miscarriage • Risk of preterm labor • Risk of low birth weight • Risk of preeclampsia • Increase rate of C-section • Risk of worsening mental health symptoms (sx) postpartum and difficulty bonding	• Likely the same risk of PNAS as SSRIs • Neonatal adaptation syndrome up to 30% risk

Table 5
Bupropion versus depression

Adverse Outcome	Untreated Depression	Bupropion
Risk of congenital malformations (3%–5% risk in general population)[39]	• Unknown: May be a marker for behaviors, environmental or behavioral factors that could increase risk for congenital malformations	• Fewer studies compared to the SSRIs • Conflicting literature with some suggesting increased risk for cardiovascular defects that cannot be ruled out as due to underlying mental illness. If true association, small absolute risk
Risk of poor developmental outcomes	• Increased risk of negative intellectual and behavioral functioning in childhood • Increased risk of mental health disorders in offspring	• No evidence of lower IQ or behavioral consequences
Complications at delivery	• Risk of miscarriage • Risk of preterm labor • Risk of low birth weight • Risk of preeclampsia • Increase rate of C-section • Risk of worsening mental health sx postpartum and difficulty bonding	• Theoretically less risk of PNAS if related to serotonin

Table 6
Tricyclic antidepressant versus depression

Adverse Outcome	Untreated Depression	TCAs
Risk of congenital malformations (3%–5% risk in general population)[39]	• Unknown: May be a marker for behaviors, environmental or behavioral factors that could increase risk for congenital malformations	• Fewer studies compared to the SSRIs • No evidence of increased risk
Risk of poor developmental outcomes	• Increased risk of negative intellectual and behavioral functioning in childhood • Increased risk of mental health disorders in offspring	• No evidence of lower IQ or behavioral consequences
Complications at delivery	• Risk of miscarriage • Risk of preterm labor • Risk of low birth weight • Risk of preeclampsia • Increase rate of C-section • Risk of worsening mental health sx postpartum and difficulty bonding	• Risk of PNAS likely similar to SSRIs • Neonatal adaptation syndrome up to 30% risk

milestones.[52] We recommend working collaboratively with a pediatrician to help with monitoring. The anticholinergic properties of TCAs warrant monitoring for constipation and urinary retention.[52] Of note, there are two case reports of breastfed babies with exposure to bupropion having seizures with subsequent resolution on cessation of breastfeeding.[53,54] Given these are case reports, studies with less rigorous methodology, bupropion is still considered compatible with breastfeeding. We also recommend consultation with a pediatrician or neonatologist regarding safety of breastfeeding with medication if an infant is premature or has a medical condition.

Integrative medicine or adjunctive treatments

Although there are less robust studies of complementary and alternative medicine, there are several methods that have safety data in pregnancy and could be helpful.[55] Most notably, it may be useful to consider supplementation with vitamin D, omega-3 fatty acids, or utilization of bright light therapy.

Vitamin D deficiency has been linked with perinatal depression; vitamin D levels less than 32 ng/mL are considered deficient, though guidelines vary.[55] In pregnant people with vitamin D deficiency, supplementation of 1000 to 2000 international units (IU) is recommended, with the upper safe limit being 4000 IU.[56] Decreased postpartum depression symptoms have been reported with supplementation of 50,000 IU every 14 days for 8 weeks, which is equivalent to 3600 UI per day.[57] It is unknown if supplementation with vitamin D is beneficial for those who do not have an underlying deficiency.

Omega-3 polyunsaturated fatty acids which include eicosapentaenoic acid (EPA) and docosahexaenoic acid (DHA) have shown a small positive effect on the prevention and treatment of perinatal depression as a stand-alone agent[58]; effectiveness increases when used adjunctively with pharmacologic treatment.[58] It should also be considered in treating PMADs in birthing people with dietary deficiency, elevated BMI, or inflammatory disorders.[58,59] The recommended dose is 1000 to 2000 mg per day of EPA with an EPA/DHA ratio of 2:1.[60]

Bright light therapy has been shown to be effective in creating and maintaining depression remission and is well tolerated. Although protocols vary, the use of 10,000 lux for 45 minutes each morning over 3 weeks was found to be more effective than placebo.[61]

Referring to higher level of psychiatric care

Although it is important that first-line providers feel comfortable having risk versus risk conversations and starting medication treatment with patients with perinatal depression, there will be patients who are more complex and require further psychiatric consultation.

Bipolar Disorder

Patients with diagnosed or suspected bipolar disorders should be referred to specialty psychiatric care. Monotherapy with an antidepressant would likely be ineffective for depression in this population and could increase risk of inducing a manic episode, which could be dangerous in pregnancy and postpartum.[62,63] In addition to more complex medication management, patients with bipolar disorder are at an increased risk of postpartum psychosis.[63,64] Specialized care for these patients is imperative as postpartum psychosis is a psychiatric emergency that has a suicide rate of 5% and infanticide rate of 4%.[64,65] Reproductive psychiatry can be helpful to patients with bipolar disorders and their first-line providers, preventatively in the pregnancy planning stages as well.

Psychosis

Another set of patients who require additional psychiatric consultation are those patients with psychotic symptoms including auditory or visual hallucinations, delusions, ideas of reference, or paranoia. Psychotic symptoms during pregnancy should be evaluated by a psychiatric provider who can discuss treatment options versus risks of psychotic symptoms. Postpartum psychotic symptoms, especially delusions related to the baby, are the most concerning; they can be dangerous and should be evaluated by a psychiatric provider emergently to rule out postpartum psychosis and create a safety plan for the family.[64] In addition, prior personal history of postpartum psychosis is a risk factor for future postpartum psychosis; psychiatric consultation should be sought early in pregnancy or before pregnancy for patients with such history.

Additional Psychiatric Referral Guidance

Psychiatric consultation is recommended for patients with unclear psychiatric diagnosis, patients with psychiatric polypharmacy, or those who are not responding to a maximized dose of first-line agents.

PSYCHOTHERAPY

Psychotherapy is a first-line treatment for mild to severe depression and should be considered that perinatal depression is first identified.[66] Referral to psychotherapy can be part of the risk versus risk conversation recommended above, as some patients will prefer a non-pharmacologic approach. Research shows that matching treatment modality with patient preferences contributes positively to treatment engagement and outcomes.[67,68]

Cognitive behavioral therapy (CBT) and interpersonal psychotherapy (IPT) are manualized evidence-based psychological treatments for perinatal depression. A Cochrane review found that both effectively treat postpartum depression.[69] Evidence-based interventions, while often time-limited and structured, include the use of effective common factors such as unconditional positive regard and reflective listening and take into account the individual's clinical presentation.

CBT is one of the most widely studied effective psychotherapies for depression including for perinatal depression.[69–72] CBT focuses on the role of negative thoughts on maintenance of negative emotions and behaviors, targeting changes in cognition and behavior to improve symptoms. CBT is appropriate for mild to severe depression, can be used with or without adjunctive medication, and has demonstrated lasting effects.[71] CBT is effective in individual, group, and Internet-based modalities.[71]

IPT[73] is a structured, manualized, idiographic approach that focuses on the role of interpersonal relationships on functioning. IPT provides tools for addressing interpersonal conflicts, transitions (eg, having a baby), and grief and loss. IPT is evidence-based both for prevention and treatment of perinatal depression.[69,70]

Recent efforts to expand the number of evidence-based psychotherapies studied in the perinatal period include work applying third-wave behavioral interventions such as acceptance and commitment therapy (ACT)[74] and dialectical behavioral therapy (DBT)[75] to PMADs.

The Cochrane review also found some evidence for the positive effects of psychosocial interventions, such as peer-to-peer and nondirective counseling.[69] Compared with postpartum care as usual (nonmental health care), these interventions were better than nothing at reducing postpartum depression.[69]

In response to COVID-19, utilization of telehealth increased broadly and in response to the needs of perinatal populations. Although additional research is needed, telehealth seems to be an effective delivery modality for perinatal focused psychotherapies and may even be preferred due to a reduction in barriers to care.[76]

In sum, referral to psychotherapy should prioritize referral to evidence-based treatments for depression, particularly CBT and IPT. However, other evidence-based treatments may be helpful including ACT and DBT. When psychological treatments are not available, psychosocial interventions may be more beneficial than nothing (supportive counseling, peer-to-peer support, and so forth).

Referral Challenges and Solutions

Referral to behavioral health treatment can itself become a barrier to care. Referring providers may often rely on outdated local referral lists, waitlists may be long in the community, and specialized care in perinatal psychiatry and mental health may be particularly difficult to find. Partnering with behavioral health providers within one's institution, building relationships with community providers, and using online referral platforms (eg, Psychology Today *Find a Therapist* search) may all contribute to more robust referral networks.

Patients themselves face financial and logistic barriers to engaging in care, including cost, insurance, transportation, mental health stigma, and lack of access to care, and these barriers are reported more often by women with more severe depression symptoms.[77] A recent study found that only 34% of women with diagnosable depression at their first antepartum visit receive any mental health care during pregnancy or up to 3 months postpartum.[78] A meta-analysis of referral uptake after perinatal depression screening suggests that referral to on-site assessment and treatment can improve engagement.[79]

The following section provides a brief overview of our own colocated clinic and what we believe are the strengths and benefits of such an approach.

OUR EXPERIENCE: COLOCATED COLLABORATIVE CARE FOR PERINATAL DEPRESSION

The authors provide, or have provided, services in a colocated, collaborative perinatal mental health clinic within an outpatient women's specialty clinic in an academic medical center. The clinic was founded out of a need for greater referral access and reliability recognized by certified nurse midwives, pediatricians, and obstetricians.

The Journeys Clinic accepts internal referrals primarily through a formal ad hoc referral process. Patients who are pregnant or recently pregnant are eligible for referral for a range of mental health conditions, most frequently PMADs. Patients remain eligible for up to 12 months postpartum. Patients who are trying to get pregnant and those who have experienced pregnancy-related loss are also eligible.

The current core providers include psychiatrists and psychologists, and referrals primarily are placed by women's health providers. Psychiatric consultation to patients and providers is provided on a one-time basis, supporting referring providers' ability to manage psychotropic medications during the perinatal period. This includes formal assessment and management of medication directly with patients as well as curbside and e-consult support for referring providers. Psychologists provide assessment, treatment planning, and psychotherapy. Patient care is shared and collaborative within the clinic and with referring providers, creating an ideal context in which to monitor progress, adjust treatment, and coordinate care. A key benefit is consistency across the patient's care team, reducing patient confusion about treatment options and recommendations, particularly with regard to medications.

Although the clinic model is not fully integrated like one might see in primary care, the colocated and collaborative coordinated care approach is one type of integrated care.[80] Anecdotally, we find that patients are able to see a psychiatrist and/or psychologist much more quickly due the existence of this clinic, rather than waiting for general behavioral health services within our institution. Research on a similar colocated program found that having a psychologist on the team, reduced wait time for a psychiatrist and increased the number of unique patients seen by a psychiatrist, likely due to matching care to patient needs and preferences.[81] In addition, patients and providers have reported decreased stigma around accessing mental health services in our clinic, as the location is not designated as a mental health facility.

The program is also focused on building reproductive behavioral health workforce capacity through training, including a reproductive psychiatry fellowship, predoctoral psychology internship rotations, and psychology postdoctoral rotations. The reproductive psychiatry fellowship addresses calls for more specialty care within psychiatry for perinatal patients.[82] One author provides supervision of quality improvement, program development, and research projects among trainees, developing capacity for much needed perinatal mental health research in a rural/frontier and urban-serving public safety net hospital.

There has been a call for greater development of and research on integrated behavioral health in women's health settings, and we believe that a colocated perinatal mental health clinic is a powerful tool for addressing the needs of women during the perinatal stage.[83] Although we expect a more formal evaluation of our clinic's practices and benefits will be forthcoming in the literature, we hope that this brief description will be beneficial to readers considering adding behavioral health providers to their women's health medical teams. Certainly, there are complexities such as space, billing, recruitment and retention, cultural responsiveness, evidence-based practices, and interprofessional training to consider, which are beyond the scope of this update. A recent study authored by one of the current authors provides a framework for integrating behavioral health into women's specialty settings and may provide helpful additional information.[83]

SUMMARY

Perinatal depression has many negative consequences for pregnant persons and their babies, but evidence-based treatments exist. Obstetric providers are often the first to identify perinatal depression and are instrumental in decreasing time to treatment. Increasing access is especially important in addressing the health disparities apparent in recent maternal mortality and morbidity rates. We encourage obstetric providers to believe empowered to recognize depression symptoms in their patients, refer to psychotherapy, have risk versus risk conversations about medications, and start treatment that is acceptable to the patient.

CLINICS CARE POINTS

- Psychiatric medication for perinatal depression can successfully be managed by front-line providers and should be considered when depression is first identified.
- Risks of medication should be weighed against the risks of untreated mental illness in the perinatal period. Risk versus risk tables provided in this article may facilitate more effective shared decision-making conversations with patients.

- Psychotherapy for depression should also be considered at the time of diagnosis; effective treatments are available.
- Referral to psychiatric and psychological assessment and treatment can be aided by on-site availability of behavioral health providers.

DISCLOSURE

No conflicts of interest to disclose.

REFERENCES

1. Biaggi A, Conroy S, Pawlby S, et al. Identifying the women at risk of antenatal anxiety and depression: A systematic review. J Affect Disord 2016;191:62–77.
2. Osborne LM, Voegtline K, Standeven LR, et al. High worry in pregnancy predicts postpartum depression. J Affect Disord 2021;294:701–6.
3. Woody CA, Ferrari AJ, Siskind DJ, et al. A systematic review and meta-regression of the prevalence and incidence of perinatal depression. J Affect Disord 2017; 219:86–92.
4. Van Niel MS, Payne JL. Perinatal depression: A review. Cleve Clin J Med 2020; 87(5):273–7.
5. Jarde A, Morais M, Kingston D, et al. Neonatal Outcomes in Women With Untreated Antenatal Depression Compared With Women Without Depression: A Systematic Review and Meta-analysis. JAMA Psychiatr 2016;73(8):826.
6. Zou R, Tiemeier H, van der Ende J, et al. Exposure to Maternal Depressive Symptoms in Fetal Life or Childhood and Offspring Brain Development: A Population-Based Imaging Study. Am J Psychiatry 2019;176(9):702–10.
7. Daglar G, Nur N. Level of mother-baby bonding and influencing factors during pregnancy and postpartum period. Psychiatr Danub 2018;30(4):433–40.
8. Trost S, Beauregard J, Chandra G, et al. Pregnancy-Related Deaths: Data from Maternal Mortality Review Committees in 36 US States, 2017-2019.
9. Bonari L, Pinto N, Ahn E, et al. Perinatal Risks of Untreated Depression during Pregnancy. Can J Psychiatry 2004;49(11):726–35.
10. Henry AL, Beach AJ, Stowe ZN, et al. The Fetus and Maternal Depression: Implications for Antenatal Treatment Guidelines. Clin Obstet Gynecol 2004;47(3): 535–46.
11. Allister L, Lester BM, Carr S, et al. The Effects of Maternal Depression on Fetal Heart Rate Response to Vibroacoustic Stimulation. Dev Neuropsychol 2001; 20(3):639–51.
12. Chung TKH, Lau TK, Yip ASK, et al. Antepartum Depressive Symptomatology Is Associated With Adverse Obstetric and Neonatal Outcomes. Psychosom Med 2001;63(5):830–4.
13. Rauh C, Beetz A, Burger P, et al. Delivery mode and the course of pre- and postpartum depression. Arch Gynecol Obstet 2012;286(6):1407–12.
14. Kurki T. Depression and anxiety in early pregnancy and risk for preeclampsia. Obstet Gynecol 2000;95(4):487–90.
15. Steer RA, Scholl TO, Hediger ML, et al. Self-reported depression and negative pregnancy outcomes. J Clin Epidemiol 1992;45(10):1093–9.
16. Butler MS, Young SL, Tuthill EL. Perinatal depressive symptoms and breastfeeding behaviors: A systematic literature review and biosocial research agenda. J Affect Disord 2021;283:441–71.

17. American College of Obstetricians and Gynecologists. Screening for Perinatal Depression 2018;132(5).
18. McGuire TG, Miranda J. New Evidence Regarding Racial And Ethnic Disparities In Mental Health: Policy Implications. Health Aff 2008;27(2):393–403.
19. Sidebottom A, Vacquier M, LaRusso E, et al. Perinatal depression screening practices in a large health system: identifying current state and assessing opportunities to provide more equitable care. Arch Womens Ment Health 2021;24(1):133–44.
20. Atkins R. Coping with Depression in Single Black Mother s. Issues Ment Health Nurs 2016;37(3):172–81.
21. Andrade C. Valproate in Pregnancy: Recent Research and Regulatory Responses. J Clin Psychiatry 2018;79(3). https://doi.org/10.4088/JCP.18f12351.
22. Kimmel MC, Cox E, Schiller C, et al. Pharmacologic Treatment of Perinatal Depression. Obstet Gynecol Clin North Am 2018;45(3):419–40.
23. Jones A. Help Seeking in the Perinatal Period: A Review of Barriers and Facilitators. Soc Work Public Health 2019;34(7):596–605.
24. Payne JL. Psychopharmacology in Pregnancy and Breastfeeding. Psychiatr Clin North Am 2017;40(2):217–38.
25. Betcher HK, Wisner KL. Psychotropic Treatment During Pregnancy: Research Synthesis and Clinical Care Principles. J Womens Health (Larchmt) 2020;29(3):310–8.
26. Raffi ER, Nonacs R, Cohen LS. Safety of Psychotropic Medications During Pregnancy. Clin Perinatol 2019;46(2):215–34.
27. Alwan S, Reefhuis J, Rasmussen SA, et al. Use of Selective Serotonin-Reuptake Inhibitors in Pregnancy and the Risk of Birth Defects. N Engl J Med 2007;356(26):2684–92. https://doi.org/10.1056/NEJMoa066584.
28. Wisner KL, Sit DKY, Hanusa BH, et al. Major Depression and Antidepressant Treatment: Impact on Pregnancy and Neonatal Outcomes. Am J Psychiatry 2009;166(5):557–66.
29. Huybrechts KF, Palmsten K, Avorn J, et al. Antidepressant Use in Pregnancy and the Risk of Cardiac Defects. N Engl J Med 2014;370(25):2397–407.
30. Suarez EA, Bateman BT, Hernández-Díaz S, et al. Association of Antidepressant Use During Pregnancy With Risk of Neurodevelopmental Disorders in Children. JAMA Intern Med 2022;182(11):1149.
31. Andrade C. Gestational Exposure to Antidepressant Drugs and Neurodevelopment: An Examination of Language, Mathematics, Intelligence, and Other Cognitive Outcomes. J Clin Psychiatry 2022;83(1). https://doi.org/10.4088/JCP.22f14388.
32. Levinson-Castiel R, Merlob P, Linder N, et al. Neonatal Abstinence Syndrome After In Utero Exposure to Selective Serotonin Reuptake Inhibitors in Term Infants. Arch Pediatr Adolesc Med 2006;160(2):173.
33. Nulman I, Koren G, Rovet J, et al. Neurodevelopment of Children Following Prenatal Exposure to Venlafaxine, Selective Serotonin Reuptake Inhibitors, or Untreated Maternal Depression. Am J Psychiatry 2012;169(11):1165–74.
34. Misri S, Reebye P, Kendrick K, et al. Internalizing Behaviors in 4-Year-Old Children Exposed in Utero to Psychotropic Medications. Am J Psychiatry 2006;163(6):1026–32.
35. Warburton W, Hertzman C, Oberlander TF. A register study of the impact of stopping third trimester selective serotonin reuptake inhibitor exposure on neonatal health: Gestational SSRI exposure and neonatal health. Acta Psychiatr Scand 2009;121(6):471–9.

36. Huybrechts KF, Bateman BT, Palmsten K, et al. Antidepressant Use Late in Pregnancy and Risk of Persistent Pulmonary Hypertension of the Newborn. JAMA 2015;313(21):2142.

37. Center for Drug Evaluation. FDA Drug Safety Communication: Selective serotonin reuptake inhibitor (SSRI) antidepressant use during pregnancy and reports of a rare heart and lung condition in newborn babies. FDA. 2019. https://www.fda.gov/drugs/drug-safety-and-availability/fda-drug-safety-communication-selective-serotonin-reuptake-inhibitor-ssri-antidepressant-use-during. Accessed December 19, 2022.

38. Palmsten K, Chambers CD, Wells A, et al. Patterns of prenatal antidepressant exposure and risk of preeclampsia and postpartum haemorrhage. Paediatr Perinat Epidemiol 2020;34(5):597–606.

39. Mai CT, Isenburg JL, Canfield MA, et al. National population-based estimates for major birth defects, 2010–2014. Birth Defects Res 2019;111(18):1420–35.

40. Huybrechts KF, Bateman BT, Pawar A, et al. Maternal and fetal outcomes following exposure to duloxetine in pregnancy: cohort study. BMJ 2020;368:m237.

41. Lassen D, Ennis ZN, Damkier P. First-Trimester Pregnancy Exposure to Venlafaxine or Duloxetine and Risk of Major Congenital Malformations: A Systematic Review. Basic Clin Pharmacol Toxicol 2016;118(1):32–6.

42. Wisner KL, Oberlander TF, Huybrechts KF. The Association Between Antidepressant Exposure and Birth Defects—Are We There Yet? JAMA Psychiatr 2020;77(12):1215.

43. Zhong Z, Wang L, Wen X, et al. A meta-analysis of effects of selective serotonin reuptake inhibitors on blood pressure in depression treatment: outcomes from placebo and serotonin and noradrenaline reuptake inhibitor controlled trials. Neuropsychiatr Dis Treat 2017;13:2781–96.

44. Orsolini L, Valchera A, De Berardis D, et al. Pregnancy and psychotropic drugs. In: Uguz F, editor. Psychotropic drugs and medical conditions. Psychiatry - theory, applications and treatments. Nova Biomedical Books; 2017. p. 181–208. https://libproxy.unm.edu/login?url=https://search.ebscohost.com/login.aspx?direct=true&db=psyh&AN=2017-31735-010&site=ehost-live.

45. Fawcett J, Barkin RL. Review of the results from clinical studies on the efficacy, safety and tolerability of mirtazapine for the treatment of patients with major depression. J Affect Disord 1998;51(3):267–85.

46. Abramowitz A, Miller ES, Wisner KL. Treatment options for hyperemesis gravidarum. Arch Womens Ment Health 2017;20(3):363–72.

47. Ostenfeld A, Petersen TS, Pedersen LH, et al. Mirtazapine exposure in pregnancy and fetal safety: A nationwide cohort study. Acta Psychiatr Scand 2022;145(6):557–67.

48. Grigoriadis S, VonderPorten EH, Mamisashvili L, et al. The Effect of Prenatal Antidepressant Exposure on Neonatal Adaptation: A Systematic Review and Meta-Analysis. J Clin Psychiatry 2013;74(04):e309–20.

49. Hendrick V, Suri R, Gitlin MJ, et al. Bupropion Use During Pregnancy: A Systematic Review. Prim Care Companion CNS Disord 2017;19(5):17r02160.

50. Moraczewski J, Aedma KK. Tricyclic antidepressants. StatPearls Publishing; 2022. https://www.ncbi.nlm.nih.gov/books/NBK557791/. Accessed December 19, 2022.

51. Gastaldon C, Arzenton E, Raschi E, et al. Neonatal withdrawal syndrome following in utero exposure to antidepressants: a disproportionality analysis of VigiBase, the WHO spontaneous reporting database. Psychol Med. Published online September 2022;21:1–9. https://doi.org/10.1017/S0033291722002859.

52. Hale T. Hale's medications & mothers' milk. 19th edition. New York, NY: Springer Publishing Company; 2021.
53. Chaudron LH, Schoenecker CJ. Bupropion and Breastfeeding: A Case of a Possible Infant Seizure. J Clin Psychiatry 2004;65(6):881–2.
54. Neuman G, Colantonio D, Delaney S, et al. Bupropion and Escitalopram During Lactation. Ann Pharmacother 2014;48(7):928–31.
55. Deligiannidis KM, Freeman MP. Complementary and alternative medicine therapies for perinatal depression. Best Pract Res Clin Obstet Gynaecol 2014;28(1): 85–95.
56. ACOG. Committee. Opinion No. 495: Vitamin D: Screening and Supplementation During Pregnancy. Obstet Gynecol 2011;118(1):197–8.
57. Amini S, Amani R, Jafarirad S, et al. The effect of vitamin D and calcium supplementation on inflammatory biomarkers, estradiol levels and severity of symptoms in women with postpartum depression: a randomized double-blind clinical trial. Nutr Neurosci 2022;25(1):22–32.
58. RJT Mocking, Steijn K, Roos C, et al. Omega-3 Fatty Acid Supplementation for Perinatal Depression: A Meta-Analysis. J Clin Psychiatry 2020;81(5):19r13106.
59. Sarris J, Freeman MP. Omega-3 Fatty Acid Supplementation for Perinatal Depression and Other Subpopulations? J Clin Psychiatry 2020;81(5):20com13489.
60. Guu TW, Mischoulon D, Sarris J, et al. International Society for Nutritional Psychiatry Research Practice Guidelines for Omega-3 Fatty Acids in the Treatment of Major Depressive Disorder. Psychother Psychosom 2019;88(5):263–73.
61. Donmez M, Yorguner N, Kora K, et al. Efficacy of bright light therapy in perinatal depression: A randomized, double-blind, placebo-controlled study. J Psychiatr Res 2022;149:315–22.
62. Sachs GS, Nierenberg AA, Calabrese JR, et al. Effectiveness of Adjunctive Antidepressant Treatment for Bipolar Depression. N Engl J Med 2007;356(17):1711–22.
63. Clark CT, Wisner KL. Treatment of Peripartum Bipolar Disorder. Obstet Gynecol Clin North Am 2018;45(3):403–17.
64. Spinelli MG. Postpartum Psychosis: Detection of Risk and Management. Am J Psychiatry 2009;166(4):405–8.
65. Perry A, Gordon-Smith K, Jones L, et al. Phenomenology, Epidemiology and Aetiology of Postpartum Psychosis: A Review. Brain Sci 2021;11(1):47.
66. Stuart S, Koleva H. Psychological treatments for perinatal depression. Best Pract Res Clin Obstet Gynaecol 2014;28(1):61–70.
67. Windle E, Tee H, Sabitova A, et al. Association of Patient Treatment Preference With Dropout and Clinical Outcomes in Adult Psychosocial Mental Health Interventions: A Systematic Review and Meta-analysis. JAMA Psychiatr 2020;77(3):294.
68. Henshaw EJ, Flynn HA, Himle JA, et al. Patient Preferences for Clinician Interactional Style in Treatment of Perinatal Depression. Qual Health Res 2011;21(7): 936–51.
69. Dennis CL, Hodnett ED. Psychosocial and psychological interventions for treating postpartum depression. Cochrane Common Mental Disorders Group. Cochrane database syst rev 2007. https://doi.org/10.1002/14651858.CD006116.pub2.
70. Dennis CL, Dowswell T. Psychosocial and psychological interventions for preventing postpartum depression. Cochrane Database Syst Rev 2013;2:CD001134.
71. Shortis E, Warrington D, Whittaker P. The efficacy of cognitive behavioral therapy for the treatment of antenatal depression: A systematic review. J Affect Disord 2020;272:485–95.
72. Sockol LE. A systematic review of the efficacy of cognitive behavioral therapy for treating and preventing perinatal depression. J Affect Disord 2015;177:7–21.

73. Stuart S. Interpersonal Psychotherapy for Postpartum Depression. Clin Psychol Psychother 2012;19(2):134–40.

74. Waters CS, Annear B, Flockhart G, et al. Acceptance and Commitment Therapy for perinatal mood and anxiety disorders: A feasibility and proof of concept study. Br J Clin Psychol 2020;59(4):461–79.

75. Agako A, Burckell L, McCabe RE, et al. A pilot study examining the effectiveness of a short-term, DBT informed, skills group for emotion dysregulation during the perinatal period. Psychol Serv 2022. https://doi.org/10.1037/ser0000662.

76. Singla DR, Hossain S, Andrejek N, et al. Culturally sensitive psychotherapy for perinatal women: A mixed methods study. J Consult Clin Psychol 2022; 90(10):770.

77. Kopelman RC, Moel J, Mertens C, et al. Barriers to Care for Antenatal Depression. Psychiatr Serv Wash DC 2008;59(4):429–32.

78. Lee-Carbon L, Nath S, Trevillion K, et al. Mental health service use among pregnant and early postpartum women. Soc Psychiatry Psychiatr Epidemiol 2022; 57(11):2229–40.

79. Xue W, Cheng K, Xu D, et al. Uptake of referrals for women with positive perinatal depression screening results and the effectiveness of interventions to increase uptake: a systematic review and meta-analysis. Epidemiol Psychiatr Sci 2020; 29:e143.

80. SAMHSA-HRSA. Advancing behavioral health integration within NCQA recognized patient-Centered medical homes 2014. www.integration.samhsa.gov.

81. Pawar D, Huang CC, Wichman C. Co-located Perinatal Psychiatry Clinic: Impact of Adding a Psychologist on Clinical Quality Improvement Metrics. J Psychosom Obstet Gynaecol 2019;40(2):123–7.

82. Payne JL. Reproductive psychiatry: giving birth to a new subspecialty. Int Rev Psychiatry 2019;31(3):207–9.

83. Crawford JN, Weitzen SH, Schulkin J. Integrated women's behavioral health: Recent literature and proposed framework. Prof Psychol Res Pract 2022;53:50–8.

Office-Based Management of Perinatal Substance Use and Substance Use Disorder for the General Obstetrician-Gynecologist

Theresa Kurtz, MD[a],*, Marcela C. Smid, MD, MS[a]

KEYWORDS

- Addiction • Substance use • Pregnancy • Substance use disorder

KEY POINTS

- Individuals should be screened for alcohol, tobacco, and drug use before, during, and after pregnancy using validated screening tools.
- Urinary toxicology tests should only be obtained after receiving patient consent and with a transparent plan for the purpose of the test and actions to be taken based on results.
- All individuals with substance use disorder (SUD) should be screened for intimate partner violence, depression, hepatitis B and C, HIV, syphilis, gonorrhea, and chlamydia. Tuberculosis screening should be performed for at-risk individuals, most commonly those with history of incarceration.
- Obstetrician-gynecologists (OB-GYNs) should know how to acutely manage individuals with SUD and be familiar with the maternal, fetal, and neonatal risks and ways to mitigate these risks.

INTRODUCTION

Substance use (SU) and substance use disorders (SUD) in pregnancy are common, underdiagnosed, and undertreated. In 2020, 8% to 11% of pregnant individuals reported past-month illicit drug, tobacco, or alcohol use,[1] and an estimated 5% to 15% of pregnant people met criteria for an SUD.[2,3] Reflecting national trends of the general population, substance-related deaths are the leading cause of maternal death.[4,5] Although office-based management of SUD is a learning objective of the American College of Obstetrics and Gynecology (ACOG)[6] and the American Board

[a] Department of Obstetrics and Gynecology, University of Utah Health, 30 North 1900 East #2B200 SOM, Salt Lake City, UT 84132, USA
* Corresponding author.
E-mail address: terri.kurtz@hsc.utah.edu

Obstet Gynecol Clin N Am 50 (2023) 609–627
https://doi.org/10.1016/j.ogc.2023.03.010
0889-8545/23/© 2023 Elsevier Inc. All rights reserved.

obgyn.theclinics.com

of Obstetrics and Gynecology,[7] obstetrician-gynecologist (OB-GYN) trainees and clinicians are often ill-prepared to care for this population owing to lack of clinician training,[8] comfort,[9] stigma,[10] and underdiagnosis.[9] Identifying individuals with SU/SUD is vital to comprehensive prenatal care and well within the capabilities of all OB-GYNs. Pregnancy is often a strong motivator for change,[11] and OB-GYNs are uniquely positioned to offer longitudinal therapeutic relationships, mental health and social resources, direct treatment or linkage to treatment, harm reduction strategies, and interventions that reduce the symptoms of SUD (eg, cravings, thoughts of use, uncontrolled use).

In this review, the authors discuss legal considerations, outline definitions, review screening tools, introduce special considerations and harm reduction, caution the use of urinary toxicology testing, and touch on the screening, brief intervention, and referral to treatment (SAMHSA) model. After this, they briefly present the most commonly used substances, associated risks, and treatments.

BACKGROUND

During pregnancy, rates of SU are lower than in the nonpregnant population and generally use declines by trimester.[12] Those with persistent SU during pregnancy likely have an SUD and merit treatment. SUD is a chronic medical condition, like diabetes or hypertension, that requires consistent medical and psychosocial interventions based on the substance or substances of use. However, unlike other chronic conditions, the treatment of SUD—particularly for pregnant and parenting individuals—is distorted by decades of systemic stigmatization and discrimination resulting in barriers to treatment. Some states have "priority access laws" for pregnant individuals with SUD that prioritize pregnant individuals in available slots at inpatient and outpatient treatment programs. However, accessing SUD treatment resources is still exceeding difficult for pregnant individuals.[13,14] Individuals not only encounter challenges in accessing treatment, but also are often deterred from doing so owing to fear of losing parental rights.[10]

Currently, 24 states and the District of Columbia mandate reporting for drug use in pregnancy, and drug use in pregnancy is grounds for civil commitment in 3 states.[15] Punitive state reporting policies are associated with an increased risk of neonatal opioid withdrawal syndrome (NOWS), likely owing to reduced engagement in prenatal care and reduced access to opioid use disorder (OUD) treatment.[16,17] Punitive policies can also destabilize individuals, triggering return to use, overdose, or exacerbation of mental illness and suicide.[18,19] Policies punishing SUD in pregnancy disproportionately affect people of color and do not improve outcomes for pregnant individuals, newborns, or families.[20,21]

Systemic racism is deeply involved in the care of pregnant people with SUD. Nonwhite women are more likely to be verbally screened for SU.[22] Nonwhite women from low-income urban areas disproportionately receive urinary toxicology testing,[23,24] despite robust evidence that demographic characteristics do not correlate with SU/SUD.[25] However, racial disparities in referral to Child Protective Services (CPS) based on SU/SUD are widely well-documented.[20,21,24] OB-GYNs must be thoughtful of racial bias in managing pregnant people with SU and reporting to CPS and must distinguish their own implicit biases. OB-GYNs should be aware of their state and institutional policies and collaborate with social workers and pediatricians to accurately articulate these policies to individuals before delivery. Acknowledging the racially inequitable care of pregnant people with SUD and the harms of punitive policies, OB-GYNs should advocate for reform of SU criminalization in pregnancy.[26]

DEFINITIONS

Application of terminology such as SU, misuse, and SUD according to the *Diagnostic and Statistical Manual of Mental Disorders* (Fifth Edition) (*DSM-V*) is imperative to communicate with colleagues, make an accurate diagnosis, and bill appropriately. Recommended terms are listed in **Table 1**. There is no *DSM-V* criteria for "addiction"; the term is often used synonymously with severe SUD.[27]

APPROACH TO INDIVIDUALS WITH SUBSTANCE USE

SUD is not a moral failing or lack of willpower; it is well-studied as a brain disorder influenced by genetics, environment, and behavior with nonadherence and complication rates akin to other chronic diseases.[28] About 40% of individuals with SUD have mental illness, and about 20% of those with mental illness have SUD.[29] Pregnant individuals with SUD have a high rate of cooccurrence with intimate partner violence (IPV),[30] trauma,[31] anxiety, depression, and bipolar disorder.[32] Individuals with SUD

Table 1	
Definitions for substance use, misuse, disorder, and recovery	
Term	**Definition**
Substance use	Sporadic use of psychoactive substances
Substance misuse	Excessive use of psychoactive substances, which may lead to physical, social, or emotional harm

Substance use disorder	*Diagnostic and Statistical Manual-V* uses the same overarching criteria for all substances to diagnosis mild (2–3 symptoms), moderate (4–5 symptoms), and severe (6 or more symptoms) states[88]:
	• Impaired control
	  ○ Use in larger amounts or longer periods than intended
	  ○ Persistent desire or unsuccessful efforts to decrease or stop use
	  ○ Craving or strong desire to use
	  ○ Excessive time spent obtaining or using substance or recovering from the effects
	• Social impairment
	  ○ Failure to fulfill major role obligations at work, school, or home
	  ○ Persistent or recurrent social or interpersonal problems exacerbated by use
	  ○ Reduction or cessation of important social, occupation, or recreational activities because of use
	• Risky use
	  ○ Use in physically hazardous situations
	  ○ Continued use despite knowledge of persistent physical or psychological problems arising from use
	• Pharmacologic properties
	  ○ Tolerance as demonstrated by increased amount needed to achieve desired effect; diminished effect with continued use of the same amount
	  ○ Withdrawal symptoms with cessation or decreased use
	Note: Solely pharmacologic symptoms are not sufficient to meet criteria for substance use disorder

Recovery[89]	A process of change through which individuals improve their health and wellness, live a self-directed life, and strive to reach their full potential

Adapted from Smid M, Terplan M. What Obstetrician–Gynecologists should know about substance use disorders in the perinatal period. Obstetrics & Gynecology. 2022;139(2):317-337. https://doi.org/10.1097/AOG.0000000000004657; with permission.

are prone to socioeconomic challenges like homelessness, poverty, incarceration, and underinsurance.[33] Systemic discrimination of individuals with SUD perpetuates their socioeconomic difficulties owing to frequent interactions with the criminal justice system and barriers finding employment[34] and housing.

Like in other settings, individuals with SUD disproportionately experience stigma while seeking medical care.[10] **Table 2** lists types of stigma. Stigma stems from prejudice and medically inaccurate views of SUD. In addition to fear of CPS involvement, pregnant individuals with SUD are often deterred from seeking prenatal care[17] because many health care and legal settings still maintain the sentiment that people who use substances are "unfit" for parenthood.[10] To reduce stigma and alienation of individuals with SUD, OB-GYNs should incorporate person-centered language into their practice. Stigmatizing language directed at people who use substances perpetuates stereotypes and assigns blame. **Table 3** outlines some terminology denounced and endorsed by the American Society of Addiction Medicine (ASAM) and the National Institute on Drug Abuse.[35]

SCREENING

OB-GYNs should adhere to universal screening recommendations for SU to reduce underreporting and bias in prenatal care.[9,36] ACOG recommends screening preconception and at the first prenatal visit. Because patterns of SU oftentimes change postpartum, screening postpartum should be considered. There are multiple validated screening tools that have been shown to be effective, and none have been identified as superior[37] (**Table 4**). Clinicians should select the screening tools and distribution (ie, verbal, paper, electronic) that fits best into their practice. Before distribution of a validated SU screening tool, OB-GYNs should ask a patient for permission to screen for SU. If the patient declines, the obstetrician should respect their wishes. If a screening tool is positive, OB-GYNs should determine if SUD criteria are met.

ADDITIONAL TESTING AND CONSIDERATIONS

All individuals seeking prenatal care should be screened for IPV[38] and depression,[39] and OB-GYNs should consider incorporating screening for anxiety, bipolar disorder, and posttraumatic stress disorder (PTSD). Any identified mood disorders should be treated. Per Centers for Disease Control and Prevention (CDC) recommendations, all pregnant people should be screened for HIV, hepatitis B and C, and syphilis. Owing to high rates of gonorrhea, chlamydia, and trichomonas in people with SUD, all pregnant individuals with SU should be tested.[40] If individuals endorse return to use of substances, retesting for infectious diseases should be considered. Individuals with risky sexual behaviors, a recent STD, a partner with HIV, or intravenous (IV) drug use who share needles should be offered HIV preexposure prophylaxis.[41] Postpartum, individuals with hepatitis C should be referred for treatment. Because of criminalization and marginalization of SU/SUD, individuals may be incarcerated, marginally housed, or living in crowded environments that place them at risk for tuberculosis (TB); therefore, TB screening should be considered in at-risk individuals.[40]

HARM REDUCTION

Harm reduction is an important public health effort in addiction medicine. It focuses on the promotion of safe use rather than the goal of abstinence. Harm reduction recommendations should be tailored to each patient depending on type of substance

Table 2
Stigma types against individuals with substance use disorder and mental health conditions

Stigma Type	Definition	Examples
Self-stigma	The internalization of public stereotypes and self-discrimination	• Belief that an individual "caused her baby to be addicted" because of substance use
Labeling avoidance	Individuals decline to engage in services to avoid labels or stereotypes	• "If I tell them about my drug use, they'll think I'm a bad mother and an addict."
Courtesy stigma	Negative behaviors or perceptions directed to family, or others close to a person with a condition	• Family and friends are shamed for association with an individual (eg, family is "enabling" substance use by allowing them to stay in the home)
Public or interpersonal stigma	Negative behaviors or perceptions directed at a person with a condition	• Using stigmatizing language in clinical setting (eg, drug addict, crack baby, clean or dirty urine test results)
Systemic or structural stigma	Rules or institutional practices that intentionally or unintentionally disadvantage individuals with certain conditions	• Criminal statutes against pregnant individuals using substances • Policy statutes mandating reporting for substance use in pregnancy

From Corrigan, P. W. (Ed.). (2014). The stigma of disease and disability: Understanding causes and overcoming injustices. American Psychological Association. https://doi.org/10.1037/14297-000; with permission.

Table 3
Stigmatizing compared with preferred substance use related terminology

Instead of...	Use...
Addict, user, junkie, alcoholic, smoker, crackhead, meth-head, stoner, drunk	Person with substance use disorder
Substance abuse	Substance use or misuse, substance use disorder
Dirty urine	Positive urine toxicology/drug screen
Clean urine	Negative urine toxicology/drug screen
Clean, sober	Abstinent, no active use, no return to use, in recovery
Habit, drug of choice, fix, hit	Substance of use
Shoot up	Injection or IV drug use
Relapse	Return to use
Opioid replacement, opioid substitution	Medication for opioid use disorder, opioid agonist treatment
Addicted baby	Baby with neonatal withdrawal, baby who was exposed to substances, baby with signs of withdrawal
Getting high, stoned, tipsy, impaired	Using, being under the influence

and mode of use. One emerging area of harm reduction relates to fentanyl, a potent opioid with enormous public health concern. In 2019, fentanyl was identified in 51.5% of overdose deaths.[42] It is commonly used intentionally and found increasingly in the drug supply of any type of illicit drug, including stimulants, heroin, counterfeit opioids, sedative-hypnotics, and synthetic cannabinoids.[42] Because of the high risk of overdose with fentanyl, all individuals with any kind of SU should be given naloxone, a life-saving opioid antagonist used for rapid reversal of opioid overdose.

Table 4
Validated screening tools for substance use in pregnancy

Substance	Tool
Alcohol	*Universal nonjudgmental screening question*: "How much beer, wine, or other alcoholic beverages do you consume in an average week?" *Positive use*: Anyone who consumes alcohol should then be further screened with either the 3-question AUDIT-C or T-ACE (both validated in pregnancy)
Benzodiazepines Cannabis Opioids Stimulants	• 4P's Plus or 5 P's • National Institute on Drug Abuse Quick Screen followed by ASSIST (modified Alcohol, Smoking, and Substance Involvement Screening Test) • Substance Use Risk Profile-Pregnancy (SURP-P) • CRAFFT (for those 26 years and younger) • Wayne Indirect Drug Use Screener (WIDUS)
Tobacco/nicotine	• 5 A's—tailored approach

Adapted from Smid M, Terplan M. What Obstetrician–Gynecologists should know about substance use disorders in the perinatal period. Obstetrics & Gynecology. 2022;139(2):317-337. https://doi.org/10.1097/AOG.0000000000004657; with permission.

OB-GYNs should also assess for safe IV drug use and direct individuals to syringe exchange programs. These programs reduce needle reuse by more than half,[43] thereby decreasing morbidity, including infectious disease acquisition and wound complications from dulled needles.

URINARY TOXICOLOGY TESTING

Urine toxicology testing should never be used in lieu of screening and should never be completed without patient consent except in very rare circumstances (eg, the patient is sedated in the intensive care unit and results would potentially change clinical management). OB-GYNs should understand that there are no national guidelines for who should undergo urinary toxicology testing and under what circumstances, oftentimes leaving the clinical decision to the individual provider.[36] Because of the lack of standardized recommendations, the use of these immunoassay screening tests is often inappropriate and racially biased.[23] This is especially true of the rapid urine tests often done in triage or office settings.

OB-GYNs must appreciate that these "rapid" immunoassay screening tests have a high rate of misinterpretation[44] and a high rate of false negatives and positives.[45] An unexpected result must be followed by confirmatory testing with gas chromatography–mass spectrometry analysis. In some cases, positive screening tests can have immense consequences by triggering CPS surveillance.[46] These tests should be used thoughtfully—with patient consent—only if the results will alter safe management of the pregnant or postpartum individual and the newborn.

EVALUATION AND TREATMENT

After completion of a standardized screening questionnaire, OB-GYNs should determine if individuals meet criteria for SUD. If they do not meet criteria for SUD but still exhibit any SU or misuse of prescription drugs during pregnancy, OB-GYNs should proceed with brief intervention and referral and/or treatment. This is in line with the SBIRT model, a technique recommended by ACOG[36] and the Substance Abuse and Mental Health Service Administration (SAMHSA) that has been shown to decrease substance misuse.[47] SBIRT uses motivational interviewing to understand patient SU, develop insight, and build motivation to change. This technique can take as little as 5 minutes and is billable time. **Table 5** provides examples of this technique.

For individuals who require treatment or meet SUD criteria, treatment and/or referral should be offered immediately. Although SUD is common, addiction treatment can be difficult to locate, and access varies vastly depending on geographic location, insurance,[14] and race.[13] Furthermore, not all treatment programs or providers will accept pregnant individuals. OB-GYNs should be comfortable with basic SUD care until a warm handoff to an addiction specialist is arranged. OB-GYNs can reference **Box 1** to find providers who treat SUD.

Polysubstance use is "the rule" rather than the exception,[48] and OB-GYNs should aim to address all SUDs synchronously. For example, if a patient has alcohol use disorder (AUD) and OUD, they should be admitted to the hospital for supervised medical withdrawal from alcohol and started on medication for opioid use disorder (MOUD).

In the following sections, the authors provide a brief overview of the prevalence, maternal and neonatal risks, and treatment approaches for each commonly used substance class. They do not provide information about breastfeeding, as the American College of Pediatrics states that SU is not an absolute contraindication to breastfeeding.[49] However, if individuals have active illicit SU or risk of infectious disease, they

Table 5
Examples of brief intervention techniques

Brief Intervention	Technique	Examples of Questions and Dialogue
Understand the patient's use	Identify pros and cons of use	"What do you like and dislike about vaping?"
Give information about use	Review maternal, fetal, and neonatal risk of use; ask permission first	"Is it okay if I discuss some of the risks of alcohol use during pregnancy with you?"
Evaluate readiness to change and build insight	Readiness scale from 0 to 10 Interrogate degree of readiness and inquire why not lower number	"So after our discussion about the risks of cocaine use, how ready do you feel to change on a scale from 0-10? 10 would mean completely ready and 0 would mean not ready at all." "Why didn't you choose a lower number?"
Evaluate confidence to change and identify intrinsic motivation	Confidence from 0 to 10 Interrogate degree of confidence and inquire why not higher number	"So you said you are very ready to change. How confident are you that you can do this from 0-10?" "What might take you from a confidence of 5 to a 7?"
Advise and plan	Summarize shared objectives, recommend future direction, and create a plan	"Now that we've identified you feel ready and confident to completely stop using cannabis, I would recommend we work toward that goal. If, at our next appointment, you are not quite meeting the goal, I would recommend a referral to a specialist for more help."

Box 1
Resources for management and referral for substance use disorder treatment

- SAMHSA Treatment Locator: search by ZIP code to find inpatient and outpatient treatment providers (https://findtreatment.gov)

- National Clinical Consultation Center: free confidential clinician-to-clinician telephone or email consultation focusing on SUD management (Substance Use Warmline (855) 300-3595 from 9 AM to 8 PM ET Monday through Friday; https://nccc.ucsf.edu/clinician-consultation/substance-use-management/).

- Perinatal Quality Collaboratives: resources for community referrals (https://www.cdc.gov/reproductivehealth/maternalinfanthealth/pqc-states.html).

Adapted from Smid M, Terplan M. What Obstetrician–Gynecologists should know about substance use disorders in the perinatal period. Obstetrics & Gynecology. 2022;139(2):317-337. https://doi.org/10.1097/AOG.0000000000004657; with permission.

---

should not breastfeed until SUD is stabilized and infectious disease workup, specifically HIV, has been ruled out.[50]

ALCOHOL

Alcohol is the most commonly used substance in the United States.[1] Approximately 10% of Americans have AUD, and 10.6% of pregnant individuals reported last month use in 2020.[1] Although alcohol was identified as a teratogen in 1973, it remains the leading cause of preventable intellectual disability and birth defects in the United States today.[51] All pregnant individuals should be educated that there is no safe amount of alcohol consumption during pregnancy.[52]

Individuals with AUD should be assessed for safety, as complicated alcohol withdrawal can be fatal. The Clinical Institute Withdrawal Assessment of Alcohol Scale, Revised (CIWA-Ar) is a reliable risk calculator for the severity of alcohol withdrawal. ASAM recommends any pregnant patient with a CIWA-Ar score of ≥10 should be admitted to the hospital for medically supervised withdrawal on a psychiatric or medicine unit.[53] Medically supervised withdrawal includes vitamin supplementation to prevent Wernicke-Korsakoff syndrome and administration of benzodiazepine or phenobarbital taper to prevent complicated withdrawal.

After admission for supervised withdrawal, individuals should be referred for AUD treatment. Psychosocial interventions like Alcoholics Anonymous, inpatient and outpatient treatments, and individual therapy alone have high rates of return to use,[54] and so all pregnant individuals should be considered for medication treatment. The 3 Food and Drug Administration (FDA) -approved medications for AUD treatment are disulfiram, acamprosate, and naltrexone. Although AUD is pervasive, multiple studies have shown that less than 10% of individuals with AUD receive evidence-based treatment.[55] The rate is likely lower in pregnant individuals with AUD. There are no rigorous studies of medication treatment for AUD in pregnancy,[56] but the risks of ongoing AUD outweigh the fetal harms of these medications.[57]

BENZODIAZEPINES

Benzodiazepines are a commonly prescribed class of medication. Because of lack of information regarding best clinical practice, benzodiazepines are often overprescribed with potentially little consideration of their addictive and dangerous potential.[58] Women are twice as likely to be prescribed benzodiazepines than men,[59] and worldwide, 1% to 3% of pregnant individuals were found to have a benzodiazepine prescription.[60] When combined with opioids and/or alcohol, benzodiazepine use can be lethal, and they are often implicated in intentional and unintentional drug overdoses.[59]

SBIRT should be used to universally screen and counsel any individuals with benzodiazepine prescription misuse or benzodiazepine use disorder about risks. Individuals should be made aware that benzodiazepines are not teratogenic, but that neonates can exhibit neonatal withdrawal symptoms.

Individuals taking benzodiazepines should be evaluated for withdrawal symptoms because benzodiazepine withdrawal can be fatal. Those at risk for complicated withdrawal should be admitted for inpatient benzodiazepine or phenobarbital taper. Generally, most individuals should undergo a prolonged outpatient taper. There are no recommended pharmacotherapies for benzodiazepine use disorder after completely tapering off of them; however, stabilizing frequently co-occurring anxiety disorders is paramount. Cognitive behavioral therapy is the foundation of long-term treatment.[59]

CANNABIS

Cannabis use is common, with 18% of Americans reportedly using in the last 12 months.[1] Legalization of cannabis for medical and/or recreational purposes is a rapidly changing political issue. It is currently approved for medical use in 37 states.[61] There are many advertised uses of medical marijuana, and few of these have been extensively investigated. Some of these include the following: chronic pain, anxiety disorders, irritable bowel syndrome, and PTSD.[62] One 2018 study showed that nearly 70% of surveyed cannabis dispensaries in Colorado recommended cannabis products for nausea and vomiting of pregnancy,[63] although this indication has not been supported. In pregnancy, 8% of individuals report last month use[1] for perceived medicinal or recreational purposes. OB-GYNs should discourage any marijuana use and offer alternative, medically proven treatments with better pregnancy-specific safety data. Effects of marijuana on the developing fetus are difficult to study owing to confounders; however, multiple studies point toward lasting neurocognitive effects.[64] There is no known safe amount of cannabis use during pregnancy.[64] About 10% of individuals who use cannabis will develop a cannabis use disorder,[1] for which there are no FDA-approved medications. Clinical trials support the use of psychotherapy techniques[65] in nonpregnant people, although data for pregnant and lactating individuals are limited.

OPIOIDS

A total of 3.4% of people report misuse of opioids in 2020, with an estimated 1% of the US population having OUD.[1] Between 2010 and 2017, opioid-related diagnoses at delivery increased 131%.[66] Individuals should be made aware that prenatal exposure of illicit or prescription opioids or buprenorphine and methadone has not been strongly associated with birth defects.[67,68] Illicit opioid use during pregnancy, which is indicative of an untreated or undertreated OUD, is associated with fetal growth restriction, preterm labor, and stillbirth.[68] Historically, maternal opioid withdrawal was thought to be associated with harm to the fetus, but recent studies have not supported the link between opioid withdrawal and stillbirth.[69]

OB-GYNs should be comfortable discussing NOWS with individuals. NOWS is diagnosed in 30% to 80% of neonates with fetal opioid exposure and is influenced by various factors (see https://www.vumc.org/childhealthpolicy/nasrisk for more details).[70] NOWS is diagnosed based on symptoms such as neonatal irritability, high-pitched cry, sleep disturbance, and feeding difficulties. Initial management involves breastfeeding, skin to skin, low stimulation environment, and rooming-in. These interventions decrease the severity of symptoms and duration of neonatal admission.[71] Severe symptoms are managed with neonatal opioid taper.

OB-GYNs should be familiar with MOUD. **Table 6** provides more details. MOUD are life-saving medications that should be offered to everyone with OUD. Use of MOUD in pregnancy reduces the risk of return to use, overdose, hospital admissions, and obstetric and infectious complications.[68] It also improves engagement in prenatal care[68] and continued MOUD use in subsequent pregnancies with a reduction in illicit SU.[72]

Unfortunately, there are still significant barriers to the access of MOUD. Previously, to prescribe buprenorphine, a Drug Enforcement Administration (DEA) X-waiver was required. The X-waiver may have created substantial obstacles for pregnant people to access MOUD, as a study showed that less than 2% of nationally surveyed OB-GYNs in 2019 had an X-waiver.[73] However, in January 2023, the federal government took meaningful steps to improving OUD treatment access by removing the X-waiver requirement. Now, barring state laws, any provider with an active DEA license may prescribe buprenorphine to an unlimited number of patients.

OB-GYNs should be knowledgeable about recognizing and treating opioid withdrawal. Withdrawal is characterized by flulike symptoms and can start within hours of recent use and last for weeks. Opioid withdrawal is generally not fatal, but it is extraordinarily uncomfortable for individuals. The Clinical Opioid Withdrawal Scale should be used to determine severity of withdrawal. Any individual admitted to the hospital in withdrawal should be treated with MOUD to control symptoms. Medically supervised withdrawal and "detoxification" from opioids without transition to MOUD is not recommended during pregnancy, as it does not improve maternal or newborn outcomes.[74] Hospitalization offers an important opportunity for treatment initiation, and individuals with untreated withdrawal symptoms are at high risk for leaving against medical advice.[75]

STIMULANTS

In 2020, 1% to 2% of the general population reported stimulant use within the last year.[1] One study found less than 1% of individuals had stimulant use disorder during delivery.[48] There are no known teratogenic or neurodevelopmental effects of prenatal cocaine or methamphetamine exposure.[76] Some studies suggest fetuses exposed to stimulants are at risk for growth restriction and preterm delivery,[77] so fetal growth scans are reasonable.

OB-GYNs should be aware of maternal risks of stimulant use, including hypertensive emergency, cardiac dysfunction, and placental abruption. Individuals with chronic cocaine or methamphetamine use should have a comprehensive cardiac workup to rule out cardiomyopathy or arrythmia.[78] Beta-blockers for treatment of cocaine-induced hypertension are contraindicated. Hydralazine is the recommended alternative.[79]

There are no FDA-approved treatments for cocaine or methamphetamine use disorder, although there are multiple studies investigating use of prescription stimulants, topiramate, naltrexone, and bupropion. Psychotherapy, especially contingency management, is the cornerstone of treatment.[79]

TOBACCO AND NICOTINE-CONTAINING PRODUCTS

In 2020, 8% of pregnant individuals used tobacco products within the last month.[1] Although, nationally, cigarette smoking is declining, use of electronic nicotine delivery

Table 6
Food and Drug Administration–approved medications for the treatment of opioid use disorder

Medication	Mechanism	Dose	Special Considerations	Pregnancy Considerations
Methadone	Full opioid agonist	Generally 10–30 mg/d initially Slow titration within first 2 wk (usually 5–10 mg every few days) due to long half-life	Must be dispensed by federally licensed opioid treatment program; do not initiate if no local resource available Risk of QT prolongation Significant drug interactions due to cytochrome P450 metabolism	Split dosing in pregnancy associated with decrease in maternal withdrawal symptoms Restricting dose in an attempt to decrease NOWS is discouraged
Buprenorphine	Partial opioid agonist	Classical initiation uses 2–4 mg sublingual testing dose after onset of withdrawal symptoms Give additional 2- to 4-mg dose for continued withdrawal and no sedation Multiple initiation protocols exist	Any provider with an active DEA may prescribe Risk of precipitated withdrawal in individuals using fentanyl	Symptoms may be improved with bid or tid dosing in pregnancy This medication should not be discontinued during delivery, regardless of delivery mode Both monoproduct and combination product (buprenorphine/naloxone) are safe
Naltrexone	Competitive opioid receptor antagonist	Consider trial of oral naltrexone or naloxone before initiation of 380-mg injection of extended release naltrexone	Will precipitate withdrawal if administered within 7–14 d of opioid use Oral medication not recommended and associated with poor retention and increased risk of continued use and overdose	Limited data on maternal, fetal, and child outcomes

Adapted from Smid M, Terplan M. What Obstetrician–Gynecologists should know about substance use disorders in the perinatal period. Obstetrics & Gynecology. 2022;139(2):317-337. https://doi.org/10.1097/AOG.0000000000004657; with permission.

systems (ENDS) like vape pens and vaporizers is on the rise, even in the pregnant population.[80] ENDS are oftentimes perceived as more safe in pregnancy than cigarettes[81]; however, this is a misconception. ENDS oftentimes contain high nicotine concentrations along with other harmful chemicals (particularly vitamin E acetate) that have been linked to a serious respiratory illness known as vaping-associated lung injury.[82] The effects of nicotine-containing ENDS on pregnancy are similar to those of tobacco.[83] All nicotine and tobacco-containing products pose a threat not only to maternal health but also to fetal and newborn health. Nicotine is associated with a dramatic increase in risk of miscarriage, low birth weight, preterm delivery, placental abruption, placenta previa, and stillbirth.[83] After delivery, the infant is at increased risk for sudden infant death syndrome, colic, obesity, bone fractures, pulmonary and ear infections, asthma, and possibly decreased cognitive-behavioral function.[83]

Nearly half of pregnant individuals who smoke completely stop by the end of pregnancy,[84] although there is a high rate of return to use postpartum.[85] The SBIRT model, when applied to pregnant and postpartum individuals who smoke, can effectively reduce tobacco use.[86] Individuals should be referred to ongoing behavioral interventions to help achieve abstinence. The various behavioral interventions for tobacco and nicotine cessation include the following: motivational interviewing, cognitive behavioral therapy, mindfulness, contingency management, call or cell phone application–based quit lines, and many more.

Current FDA-approved medications for tobacco cessation are nicotine replacement therapies (NRT), bupropion, and varenicline. Small studies suggest NRT in pregnancy is safe and effective, and the general consensus is that it is safer than smoking in pregnancy.[87] There are few data about the use of bupropion and varenicline in pregnant individuals. Given the lack of data, the United States Preventive Services Task Force (USPSTF) recommends use of shared decision making when recommending bupropion or varenicline.[87]

SUMMARY

SU is common in pregnancy and postpartum and will be regularly encountered in an OB-GYN office. Familiarity with SBIRT and the basics of initiating treatment while awaiting a referral to an addiction specialist is crucial for all OB-GYNs. Pregnant individuals with SUD require considerate and comprehensive care owing to the high rate of comorbid socioeconomic difficulties, IPV, mood disorders, infectious diseases, and polysubstance use. Further complicating their care, individuals are confronted by stigma, unequitable CPS surveillance, punitive reporting policies, provider inexperience with best management, lack of evidence-based treatments in pregnancy, and difficulty accessing addiction services. Improving the outcomes for these individuals and their families requires a multidisciplinary, patient-centered approach led by the OB-GYN.

CLINICS CARE POINTS

- As there is a high rate of illicit drug contamination with fentanyl, individuals with any substance use should be offered a prescription for naloxone.
- Individuals at risk for complicated withdrawal from alcohol or benzodiazepines must be admitted to the hospital.
- Individuals using stimulants such as cocaine and methamphetamine are at risk for hypertensive emergencies, cardiac dysfunction, and placental abruption.

- Medication for opiate use disorder is the standard of care for OUD.
- OB-GYNs should counsel patients about risks of tobacco use and consider pharmacotherapy.

DISCLOSURES

M.C. Smid serves as a medical consultant for Gilead Science Inc for hepatitis C treatment in pregnancy and RH Capital. M.C. Smid's institution receives research funding from Gilead Science Inc and Alydia/Organon. M.C. Smid receives research funding from NIH, United States, NIDA, United States, and CDC, United States.

CONFLICTS OF INTEREST

None.

REFERENCES

1. 2020 National Survey on Drug Use and Health: Detailed Tables. Substance Abuse and Mental Health Services Administration. Available at: https://www.samhsa.gov/data/release/2020-national-survey-drug-use-and-health-nsduh-releases. Accessed November 14, 2022.
2. Vesga-López O, Blanco C, Keyes K, et al. Psychiatric disorders in pregnant and postpartum women in the United States. Arch Gen Psychiatry 2008;65(7):805–15.
3. Kotelchuck M, Cheng E, Belanoff C, et al. The prevalence and impact of substance use disorder and treatment on maternal obstetric experiences and birth outcomes among singleton deliveries in Massachusetts. Matern Child Health J 2017;21(4):893–902.
4. Trost SL, Beauregard JL, Smoots AN, et al. Preventing Pregnancy-Related Mental Health Deaths: Insights From 14 US Maternal Mortality Review Committees, 2008-17. Health Aff 2021;40(10):1551–9.
5. Pregnancy-related deaths: data from maternal mortality review committees in 36 US states, 2017-2019. Centers for Disease Control. 2022. Available at: https://www.cdc.gov/reproductivehealth/maternal-mortality/docs/pdf/Pregnancy-Related-Deaths-Data-MMRCs-2017-2019-H.pdf. Accessed January 15, 2023.
6. Educational objectives: core curriculum in obstetrics and gynecology, 12th ed. Council on Resident Education in Obstetrics and Gynecology. 2020. Available at: https://www.acog.org/-/media/project/acog/acogorg/files/creog/creog-educational-objectives-12th-edition-secured.pdf. Accessed November 16, 2022.
7. Appendix B: specialty certifying examination topics. 2021. Available at: https://www.abog.org/docs/default-source/bulletins/2021/2021-ce-exam-topics.pdf. Accessed November 16, 2022.
8. Isaacson JH, Fleming M, Kraus M, et al. A national survey of training in substance use disorders in residency programs. J Stud Alcohol 2015;61(6):912–5.
9. Ko J, Tong V, Haight S, et al. Obstetrician-gynecologists' practices and attitudes on substance use screening during pregnancy. J Perinatol 2020;40(3):422–32.
10. Weber A, Miskle B, Lynch A, et al. Substance Use in Pregnancy: Identifying Stigma and Improving Care. Subst Abuse Rehabil 2021;12:105–21.
11. Frazer Z, McConnell K, Jansson L. Treatment for substance use disorders in pregnant women: Motivators and barriers. Drug Alchol Depend 2019;2015:107652.
12. Terplan M, McNamara E, Chisolm M. Pregnant and non-pregnant women with substance use disorders: the gap between treatment need and receipt. J Addict Dis 2012;31(4):342–9.

13. Martin C, Scialli A, Terplan M. Unmet substance use disorder treatment need among reproductive age women. Drug Alcohol Depend 2020;206:107679.
14. Patrick S, Richards M, Dupont W, et al. Association of Pregnancy and Insurance Status With Treatment Access for Opioid Use Disorder. JAMA Netw Open 2020; 3(8):e2013456.
15. Substance Use During Pregnancy: State Laws and Policies. Guttmacher Institute. 2022. Available at: https://www.guttmacher.org/state-policy/explore/substance-use-during-pregnancy. Accessed December 28, 2022.
16. Faherty LJ, Kranz AM, Russell-Fritch J, et al. Association of Punitive and Reporting State Policies Related to Substance Use in Pregnancy With Rates of Neonatal Abstinence Syndrome. JAMA Netw Open 2019;2(11):e1914078.
17. Austin A, Naumann R, Simmons E. Association of state child abuse policies and mandated reporting policies with prenatal and postpartum care among women who engaged in substance use during pregnancy. JAMA Pediatr 2022;1123–30.
18. Schiff DM, Nielsen T, Terplan M, et al. Fatal and Nonfatal Overdose Among Pregnant and Postpartum Women in Massachusetts. Obstet Gynecol 2018.
19. Smid MC, Maeda J, Stone NM, et al. Standardized Criteria for Review of Perinatal Suicides and Accidental Drug-Related Deaths. Obstet Gynecol 2020;136(4): 645–53.
20. Roberts D. Shattered bonds: the color of child welfare. New York: Civitas Books; 2002.
21. Edmonds BT. Mandated Reporting of Perinatal Substance Use: The Root of Inequity. JAMA Pediatr 2022;176(11):1073–5.
22. Patel E, Bandara S, Saloner B, et al. Heterogeneity in prenatal substance use screening despite universal screening recommendations: findings from the Pregnancy Risk Assessment Monitoring System, 2016-2018. Am J Obstet Gynecol MFM 2021;3(5):100419.
23. Perlman NC, Cantonwine DE, Smith NA. Racial differences in indications for obstetric toxicology testing, and relationship of indications to test results. Am J Obstet Gynecol MFM 2021;4(1):100453.
24. Rubin A, Zhong L, Nacke L, et al. Urine Drug Screening for Isolated Marijuana Use in Labor and Delivery Units. Obstet Gynecol 2022;140(4):607–9.
25. Substance Abuse and Mental Health Services Administration. Racial/Ethnic Differences in Substance Use, Substance Use Disorders, and Substance Use Treatment Utilization among People Aged 12 or Older (2015-2019). Substance Abuse and Mental Health Services Administration. Available at: https://www.samhsa. gov/data/sites/default/files/reports/rpt35326/2021NSDUHSUChartbook102221B. pdf. Accessed November 5, 2022.
26. Substance Abuse Reporting and Pregnancy: The Role of the Obstetrician–Gynecologist. ACOG Committee Opinion No. 473. American College of Obstetricians and Gynecologists. Obstet Gynecol 2011;117(1):200–1. Reaffirmed 2014.
27. Medications for opioid use disorder: for healthcare and addiction professionals, policymakers, patients, and families. Substance Abuse and Mental Health Services Administration. Department of Health and Human Services. Available at: https://store.samhsa.gov/sites/default/files/SAMHSA_Digital_Download/PEP21-02-01-002.pdf. Accessed December 18, 2022.
28. McLellan A, Lewis D, O'Brien C, et al. Drug Dependence, a Chronic Medical Illness: Implications for Treatment, Insurance, and Outcomes Evaluation. JAMA 2000;284(13):1689–95.
29. Comorbidity: substance use and other mental disorders. National Institute on Drug Abuse. 2018. Available at: https://nida.nih.gov/research-topics/trends-statistics/info

graphics/comorbidity-substance-use-other-mental-disorders. Accessed December 13, 2022.

30. Gibbs A, Jewkes R, Willan S, et al. Associations between poverty, mental health and substance use, gender power, and intimate partner violence amongst young (18-30) women and men in urban informal settlements in South Africa: A cross-sectional study and structural equation model. PLoS One 2018;13(10):e0204956.

31. Chandler GE, Kalmakis KA, Murtha T. Screening Adults With Substance Use Disorder for Adverse Childhood Experiences. J Addict Nurs 2018;29(3):172–8.

32. Jones CM, McCance-Katz EF. Co-occurring substance use and mental disorders among adults with opioid use disorder. Drug Alcohol Depend 2019;197:78–82.

33. Clinical guidance for treating pregnant and parenting women with opioid use disorder and their infant. Substance Abuse and Mental Health Services Administration. 2018. Available at: https://store.samhsa.gov/sites/default/files/d7/priv/sma18-5054.pdf. Accessed November 5, 2022.

34. Laudet A. Rate and Predictors of Employment among Formerly Polysubstance Dependent Urban Individuals in Recovery. J Addict Dis 2012;31(3):288–302.

35. Words matter: terms to use and avoid when talking about addiction. National Institute on Drug Abuse. Available at: https://www.asam.org/docs/default-source/default-document-library/nidamed_wordsmatter3_508.pdf?sfvrsn=5cf550c2_2. Accessed November 5, 2022.

36. Ecker J, Abuhamad A, Hill W, et al. Substance use disorders in pregnancy: clinical, ethical, and research imperatives of the opioid epidemic: a report of a joint workshop of the Society for Maternal-Fetal Medicine, American College of Obstetricians and Gynecologists, and American Society of Addiction Medicine. Am J Obstet Gynecol 2019;221(1):B5–28.

37. Ondersma SJ, Chang G, Blake-Lamb T, et al. Accuracy of five self-report screening instruments for substance use in pregnancy. Addiction 2019;114(9):1683–93.

38. Intimate Partner Violence Screening. Agency for Healthcare Research and Quality. 2015. Available at: https://www.ahrq.gov/ncepcr/tools/healthier-pregnancy/fact-sheets/partner-violence.html. Accessed November 6, 2022.

39. ACOG Committee Opinion No. 757: Screening for Perinatal Depression. Obstet Gynecol 2018;132(5):e208–12.

40. Pregnancy and HIV, Viral Hepatitis, STD & TB Prevention. Centers for Disease Control and Prevention. 2022. Available at: https://www.cdc.gov/nchhstp/pregnancy/screening/index.html. Accessed November 6, 2022.

41. Pre-Exposure Prophylaxis (PrEP). Centers for Disease Control and Prevention. 2022. Available at: https://www.cdc.gov/hiv/clinicians/prevention/prep.html. Accessed November 6, 2022.

42. Mattson C, Tanz L, Quinn K, et al. Trends and Geographic Patterns in Drug and Synthetic Opioid Overdose Deaths — United States, 2013–2019. MMWR Morb Mortal Wkly Rep 2021;70(5):202–7.

43. Marotta PL, Stringer K, Beletsky L, et al. Assessing the relationship between syringe exchange, pharmacy, and street sources of accessing syringes and injection drug use behavior in a pooled nationally representative sample of people who inject drugs in the United States from 2002 to 2019. Harm Reduct J 2021;18:115.

44. Reisfield GM, Bertholf R, Barkin RL, et al. Urine drug test interpretation: what do physicians know? J Opioid Manag 2007;3(2):80–6.

45. Moeller KE, Kissack JC, Atayee RS, et al. Clinical interpretation of urine drug tests: what clinicians need to know about urine drug screens. Mayo Clin Proc 2017;92(5):774–96.
46. Branigin A. A false positive on a drug test upended these mothers' lives. Washington Post. 7/2/22. Available at: https://www.washingtonpost.com/lifestyle/2022/07/02/false-positive-drug-test-mothers/. Accessed November 13, 2022.
47. Screening, Brief Intervention and Referral to Treatment (SBIRT) in Behavioral Healthcare.Substance Abuse and Mental Health Services Administration. 2011. Available at: https://www.samhsa.gov/sites/default/files/sbirtwhitepaper_0.pdf. Accessed November 13, 2022.
48. Jarlenski M, Krans EE. Co-occurring Substance Use Disorders Identified Among Delivery Hospitalizations in the United States. J Addict Med 2021;15(6):504–7.
49. American Academy of Pediatrics. Breastfeeding and the use of human milk. Pediatrics 2012;129(3):e827–41.
50. Sachs H, DRUGS CO, Frattarelli D, et al. The Transfer of Drugs and Therapeutics Into Human Breast Milk: An Update on Selected Topics. Pediatrics 2013;132(3):e796–809.
51. Williams J, Smith V, Abuse TCoS. Fetal Alcohol Spectrum Disorders. Pediatrics 2015;136(5):e20153113.
52. Alcohol and public health. Frequently Asked Questions. Centers for Disease Control. 2022. Available at: https://www.cdc.gov/alcohol/faqs.htm. Accessed December 13, 2022.
53. The ASAM clinical practice guideline on alcohol withdrawal management. American Society of Addiction Medicine. 2020. Available at: https://www.asam.org/docs/default-source/quality-science/the_asam_clinical_practice_guideline_on_alcohol-1.pdf?sfvrsn=ba255c2_2. Accessed November 16, 2022.
54. Anton RF, O'Malley SS, Ciraulo DA, et al. Combined pharmacotherapies and behavioral interventions for alcohol dependence: the COMBINE study: a randomized controlled trial. JAMA 2006;295(17):2003–17.
55. Kranzler H, Soyka M. Diagnosis and pharmacotherapy of alcohol use disorder. JAMA 2018;320(8):815–24.
56. Smith E, Lui S, Terplan M. Pharmacologic interventions for pregnant women enrolled in alcohol treatment. Cochrane Database Syst Rev 2009;2009(3):Cd007361.
57. DeVido J, Bogunovic O, Weiss RD. Alcohol use disorders in pregnancy. Harv Rev Psychiatr 2015;23(2):112–21.
58. Cuevas Cdl, Sanz E, Jdl Fuente. Benzodiazepines: more "behavioural" addiction than dependence. Psychopharmacology (Berl) 2003;167(3):297–303.
59. Soyka M. Treatment of Benzodiazepine Dependence. N Engl J Med 2017;376(12):1147–57.
60. Bais B, Molenaar NM, Bijma HH, et al. Prevalence of benzodiazepines and benzodiazepine-related drugs exposure before, during and after pregnancy: A systematic review and meta-analysis. J Affect Disord 2020;269:18–27.
61. State medical cannabis laws. National Conference of State Legislatures. 2022. Available at: https://www.ncsl.org/research/health/state-medical-marijuana-laws.aspx. Accessed November 14, 2022.
62. Cannabis (Marijuana) and Cannabinoids: What you need to know. US Department of Health and Human Services National Center for Complementary Integrative Health. 2023. Available at: https://www.nccih.nih.gov/health/cannabis-marijuana-and-cannabinoids-what-you-need-to-know. Accessed January 16. 2023.

63. Dickson B, Mansfield C, Guiahi M, et al. Recommendations From Cannabis Dispensaries About First-Trimester Cannabis Use. *Obstet Gynecol.* Jun 2018;131(6): 1031–8.
64. Marijuana use during pregnancy and lactation. Committee Opinion No. 722. American College of Obstetricians and Gynecologists. Obstet Gynecol 2017; 130(4):e205–9.
65. Sherman B, McRae-Clark A. Treatment of Cannabis Use Disorder: Current Science and Future Outlook. Pharmacotherapy 2016;36(5):511–35.
66. Hirai AH, Ko JY, Owens PL, et al. Neonatal Abstinence Syndrome and Maternal Opioid-Related Diagnoses in the US, 2010-2017. JAMA 2021;325(2):146–55.
67. Zedler BK, Mann AL, Kim MM, et al. Buprenorphine compared with methadone to treat pregnant women with opioid use disorder: a systematic review and meta-analysis of safety in the mother, fetus and child. Addiction 2016;111(12):2115–28.
68. Opioid use and opioid use disorder in pregnancy. Committee Opinion No. 711. American College of Obstetrics and Gynecology. Obstet Gynecol 2017;130: 81–94.
69. Bell J, Towers CV, Hennessy MD, et al. Detoxification from opiate drugs during pregnancy. Am J Obstet Gynecol 2016;215(3):374.e1–6.
70. Patrick SW, Slaughter JC, Harrell FE Jr, et al. Development and Validation of a Model to Predict Neonatal Abstinence Syndrome. J Pediatr 2021;229:154–60.
71. Wachman EM, Schiff DM, Silverstein M. Neonatal abstinence syndrome: advances in diagnosis and treatment. JAMA 2018;319(13):1362–74.
72. Mason I, Mashburn S, Cleary E, et al. Outcomes in subsequent pregnancies of individuals with opioid use disorder treated in multidisciplinary clinic in prior pregnancy. J Addiction Med 2022;16(4):420–4.
73. Tiako MJN, Culhane J, South E, et al. Prevalence and Geographic Distribution of Obstetrician-Gynecologists Who Treat Medicaid Enrollees and Are Trained to Prescribe Buprenorphine. JAMA Netw Open 2020;3(12):e3039043.
74. Terplan M, Laird HJ, Hand DJ, et al. Opioid Detoxification During Pregnancy: A Systematic Review. Obstet Gynecol 2018;131(5):803–14.
75. Nolan NS, Marks LR, Liang SY, et al. Medications for Opioid use Disorder Associated With Less Against Medical Advice Discharge Among Persons Who Inject Drugs Hospitalized With an Invasive Infection. J Addict Med 2021;15(2):155–8.
76. Chavkin W. Cocaine and pregnancy—time to look at the evidence. JAMA 2001; 285(12):1626–8.
77. Eriksson M, Jonsson B, Steneroth G, et al. Cross-sectional growth of children whose mothers abused amphetamines during pregnancy. Acta paediatrica (Oslo, Norway : 1992) 1994;83(6):612–7.
78. Afonso L, Mohammad T, Thatai D. Crack whips the heart: a review of the cardiovascular toxicity of cocaine. Am J Cardiol 2007;100(6):1040–3.
79. Smid M, Metz T, Gordon A. Stimulant use in pregnancy — an under-recognized epidemic among pregnant women. Clin Obstet Gynecol 2019;62(1):168–82.
80. Kurti AN, Redner R, Lopez AA, et al. Tobacco and nicotine delivery product use in a national sample of pregnant women. Prev Med 2017;104:50–6.
81. Breland A, McCubbin A, Ashford K. Electronic nicotine delivery systems and pregnancy: Recent research on perceptions, cessation, and toxicant delivery. Birth Defects Res 2019;111(17):1284–93.
82. Layden JE, Ghinai I, Pray I, et al. Pulmonary Illness Related to E-Cigarette Use in Illinois and Wisconsin — Final Report. N Engl J Med 2019;382(10):903–16.

83. American College of Obstetricians and Gynecologists. Committee Opinion, Number 807: Tobacco and Nicotine Cessation During Pregnancy. Obstet Gynecol 2020;135(5):e221–9.
84. Tong VTJJ, Dietz PM, D'Angelo D, et al. Trends in smoking before, during, and after pregnancy—Pregnancy Risk Assessment Monitoring System (PRAMS), United States, 31 sites, 2000–2005. Morb Mortal Wkly Rep - Surveillance Summ 2009;58(4):1–31.
85. Rockhill K, Tong V, Farr S, et al. Postpartum smoking relapse after quitting during pregnancy: Pregnancy Risk Assessment Monitoring System, 2000–2011. J Wom Health 2016;25(5):480–8.
86. Lumley J, Chamberlain C, Dowswell T, et al. Interventions for promoting smoking cessation during pregnancy. Cochrane Database Syst Rev 2009;(3):Cd001055.
87. US Preventative Task Force Recommendation Statement. Interventions for tobacco smoking cessation in adults, including pregnant persons. JAMA 2021; 325(3):265–79.
88. American Psychiatric Association. Diagnostic and statistical manual of mental disorders (DSM-5®). Arlington, VA: American Psychiatric Pub; 2013.
89. SAMHSA's Working Definition of recovery. Substance Abuse Mental Health Services Administration. Rockville, MD. Updated July 5th, 2021. Available at: https://store.samhsa.gov/sites/default/files/d7/priv/pep12-recdef.pdf. Accessed November 16, 2022.

Screening for Social Determinants of Health During Prenatal Care
Why, What, and How

Sharon T. Phelan, MD*

KEYWORDS

- Prenatal screening • Social determinants of health • Implementing screening tools

KEY POINTS

- The foundation of comprehensive prenatal care is screening patients for their risk of having or developing conditions that will negatively impact the patient or pregnancy.
- Social determinants of health (SDOH) are acknowledged as a significant force in pregnancy outcomes.
- Implementing screening for SDOH requires decisions around what tools will be used, how to incorporate into clinical processes, and how to respond to a positive screen.

INTRODUCTION AND BACKGROUND

Standard prenatal care has expanded greatly from the original approach of focusing on fetal growth and maternal well-being. Over the past 50-plus years an increasing number of tests were developed that look at the risks of fetal anomalies, maternal pre-existing conditions (eg, diabetes, cancer screening, obesity), infectious risks (sexually transmitted infections, rubella, group B streptococcus), and the development of clinical pathology during the course of a pregnancy (gestational diabetes mellitus, abnormal fetal growth). Over the past three decades, there has been a rapid increase in the medical testing availability (eg, three-dimensional ultrasound, noninvasive genetic testing of the fetus, carrier testing for the birth parents). These are quickly incorporated into the structure of standard prenatal care.

Despite the increased medical surveillance of and intervention during a pregnancy, the maternal mortality rate in the United States continues to increase.[1] In 2017 the Centers for Disease Control and Prevention (CDC) launched a new system for recording deidentified comprehensive data. This program, the Maternal Mortality

University of New Mexico
* 601 Park Lake Circle, Helena, AL 35080.
E-mail address: Stphelan@salud.unm.edu

Obstet Gynecol Clin N Am 50 (2023) 629–638
https://doi.org/10.1016/j.ogc.2023.03.011
0889-8545/23/© 2023 Elsevier Inc. All rights reserved.

obgyn.theclinics.com

Review Information Application (MMRIA), facilitates the consistent recording of detailed deidentified data from each death reviewed by the states' Maternal Mortality Committees. This in turn has provided extensive comparable data on maternal deaths from across the nation including cause of death, preexisting conditions, timing of death relative to the pregnancy, and locations of residence versus site of death. Findings yielded the following data:

- 21.6% of maternal pregnancy-related deaths occurred during the pregnancy with another 13.3% occurring on the day of delivery.[2]
- Mental health disorders (including suicides and overdoses from substance use disorder) are the underlying cause of more than 20% of all pregnancy-related deaths.[2]
- Living in a rural setting increased the risk of maternal death almost two-fold when compared with living in an urban area.[3,4]

The data made it clear that there were social determinants of health (SDOH) that greatly affect pregnancies and their outcome. In fact, many believe that the challenge of addressing SDOH is one of the most important issues in reproductive health.[5] The Joint Commission's Division of Healthcare Improvement published a Sentinel Event Alert stressing the need to eliminate disparities in care.[6] It has been found that all-cause mortality rates for recently pregnant women increased 4.4% annually from 2015 to 2019, mostly attributable to causes other than pregnancy-specific complications including drug and alcohol poisoning.[7] As national organizations begin to emphasize the importance of screening for SDOH, primary care settings are looking to improve their screening approaches.[5,8] Because of this greater interest in acknowledging SDOH within the primary care setting more screening tools and interventions have been and continue to be developed and tested.

With the help of the US Preventive Services Task Force (USPSTF) there is a greater understanding of the importance of screening for SDOH.[9] By 2019 the USPSTF reviewed only two screening recommendations specifically for SDOH (eg, screening for intimate partner violence [IPV] and for child maltreatment).[9] The USPSTF undertook a review of their 85 currently active recommendations in 2021. That review found that 57 of the 85 identified screening recommendations included social determinants as part of the risk assessment even though the screening tools were not specifically directed at an SDOH.[10]

PRINCIPLES BEHIND IMPLEMENTING SCREENING PROGRAMS

Screening is the evaluation of a patient for a disease or adverse social situation before it becomes clinically evident. The key to treatment is often early diagnosis and management to decrease maternal morbidity and mortality. Screening is done when there is no history or physical findings for a problem in need of an intervention (**Box 1**).[11]

Box 1
Components of screening tests or tools

- To detect potential disease indicators that may merit more diagnostic testing
- Designed to be used in a large number of asymptomatic individuals
- Simple and acceptable to staff and patient
- Generally desires a high sensitivity to not miss a potential disease
- Inexpensive

USPSTF states that before routine screening for SDOH can be recommended there needs to be:[9]

1. An accurate screening test to identify patients with SDOH
2. Effective treatment to address the need, once identified
3. Evidence demonstrating a meaningful health outcome improvement

Currently, most of the more "accurate" general screening questionnaires for SDOH developed are lengthy and detailed.[12] This makes using them too time consuming for most medical practices. There are efforts to see if the most comprehensive tools can be pared down to more manageable options while still having acceptable accuracy.

However, effective screenings mean little if there are no existing meaningful interventions. SDOH is complex, requiring interventions outside of the traditional office setting. There are few feasible interventions for a provider that make a difference for many of the acknowledged SDOH. This concern raises the question as to whether it is ethical to screen for an issue if there is no intervention or treatment available. There are studies ongoing that will address this last concern.[13] Preliminary reports indicate that in most cases patients are still pleased that their SDOH issues are identified. The fact that the only "interventions" are acknowledgment and emotional support is acceptable to many patients. One significant patient concern with screening for some SDOH, such as substance use disorder or domestic violence, is confidentiality. Patients might fear that a positive screen could result in loss of custody of their children or loss of employment, depending on local laws and regulations.

The previously mentioned criteria become more problematic for SDOH screening in obstetrics. General SDOH screening questionnaires are created and validated in nonpregnant populations, not those that are pregnant. Thus one cannot be certain as to how the tool will perform when used with pregnant populations. Some questionnaires have been validated for pregnancy that screen for depression, alcohol abuse, and tobacco/nicotine use. The recent awareness of the impact of SDOH on pregnancy outcome has come to the forefront based on the MMRIA data from the CDC. These findings have resulted in recommendations from numerous agencies and national organizations to screen more broadly for SDOH as part of basic health care, including prenatal care. The validated screening tools for pregnancy primarily concentrate on single issues, such as alcohol or tobacco use. Nevertheless, there is reason to believe that the general screening surveys should work well for the pregnant population. Some of the screening tools even include effective recommended office management approaches, such as the 5 A's for tobacco use.[14] Most positive screens for SDOH require a referral out of the obstetrics-gynecology practice to community programs or a case manager/social worker for intervention or support. It is suggested that, when screening for SDOH, one must realize that the screening is not to direct an immediate treatment or intervention. Instead, screening for SDOH is a practice to identify patients that might benefit with referrals to community organizations to address their recurrent social need.[9] Unique aspect of using these questionnaires is that they are effectively cost neutral for the patient, can be implemented universally (not just in pregnancy), and have flexibility as to how they are incorporated into a practice.

IMPLEMENTING A SCREENING PROGRAM WITHIN A CLINICAL SETTING

Although there are several validated screening tools for use in pregnancy, the initial incorporation of such a tool is complicated and time consuming. Experts recommend the following steps.[15,16]

Step 1: Choose the Questionnaire to Be Used

It is best to identify an SDOH that seems to be common in your practice and to choose a questionnaire addressing that issue. The benefits of a high yield from the tool will encourage more buy-in for the process from staff and patients, thus maintaining enthusiasm for continuing use. Start small by choosing one that is short and easy to score.[15,16] Many practices find that pregnancy-related depression, substance use, alcohol misuse, or tobacco/nicotine use may be a good first step for a screening initiation. There are specific tools endorsed by American College of Obstetricians and Gynecologists (ACOG) and other professional groups (see **Box 2** for examples). For clinical practices using an electronic medical record system, there may be an acknowledged tool already embedded within the system.

Step 2: Determine Workflow

Workflow issues must be addressed, such as the following:

- Who will complete the screening? (Patient before being seen? Front desk staff? Medical assistant while "rooming" patient? Provider?)
- When will screening be done? (At every visit? Only at initial prenatal visit? Every trimester?)
- Who will score the screening tool and enter results into the medical record?
- How is the provider alerted to a positive screen?
- Who informs the patient of the results?
- What is the process for treatment or referral for a positive screen?
- How is the positive screen documented to allow the provider to follow up at subsequent visits while still providing confidentiality?

Step 3: Use an Established Work Group

Establish a work group that does the following:

- Represents each of the groups that will participate in the process, including selection of the screening survey to be used
- Develops the workflow plan within the clinic
- Quickly addresses any sudden difficulty or problem with the work plan
- Tracks results ensuring that screening is done consistently and that all positive screens are identified to provider
- Verifies that the management plan (treatment or referral) is happening and is effective
- Keeps clinical staff engaged, informed, and participating
- Identifies the referral resources within the health care system and community. Ensures that the list is current with frequent verifications of contact information. This listing can include community programs, care coordinators, social workers, food banks, housing authority, safe houses and so forth, and specialists within health care.

ROLE OF PRENATAL SCREENING FOR SOCIAL DETERMINANTS OF HEALTH

Currently, routine screening during prenatal care is offered for issues with a prevalence rate that is much lower than many of the SDOH. The following screening activities are encouraged for pregnant patients. Each is listed with the prevalence of a positive screen: cystic fibrosis less than 1%, preeclampsia less than 5%, and anemia 15%. Yet illicit substance use has a prevalence of 15% and is not part of routine screening.[17]

Box 2

Common screening tools for prenatal patients (number of questions)

Mental health focus
- Edinburgh postnatal depression screen (10)* https://perinatology.com/calculators/Edinburgh%20Depression%20Scale.htm

Substance use: alcohol and/or illicit substances
- 5Ps (5)*
  https://ilpqc.org/wp-content/docs/toolkits/MNO-OB/5Ps-Screening-Tool-and-Follow-Up-Questions.pdf
- 4Ps (5)*
  https://oasas.ny.gov/system/files/documents/2019/09/4Ps.pdf
- CRAFFT (5–17 tiered approach)*
  https://crafft.org/
- AUDIT (10)
  https://auditscreen.org/check-your-drinking/
- ASSIST (8)
  https://apps.who.int/iris/bitstream/handle/10665/44320/9789241599382_eng.pdf;
  jsessionid=8F228E2A81357E8E0E460114543FCF00?sequence=1
- DAST (4)
  https://gwep.usc.edu/wp-content/uploads/2019/11/DAST-10-drug-abuse-screening-test.pdf
- T-ACE (4)
  https://www.healthsadvisor.com/en/guest/qs/test-t-ace-de-dependance-a-l-alcool/
- TAPS (4)
  https://nida.nih.gov/taps2/
- CAGE (4)
  https://pedagogyeducation.com/Resources/Correctional-Nursing/CAGE-AID-Substance-Abuse-Screening-Tool
- MAST (10)
  https://preventionforme.org/wp-content/uploads/2017/09/BriefMAST.pdf
- TWEAK (5)
  http://mqic.org/pdf/TWEAK.pdf
- SURP-P (2)
  https://ilpqc.org/wp-content/docs/toolkits/MNO-OB/Substance-Use-Risk-Profile-Pregnancy-Scale.pdf

Tobacco focus
- 5As for (5)*
  https://www.ahrq.gov/prevention/guidelines/tobacco/5steps.html#:~:text=Successful%20intervention%20begins%20with%20identifying,every%20patient%20at%20every%20visit.

Intimate partner violence
- WAST or WAST short (8 or 4)
  http://womanabuse.webcanvas.ca/documents/wast.pdf

Screen for multiple issues
- Patient Health Questionnaire–9 (9)*
  https://www.apa.org/depression-guideline/patient-health-questionnaire.pdf
- PRAPARE for general social determinants of health (21)
  https://prapare.org/wp-content/uploads/2023/01/PRAPARE-English.pdf

This list is not exhaustive, and screens are not listed in any particular order. Asterisk refers to tools that are specifically mentioned in ACOG documents. Each test has the link where the tool is available. All were accessed as of February 6, 2023.

This is not acceptable if we are to decrease maternal and infant morbidity. This failure is a deficit that must be addressed.

In the in-depth reviews of maternal deaths in which substance use disorder, mental health problems, or risky behaviors caused or contributed significantly to a death, the state maternal mortality review committees (MMRC) find that often there is no indication that the provider was aware of the problem. It is unclear if screening was not done or that the provider was not informed of a positive screen. The question being asked by the MMRCs is: If the provider knew of the problems and mobilized the health care system or community resources to address them, could the woman's death have been prevented? The data from MMRIA indicate that 80% of pregnancy-related maternal deaths are deemed preventable by state MMRCs.[2] In this context "preventable" means that some reasonable change by the patient, community, provider, facility, and/or health care system might have prevented the death. For an intervention to occur, the contributing factors need to be recognized or identified.

This issue of *Obstetric and Gynecologic Clinics of North America* contains articles on SDOH with a focus on substance use disorders, mental health, and living in rural/low resourced communities with suggestions on approaches to treatment. Unless providers know about these issues, they cannot be addressed. In some patients, SDOH are evident, with track marks from intravenous drug use, acting out or prior diagnosis of a psychiatric condition, strong smell of tobacco on the patient, or clothing and hygiene that imply insecure housing. But many women experiencing such challenges do not volunteer information unless asked. This is why it is critical to start or expand current screening for these conditions with all pregnant women. Without recognizing the problem, health care providers cannot help their patients with support or treatment within the practice and/or a facilitated referral to another community or health care group to provide treatments.

Review of Some Screening Instruments for Common Social Determinants of Health in Pregnancy

There are numerous screening tools available (see **Box 2**). Many of the tools regarding tobacco, alcohol, and illicit substances are validated in the pregnant population. These structured screening tools ask difficult questions in a more socially accepted way that does not stigmatize the activity in a way that might promote false reporting or not returning for further care. Each medical practice needs to determine which is best for them. Do they want a tool that is issue-specific, such as depression in pregnancy, or a tool that is more inclusive of all substance use? Perhaps a tool that is very short? One that is proven useful for screening in all populations and not just those who are pregnant? These should be considerations when adopting a screening tool.

Depression and Mental Health Focused

The risk of depression, especially postpartum, has been commonly acknowledged for decades. Media coverage of tragic outcomes and celebrities sharing their own personal stories of postpartum depression have increased general awareness. There are several screening tools that are validated for pregnancy but two are the most practical for a busy obstetric clinic: the Edinburgh Postnatal Depression Scale, with 10 questions; and the Patient Health Questionnaire-9, with nine questions.[18] They need less than 5 minutes to administer and score, with acceptable sensitivity/specificity.

The Edinburgh Postnatal Depression Scale is most often used in research and clinical practice. It has been translated into more than 50 languages. It is noted to be "health literacy appropriate." It focuses only on depression.[18]

The Patient Health Questionnaire-9 includes questions about constitutional symptoms of depression and anxiety and may identify patients with other mental health concerns.[18]

Substance Use/Misuse Including Alcohol and Illicit Substances Focused

The ACOG has numerous statements regarding the dangers of illicit substances and/or alcohol use during pregnancy. These statements include recommendations regarding screening and management.[19] Many screening tools that were initially focused on alcohol misuse have since been found to be effective screens for illicit substance use. Some of these are listed in **Box 2**. A recent study compared five self-reporting screening instruments for substance use/misuse in pregnancy with findings that none showed high sensitivity or specificity.[17] Another study found that the 4P and SURP-P were accurate, although patients showed a preference for the 4P tool.[20,21] Each survey had strengths and limitations. The choice of a screening tool for a practice needs to take into consideration the patient population to be screened and setting where the screening will be done.[17]

Tobacco/Nicotine Focused

Use of tobacco or nicotine in pregnancy is well researched. Tobacco is an established risk factor for adverse pregnancy outcomes and a health issue for mother and infant later in life. ACOG produced several statements regarding tobacco use in pregnancy along with a tool kit to screen for and counsel women who smoked during pregnancy and postpartum.[14] It seems that these efforts along with other federal initiatives are working. A recent brief from the National Center for Health Statistics has noted a decline in tobacco use of 36% in 5 years.[22] This decline was evident across all age groups, racial/ethnic groups, and state of residency, but especially in younger women.[22] Still there are populations that continue to have a high rate of nicotine use (either smoking or vaping) during pregnancy and would benefit from ongoing screening.

Alcohol Focused

A recent study noted that approximately 20% of pregnant women had no screening or assessment for alcohol use.[23] The percentage of nonscreening was greater in populations with a higher prevalence of adverse SDOH. Although the study notes limitations regarding lack of detailed data, the lack of screening for alcohol abuse/misuse is concerning. Alcohol is a proven teratogen and all pregnant women (and ideally all women) should be screened for alcohol abuse/misuse.[23,24]

There are numerous screening tests for alcohol use (see **Box 2**). Several reviews indicate that TACE or 5Ps may be better in pregnant populations. A practice may want to make screening universal for all women and not focus on pregnant patients. In that case a different tool may be a better choice.

Intimate Partner Violence Focused

IPV is a cycle of abuse that may be broken through screening with support and referral for those with a positive screen. Commonly, there are state laws regarding whether a finding of IPV must be reported to police or similar law enforcing agency. This screening should be conducted in a safe area with only the patient. A general approach with some typical questions might be:

- Has your partner ever hit, choked, or physically hurt you?
- Has your current partner ever threatened you or made you feel afraid?
- Does your partner control who you talk to or where you go?
- Do you feel unsafe at home?

These can be asked verbally during rooming the patient or as part of the intake history completed by the patient or medical assistant. In the setting of a positive screen the provider should assess the immediate safety of the patient and any children.[25] Providing information about a local safe house or having an exit plan is important. Some practices have found it useful to have a poster in the women's restroom with "tear-offs" including the telephone numbers for local shelters.

A recent publication noted that the WAST-Short tool was found to be useful to screen for IPV during pregnancy and performed better than Abuse Assessment Screen and World Health Organization IPV questionnaire (see **Box 2**).[26]

More Global Screen for Multiple Social Determinants of Health

Many of the screening tools designed to cover most of the major determinants of health are long and cumbersome. An example is one created by the Center for Medicare and Medicaid Innovations. Although comprehensive and detailed it consists of 26 specific questions.[27] The Centers for Medicare and Medicaid Services recognizes that its length may be problematic and is currently conducting a study to see if the tool can be pared down to 10 questions or less for initial screening and still maintain acceptable sensitivity and specificity. The PRAPARE instrument is also comprehensive thus making it difficult to incorporate into a busy office practice. Studies are under way to see if this tool can be reduced in length.[28]

SUMMARY

Data from the CDC and individual research activities have clearly demonstrated that SDOH have a significant influence on poor pregnancy outcomes. It is necessary for providers to acknowledge the impact of these factors for the patient and address them by support within the clinic setting or referral to outside community resources. Many of these issues are not something that most patients will volunteer. This is an ideal situation in which screening of an asymptomatic pregnant patient may allow an intervention that can positively impact the pregnancy. The process of introducing such screening is complicated but worth the effort. The key is to start slowly with screening for one issue, and as that is established, add additional screening tools.

CLINICS CARE POINTS

- Screening tests during prenatal care need to expand beyond those accomplished with laboratory tests or imaging to include screening for SDOH, such as depression, substance use, stable housing and food, IPV, transportation, and so forth, if obstetrics-gynecology practices are to impact increasing maternal mortality rates.

- Choose issues that are most prevalent and problematic for your patients and practice. Then identify a tool that screens for that concern.

- Once a tool is selected the clinic staff must determine workflow: Who does the screening with the patient and when it occurs within the clinic visit? Is the screening done at every visit or on every patient at certain times during their prenatal care?

- Develop a protocol as to who notifies who with a positive screen and how to record it so it will be tracked/addressed at future visits during the pregnancy.

- Determine the level of management: support only, active intervention at the clinic level, or facilitated referral to another health care facility or community facility.

- Meet regularly with the staff to refine the system and determine readiness to add another screening tool. For example, the initial screen may focus on depression and now the staff wants to incorporate another on substance use disorders.

DISCLOSURE

The author has no financial conflict of interest.

REFERENCES

1. Pregnancy Mortality Surveillance Committee. Trends in Pregnancy-related deaths. CDC. Available at: www.cdc.gov/reproductivehealth/maternal-mortality/pregnancy-mortality-surveillance-system.htm#trends. Accessed on February 6, 2023.
2. Trost S, Beauregard J, Chandra G, et al. Pregnancy – related deaths: data from maternal mortality review committees in 36 states 201-2019. Available at: cdc.gov/reproductivehealth/maternal-mortality/erase-mm/data-mmrc.html. Accessed on February 6, 2023.
3. Merkt PT, Kramer MR, Goodman DA, et al. Urban-rural difference in pregnancy-related deaths, United States 2011-2016. Am J Obstet Gyncol 2021;225:183e 6.
4. Cross SH, Califf RM, Warraich HJ. Rural-urban disparities in mortality in the US from 199-2019. JAMA 2021;325:2312–4.
5. Society for Maternal-Fetal Medicine (SMFM), Greenberg MB, Gandhi M, et al. Society for Maternal-Fetal Medicine Consult Series #62: Best practices in equitable care delivery – addressing systemic racism and other social determinants of health as causes of obstetric disparities. Am J Obstet Gynecol 2022;227:B44–59.
6. Joint Commission, Division of Healthcare Improvement. Eliminating racial and ethnic disparities causing mortality and morbidity in pregnant and postpartum patients. Sentinel Event Alert 2023;66.
7. Howard JT, Sparks CS, Santos-Lozada AR, et al. Trends in mortality among pregnant and recently pregnant women in the United States 2015-2019. JAMA 2021; 326:1631–3.
8. ACOG Committee on Health Care for Underserved Women. Importance of social determinants of health and cultural awareness in the delivery of reproductive health care. ACOG Comm Opin 729. Obstet Gyn 2018;131:43.
9. Krist AH, Davidson KW, and Ngo-Metzger Q. What evidence do we need before recommending routine screening for social determinants of health? Available at: www.aafp.org/afp. Accessed February 6, 2023.
10. Davidson KW, Krist AH, Tseng CW, et al. Incorporation of social risk in US Preventive Services Task Force recommendations and identification of key challenges for primary care. JAMA 2021;326:1410–5.
11. Ruf M and Morgan O. Difference between screening and diagnostic tests and case finding. Available at: https://www.healthknowledge.org.uk/public-health-textbook/disease-causation-diagnostic/2c-diagnosis-screening/screening-diagnostic-case-finding. Accessed February 6, 2023.
12. Eder M, Henninger M, Durbin S, et al. Screening and interventions for social risk factors: Technical Brief to Support the US Preventive Service Task Force. JAMA 2021;326:1416–28.
13. Garg A, Boynton-Jarrett R, Dworkin PH. Avoiding the unintended consequences of screening for social determinants of health. JAMA 2016;316:813–4.
14. Committee on Obstetric Practice. ACOG Committee Opinion 807. Tobacco and nicotine cessation during pregnancy. Obstet Gynec 2020;135:e221.
15. Blecher H, Lyon C, Mims L. The feasibility of screening for social determinants of health: 7 lessons learned. Fam Pract Manag 2019;26:13–9.
16. O'Gurek DT, Henke C. Practical approach to screening for social determinants. Fam Pract Manag 2018;25:7–12.

17. Ondersma SJ, Chang G, Blake-Lamb T, et al. Accuracy of five self-report screening instruments for substance use in pregnancy. Addiction 2019;114: 1683–93.
18. ACOG Committee on Obstetric Practice. ACOG Committee Opinion 757 Screening on perinatal depression. Obstet Gynec 2018;132:208–11.
19. Committee on Obstetric Practice and the American Society of Addiction Medicine. ACOG Committee Opinion #711. Opioid use and opioid use disorder in pregnancy. ACOG Obstet Gynec 2017;130:e81–94.
20. Coleman-Cowger VH, Oga EA, Peters EN, et al. Accuracy of three screening tools for prenatal substance use. Obstet Gynec 2019;133:952–61.
21. Trocin KE, Oga EA, Mulatya C, et al. Patient perceptions of three substance use screening tools for use during pregnancy. Matern Child Health J 2022;26:1488–95.
22. Martin J, Osterman MJK, Drixcoll AK. Declines in cigarette smoking during pregnancy in the United States 2016-2021. NCHS Data Brief 2023;448:1-8 Available at: https://www.cdc.gov/nchs/data/databriefs/db458.pdf. Accessed February 6, 2023.
23. Luong J, Board A, Cosdin L, et al. Alcohol use, screening and brief intervention among pregnant persons – 24 US jurisdictions 2017-2019. MMWR (Morb Mortal Wkly Rep) 2023;72(3):55–62.
24. ACOG Committee on Health Care for Underserved Women. At-risk drinking and alcohol dependence: obstetric and gynecologic implications - Committee Opinion 496. Obstet Gynecol 2011;118:382–8.
25. ACOG Committee on Health Care for Underserved Women. Intimate partner violence Committee Opinion number 518. Obstet Gynecol 2012;119:412–7.
26. Zapata-Calvente AL, Megias JL, Velasco C, et al. Screening for intimate partner violence during pregnancy: a test accuracy study. Eur J Publ Health 2022;32: 429–35.
27. Center for Medicare and Medicaid Innovations. The accountable health communities health-related social needs screening tool. Available at: https://innovation.cms.gov/files/worksheets/ahcm-screeningtool.pdf. Accessed February 6, 2023.
28. Prapare Partnership. Protocols for responding to and assessing patient's assets, risks and experiences screening tool. Available at: https://prapare.org/the-prapare-screening-tool/. Accessed February 6, 2023.

Health Advocacy for Undocumented Immigrant Pregnant Patients

Reshma Khan, MD[a],*, William Rayburn, MD, MBA[b]

KEYWORDS

- Advocacy • Outpatient obstetrics care • Prenatal care • Postpartum • Underserved
- Undocumented immigrants

KEY POINTS

- Undocumented immigrant women who are pregnant should receive prenatal care tailored to their specific needs, with an emphasis on basic needs (eg, housing, safety, food, transportation to appointment).
- Financial, cultural, and language barriers can impede undocumented immigrants from receiving adequate or optimal prenatal care.
- Adverse maternal and fetal outcomes may be more common but have not been well-quantified and cannot be compared with outcomes if care had been provided in their country of origin.
- Prenatal and postpartum planning frequently involves members of an interdisciplinary team to advocate for the basic needs of the mother and baby.
- These patients provide an excellent source for understanding social determinants of health for trainees in pregnancy care.

INTRODUCTION

A comprehensive outpatient obstetrics program involves a coordinated approach to medical care and psychosocial support that ideally begins before conception and extends well beyond delivery. Three main components of prenatal care include risk assessment, health promotion and education, and therapeutic intervention when necessary.[1] Family-centered care should be integrated into prenatal and postpartum care.[2] Patients and preferably couples should be encouraged to work with their caregivers in developing support systems, education, and a birthing plan, and in making well-informed decisions about pregnancy, labor, delivery, and the postpartum period.

[a] Shifa Free Clinic, 668 Marina Drive, Unit 4A, Charleston, SC 29492, USA; [b] Department of Obstetrics and Gynecology, Medical University of South Carolina, 1721 Atlantic Avenue, Sullivan's Island, SC 294482, USA
* Corresponding author. 171 Ashley Avenue, Charleston, SC 29425.
E-mail address: rkhan@icnarelief.org

Obstet Gynecol Clin N Am 50 (2023) 639–652
https://doi.org/10.1016/j.ogc.2023.03.012
0889-8545/23/© 2023 Elsevier Inc. All rights reserved.

obgyn.theclinics.com

Women who enter the United States without proper documents and are either pregnant or become pregnant often have different languages, educational, and cultural backgrounds. Nearly 6% of citizen babies born in the United States have at least one undocumented parent. Undocumented immigrants are ineligible for most public health insurance. Prenatal care is a recommended health service that improves birth outcomes. Certain states, including both traditionally "blue" and "red" states, have opted to provide publicly funded coverage of prenatal services for people who are otherwise ineligible owing to immigration status.[3]

There may be areas where policy makers with different political orientations can converge on health policies affecting access to care for undocumented immigrants. Examples exist about how courts and legislatures in certain states have approached the question of publicly funded prenatal care for undocumented immigrants.[3] Advocating for their health brings gratification and an awareness of medical and social challenges. Generally, conditions in their disadvantaged background can lead to a higher-risk pregnancy that prohibit many clinics to offer specialized care.

In this article, the authors highlight what has been reported in the obstetric literature and report examples of a community-funded clinic designed to aid undocumented immigrant pregnant women.

INITIAL ASSESSMENT

The major goal of prenatal care is to help ensure the eventual birth of a healthy newborn while minimizing maternal risk. Respect for each mother-to-be is critical regardless of her circumstances or background. Cultivation of trust and rapport between the obstetric clinician and patient requires flexibility in providing appointments, services, and treatment approaches. Attention to basic survival can be a greater challenge in addressing a patient and her family's needs, so her health care may not be an immediate priority.

Ideally, all pregnant women should have access in their community to available and regularly scheduled outpatient care, beginning in early pregnancy and continuing into the postpartum period. Major barriers to prenatal care can be site-related, such as the distance to the clinic, lack of transportation, and long wait times for appointments. Socioeconomic constraints and a lack of insurance coverage contribute to poor compliance with visits and therapy recommendations. Health care demands compete with needs for food, clothing, and shelter. Other significant limitations are a lack of knowledge about where or how to acquire prenatal care and fears about how undocumented immigration will interfere with perceptions and provision of care. For example, women with undocumented immigrant status may fear either being reported to the authorities or having their children taken away.

At most clinics where there are immigrants, there is often a need for interpreter services. The Executive Order 13166 by the President of the United States has mandated access to a medical interpreter for all patients seeking care at any clinic that receives federal funding. Not receiving federal funding, most free clinics use untrained family members or friends to interpret, with about half of the clinics admitting that the ad hoc interpreter is typically a child. Bilingual staff members or volunteers who interpret are often inconsistently available, and only a small proportion of these individuals receive adequate health training. When a trained interpreter is not used, there may be more adverse events, longer hospital stays, higher morbidity, and higher health care costs.

Regardless of their background, women who receive early and regular prenatal care are more likely to have healthier infants. Therefore, a standard clinical performance measure is the percentage of pregnant patients who initiate their prenatal care in the first trimester.[4] In the United States, approximately 575 of federally funded community health centers met the Health People 2020 baseline (78% of patients initiating prenatal care in the first trimester). The World Health Organization estimated that 60% of pregnant people worldwide initiated prenatal care before 12 weeks. Less than 50% of pregnant people in resource-limited regions received early prenatal care.

An initial assessment often requires more than one clinic visit. Several components of the following are involved: confirmation of pregnancy, accurate estimation of gestational age, identification of risks associated with maternal or fetal morbidity and mortality, anticipation of problems and intervention to minimize morbidity, and health promotion with shared decision making.[4] This plan of care should take into consideration the medical, nutritional, psychosocial, and educational needs of the patient and her family. Plans should be periodically reevaluated and revised in accordance with the progress of the pregnancy.

Accurate dating is crucial for managing any pregnancy, especially with monitoring fetal growth and timing the delivery. Sonographic assessment of the estimated date of delivery is standard for confirming or revising gestational dating or establishing dating in clinics without last menstrual period (LMP) information in all pregnancies. Although not routinely recommended in the first trimester, transvaginal ultrasound examination is particularly important when menses are irregular, the LMP is unknown or uncertain, contraception has failed, or uterine size is discordant with menstrual dates. Scanning well before 20 weeks provides a better estimation of gestational age than menstrual dates alone, resulting in significant reductions in postdate pregnancy, more appropriate prescribing of medications for suspected preterm labor, and improved scheduling of inductions of labor or planned cesarean birth.

For a woman with an undocumented immigrant status, the initial prenatal visit may be the only opportunity to provide care before delivery. Therefore, it is important to assess what information is critical and to prioritize active problems accordingly.[5] This information should be relevant to the patient's circumstances and living situation and, if possible, addressed in small increments. A complete physical examination is performed, with attention to nutritional status, dental health, and visual acuity, as these needs may be neglected. Screening for food insecurity (being without reliable access to enough affordable, nutritious food) is particularly important. Routine prenatal laboratory tests are obtained, as well as any additional testing based on patient-specific risk factors.

A "migrant" refers to a person who moves away from their place of residence, temporarily or perhaps for a longer period. The Centers for Disease Control and Prevention has published guidelines for screening recommended for refugees arriving in the United States.[5] Assessments for completion of primary immunizations and immunity to vaccine-preventable diseases are strongly encouraged, even though immunization records are often unavailable.

Many undocumented immigrants come from countries where the prevalence of tuberculosis, hepatitis B, and hepatitis C are more common.[5] Screening for sexually transmitted disease includes a thorough medical history, physical examination, and prenatal laboratory testing. Screening for hepatitis C, tuberculosis, and illicit drugs is another important consideration, in addition to routine screening for chlamydia, gonorrhea, genital herpes/genital warts, trichomoniasis, syphilis, hepatitis B, and HIV.[5,6] Challenges related to surveillance, testing, and management strategies for COVID-19 in this population would apply to other viral infections in a setting where quarantines are usually not possible.

ONGOING PRENATAL CARE

The typical intervals for prenatal visits for nulliparous patients are every 4 weeks until 28 weeks of gestation, every 2 weeks from 28 to 36 weeks, and then weekly until delivery.[2] The authors assume that these intervals also apply to undocumented immigrants. Technology has advanced to connect more easily with patients having medical and psychosocial needs, yet individuals experiencing undocumented immigrant status much like other socioeconomically challenged groups may not have such access to telemedicine platforms.

Periodic assessments and procedures should be performed according to gestational ages listed in **Table 1**.[7] Screening and diagnostic testing performed during the second and third trimesters are reviewed in detail elsewhere.[2,7] Ongoing care should be provided without bias or prejudice and with empathy and effort to establish rapport so that a trusting relationship can be developed. Treatment regimens should be simplified whenever possible, and more cost-effective options should be offered, when available. Treatment should not be withheld because of assumptions about a lack of compliance.

All pregnant patients should be offered prenatal genetic screening or have the option of invasive genetic testing, as recommended American College of Obstetricians and Gynecologists (ACOG) guidelines.[2] Despite language and comprehension barriers, discussions about routine testing for genetic abnormalities and carrier screening and early screening for congenital anomalies require the patient's and family's general understandings about what is and is not being screened. Interpretation of screen-positive results, follow-up invasive or noninvasive testing, pregnancy termination options, and any additional costs are important considerations for open discussions. Ideally, a trained interpreter should be used for these conversations, and a community health worker (CHW) or doula might be able to develop the skills to do this for referrals in the system or perhaps for training about general counseling and prescreening.

Table 1
Periodic assessments and procedures by gestational period

Gestational Period	Assessment and Procedure
15–18 wk	• Screen for neural tube defects with maternal serum alpha fetoprotein (MSAFP) • Screen for trisomy 21 and other genetic disorders
18–22 wk	• Ultrasound for fetal anatomic anomalies, short cervix ($\leq$2.5 cm), confirm dating
24–28 wk	• Screen for gestational diabetes • Screen for red blood cell antibodies and administer anti-D immune globulin to D-negative patients • Screen for anemia (hemoglobin <10.5 g/dL)
28–36 wk	• Screen for sexually transmitted infections (HIV, syphilis, chlamydia, gonorrhea) if increased risk • Assess for fetal growth restriction if the fundal height appears to be lagging • Consider antenatal fetal surveillance along with fetal movement charting if an indication is identified
36–41 wk	• Offer external cephalic version if noncephalic >36 weeks 0 days • Obtain group B beta-hemolytic streptococcus culture • Ultrasound screen for accelerated fetal growth if suspect macrosomia
Postpartum	• Checklist for those with uncomplicated or complicated patients • Assess physical and mental well-being, referral as necessary, discuss future health risks

Prenatal care often requires referrals for other available resources and social support. It is helpful to be flexible about scheduling appointments. Many women do not have a reliable phone number; thus, part of the prenatal intake should include discussing alternate ways of reaching the patient. Pregnant patients with medical comorbidities benefit from multidisciplinary care by a team that includes their obstetric provider and appropriate medical or surgical subspecialists and specialists in genetics, anesthesia, and pediatrics. These discussions are often limited by the availability of teams and language barriers.

Analyses in low-risk populations have shown that those who received usual care versus closer monitoring (ie, repeated fetal ultrasounds, antepartum fetal surveillance) do not encounter significantly lower rates of preterm birth, very preterm birth, or stillbirth. Most interventions were unable to demonstrate a clear effect in reducing stillbirth or perinatal death. At institutions where group prenatal care is available, this option can be offered to further develop social supports for the patients and her growing families. Furthermore, the authors were unable to find any literature about these components of prenatal care in an undocumented immigrant pregnancy population. Certain principles about prenatal care for women experiencing homelessness also apply to undocumented immigrants.[8,9]

Costs of care and necessities warrants discussions with the patient. Appropriate and improper use of emergency departments should be discussed with the patient. Establishing the specific hospital for eventual delivery early in gestation will allow entry into obstetric triage areas for care of more immediate needs. During prenatal care, all women need to be instructed on labor and delivery, postpartum issues, care and breastfeeding of the newborn, and parenting. This may be even more important for the immigrants, who may have less access to family for support and be unfamiliar with the US health care system. Continued access to social workers is valuable, along with ongoing assessments of basic needs, such as proper food, clothing, safety, and shelter.

Because undocumented immigrants may not seek care until later in gestation, the following activities need more immediate attention regardless of gestational age: assessment of gestational age, routine laboratory tests, substance use, and rapid HIV testing. Retesting for sexually transmitted infections is recommended in the third trimester (28–36 weeks) and at delivery in women at increased risk.[6]

PREPARING FOR POSTPARTUM VISITS

The postpartum period or "fourth trimester" can be a challenging time for any patient, both physically and emotionally, as they recover from childbirth and adjust to the life with a newborn. Particularly for undocumented immigrants, it is best to prepare for life after delivery during the prenatal period. What was once a single office visit at 6 weeks after delivery is now being reimagined as a continuum of care that transitions patients from pregnancy to lifelong health optimization.

Women with limited resources, those on Medicaid, and those from rural communities who have challenges with access are less likely to seek postpartum care. A postpartum follow-up visit sooner rather than later permits a more objective means of assessing adjustment to physiologic changes and parenting adjustment. A lack of postpartum follow-up can contribute to maternal and infant mortality and early breast-feeding discontinuation.

The pregnant patient can be informed that the initial postpartum visit is an excellent time to reflect on recurrence risks of any pregnancy complications, such as morbid obesity, preeclampsia, prematurity, low birth weight, gestational diabetes, operative delivery, excessive hemorrhage, or prolonged hospital stay.[10] Although the initial visit between 2 to 6 weeks after delivery should address recovery from childbirth, continuation of lactation, contraception options, and vaccinations, it is an opportunity to evaluate mental health. Another, more comprehensive visit within 12 weeks postpartum can provide an opportunity for mental health assessment and reproductive life planning.[2,11]

Like during the prenatal period, counseling about nutrition and supplementation, exercise, hazardous behaviors, and the planning, spacing, and timing of any subsequent pregnancy is essential for overall health. Contraception options include long-acting reversible contraceptive methods. Any patient can also be informed that a follow-up is encouraged at 12 months for ongoing care, particularly for those women at risk of medical conditions or who experienced a pregnancy complication or a near-miss pregnancy-related morbidity that could impact long-term health.

SHIFA FREE CLINIC: A MODEL FOR PRENATAL CARE OF UNDOCUMENTED IMMIGRANTS
Overview

Located in Charleston, South Carolina, the Shifa Free Clinic ("the Clinic") was founded in January 2011 by a board-certified obstetrician-gynecologist, Reshma Khan, MD. The Clinic was originally for women and then became a primary care clinic. Obstetrics care was provided once the Clinic became established. The Clinic is a place where patients are treated with respect, dignity, and compassion in a culturally sensitive and courteous manner to enable strong and trusting relationships with providers and staff members.

The Clinic is called a free clinic because all services and many of the laboratory tests and medications are available at no charge to the patients. Any costs to patients (such as from radiologists) are mentioned to them beforehand, and an attempt at obtaining outside funding is undertaken if possible. Efforts are made to provide high-quality medical care to all uninsured persons and support efforts to reduce food insecurity in the community.

The Clinic adheres to principles by the ACOG that support the health and well-being of all who seek obstetric care and advocates to secure quality health care for all, without regard to documented or undocumented immigration status.[12] The Clinic's model of care is based on following principles.

- Patient centered: Health care decisions incorporate patients' wants, needs, and preferences, Patients receive the education and support they need to make decisions and participate in their own care. Patients are often given the opportunity to choose a provider, although this is not common in obstetrics.
- Comprehensive: The care team provides comprehensive care, including acute care, chronic care, and preventive services.
- Integrated and coordinated care: The Clinic take steps to ensure that patients receive the care and services they need, in a culturally and linguistically appropriate manner.
- Focus on quality and safety: The Clinic uses the quality improvement process and evidence-based medicine to continually improve patient outcomes.
- Access: The practices commit to enhancing patients' access to care using electronic medical records (EMR) providing patient access to email practice and having patient portal access. The patients are provided proper education and support to actively participate in their care. The Clinic is unique, having no by ZIP code restriction and multispecialty services under one roof.

At the Clinic, female and male patients have access to comprehensive care, including acute, chronic primary care, and preventative services in various specialties. Women are more likely to attend the Clinic, especially those of reproductive age. In addition, the ability to provide no-cost laboratory tests and imaging services helps in improved patient compliance and treatment. The on-site dispensary carries a limited variety of much-needed medications free of charge, completing the circle of comprehensive care.

Clinic Setup, Staffing, and Food Pantry

The Clinic consists of a waiting room, examining rooms, provider workstation, secured pharmacy dispensary, director and manager offices, corridor for 4 staff members, and large pantry for unrefrigerated and refrigerated/frozen food. Examining rooms include provisions for a portable electronic fetal heart rate monitoring, portable real-time ultrasound machine, LEEP machine and colposcope. The Clinic's EMR and data software for easy reporting are essential tools for complete and comprehensive care. The EMR at the clinic is not the same used by the hospital system; however, providers at the hospital can log into the clinic EMR, which makes it easier for communication and handoffs. There is no phlebotomy station, and the postgraduate health care students perform all blood gathering, urine reagent strips examinations, and vaginal secretion microscopic examinations. Although there are provisions for telehealth, its use in the Clinic is used much less after the COVID pandemic.

The Clinic aims to involve historically disadvantaged communities in the leadership and decision-making process by having a diverse staff who can relate to their community. The obstetric providers are informed about results from patient surveys, suggestion boxes for service modifications, and meetings that involve patients in the decision-making process of their care and treatment. Along with a medical director, office manager, and administrative assistants, the Clinic staff includes a patient navigator, food pantry assistants, dispensary and patient care coordinator, and volunteer coordinator. Having several bilingual staff members at the front desk gives patients comfort, reemphasizes attention to needs, and helps with patient satisfaction. There are no allied health professionals, lactation consultants, and obstetric health educators. Their services are provided at no cost at the preferred hospital where patients are expected to deliver.

Being a nonprofit organization, the Clinic is not held to the same standard of having medical interpreters for all patients. An attempt is made for all volunteer interpreters to complete a standardized training program; however, all patients are required to have a family member or friend they can use to interpret for them at each visit. The Clinic is working with the nearby Roper Saint Francis Hospital to establish an interpretation service through Stratus language interpretation. This service provides access to thousands of professional interpreters who are culturally competent and extensively trained. These interpreters can provide their services through either video or phone calls depending on the client's preference.

Food insecurity is a key social determinant of health that adversely impacts racial and ethnic minority groups and lower-income individuals. The Clinic's food pantry has both short- and long-term goals to not only decrease food insecurity in the community but also minimize adverse health outcomes that can result from the lack of access to adequate nutrition. The Clinic targets individuals experiencing food insecurity who often make difficult tradeoffs between food and other basic needs, including health care. Access to healthy foods can sometimes involve long distances between residences and grocery stores. The Clinic's home delivery program helps alleviate this issue through a partnership with Amazon after referral from a regional food bank, critical review every year, and adequacy of funding.

Patients

The target population is indigent and uninsured community members who have difficulty accessing health care options. Approximately 80% of the pregnant patients are Hispanic. The authors acknowledge that many patients face barriers in accessing health care: low socioeconomic status, low health literacy, lack of health insurance, limited English proficiency, lack of transportation, lack of childcare support, lack of work permits, immigration status, and often cultural mistrust of the medical system.

Before being seen for prenatal care, patients often have not attended any primary care clinics, so they may not have received preventive care and immunizations. The consequences of delayed treatment spread everywhere. The uninsured end up in emergency rooms incurring avoidable hospital costs, which are passed on to the hospitals, insured population, and overburdened taxpayers. The Clinic combats these barriers by cultivating a welcoming health care environment for persons of all races, ethnicities, cultures, and genders. Although the Clinic is not conveniently located near a citywide bus stop, personal transportation is often accessible by friends or family members on a restricted basis.

Volunteer Providers and Students

Volunteerism not only helps organizations and the community but also brings joy and happiness to the people being served. The obstetric team includes 2 retired and 2 practicing obstetrician-gynecologists, one maternal-fetal medicine subspecialist, and one CHW. A state law provided immunity from litigation for volunteers. This also applies to sudents whose actions are overseen directly by the practicing clinicians. All patients are informed and must sign a letter of understanding.

Through a grant from University of South Carolina Arnold School of Public Health Center for Community Health Alignment for participation in EACH Mom and Baby collaborative, the Clinic was able to hire a CHW to improve birth outcomes. Perinatal CHWs are professional nonclinical support providers who help pregnant and parenting families to connect with information, resources, and their capacity to improve their social determinants of health (such as housing, transportation, education, insurance, and more). They also bring insight and information from the community back to clinical services for improved understanding and quality improvement. Specialized training that CHWs receive focuses on perinatal health and child developmental milestones to help the prenatal patients. Through these trainings, the CHW is encouraged to advocate and refer for childbirth preparation, lactation, and any other needs that ultimately lead to successful pregnancy and delivery.

The Clinic is a 4- to 5-week rotation site for graduating nurse practitioner (NP) students, doctor of NP students, physician assistant (PA) students, and family medicine residents. Educational opportunities and teaching remain a huge part of the Clinic's identity. The Clinic has contracted through the Medical University of South Carolina (MUSC) Family Practice Residency Program, MUSC PA Program, South University PA Program, Charleston Southern University PA Program, and MUSC NP Program for established student rotations. Each PA and NP program offers financial support for the training of their students. The required onsite hours of all students are counted toward their successful graduation on time.

This partnership provides respectful, empowering, high-quality health care for the underserved while inspiring the next generation of health professionals. This is a great combination of autonomy and teaching. The students feel like they are taking on the primary responsibility for their patients while the attending obstetricians enjoy teaching while signing the charts.

Collaboration with community partners is essential to the success of the Clinic and requires constant justification and searching for support. The Clinic serves as a platform for collaboration with organizations in serving the needs of the community. Shown in **Table 2** are examples of local and national organizations that support the holistic health approach to the Clinic's uninsured and low-income population. Descriptions of each organization's primary contributions are described briefly. In addition, the Clinic has fulfilled standards of care to receive accreditation/certifications from the following organizations.

- State Department of Health Vaccine for Children Program: Passed the Department Health/Environmental Control inspection and became reaccredited for an additional 2 years to continue with the Clinic's Vaccine for Children program.
- State Board of Pharmacy: Obtained valid permit from State Board of Pharmacy for the onsite dispensary.
- South Carolina Free Clinic Association: Obtained level 1 recertification valid every 2 years for demonstrating a commitment to high-quality care and compliance with rigorous standards established by South Carolina Free Clinic Association.
- American Association of Diabetes Education: Obtained accreditation for the authors' Diabetes Self-Management Education program.

In addition, the Clinic is a member in good standing of the following organizations: National Association of Free Clinics, South Carolina Free Clinic Association, and Low Country Food Bank.

Prenatal and Postpartum Care at the Clinic

About 4% of all patients seen at the Clinic are women seeking prenatal care. Nearly 600 pregnant women were seen since 2017 with increasing numbers each year. More than 150 are seen annually since 2021. Nearly all are undocumented immigrants. Few patients transfer care elsewhere unless there is another "free" clinic closer to their home or there is the need to move elsewhere. The Clinic does advertise, but most referrals are by "word of mouth," and only one other clinic in the Charleston, South Carolina area offers free care to a low number of uninsured pregnant patients.

Approximately 85% speak Spanish only. Less than 5% seek prenatal care in the first trimester. Approximately 10% of patients are referred for maternal-fetal medicine consultations, and even fewer (2%–3%) have their prenatal care completely transferred to a high-risk obstetrics service before delivery. The CHW educates the patients during clinic visits about contraceptive methods, prenatal and postpartum care, mental health, nutrition and prenatal supplements, and vaccinations. She advocates and connects patients with other resources, such as WIC, emergency Medicaid, and food services.

Genetic testing is encouraged and available to all. Despite many risk factors associated with social determinants of health among undocumented immigrants, the proportion of pregnancies with fetal structural or genetic abnormalities is very low. Midgestation fetal anatomy scans are performed routinely by a very part-time obstetric sonographer paid by the Clinic, and patients are referred for maternal-fetal medicine evaluation for any suspicions on imaging or genetic testing.

Anemia and obesity are common. Morbid obesity (or a body mass index or 35 or higher) is present in 2% of the population, gestational diabetes in 2%, and gestational hypertension or preeclampsia in less than 6%. Patients with chronicm meical disorders oftern require some form of therapy, and most obstetricians feel comfortable with continuation of the treatment unless multiple medications are necessary. Behavioral and mental health illness is often difficult to assess, although the authors routinely

Table 2
Organizations providing essential services or in-kind donations to the Shifa Free Clinic

Organizations	Services Provided or In-Kind Donations
Access Health, Tri-county Network	Mutual relationship between clinics with referrals of uninsured patients for specialty care
AmeriCares	Provides free medications and medical supplies as ordered
Athena Health	Provides free electronic medical records services
Best Chance Network	Provides breast cancer screening services with mammograms
Choose Well	Provides immediately available long-acting reversible contraception or intrauterine devices
Colon Cancer Prevention Network	Provides free colorectal cancer screening and colonoscopy
Department Health/Environmental Control	Free vaccines, including the flu vaccine for adults and Advisory Committee on Immunization Practices (ACIPP)-approved vaccines for children
Direct Relief USA	Distributes medications at no cost
Each Mom and Baby Collaborative Project	Provides strategies to cocreate solutions to health inequities
Field to Families	Grows and collects fresh local fruits and vegetables
Help Me Grow	Provides support for pregnant women, others with new babies
Junior League of Charleston Diaper Bank	Collects, packages, and distributes diapers
LabCorp	Provides leading-edge laboratory tests and services at no cost
Low Country Food Bank	Provides high-quality food for no cost to eligible families
MAVEN project	Provides volunteer specialists through telehealth technology
Medical University South Carolina (MUSC)	Provides financial assistance, specialized care: surgery referrals, no cost screening mammograms, and low-cost mammograms
Merck	Provides free Gardasil, pneumococcal, shingles vaccines
New Eyes	Provides complementary eye examinations and glasses
Physicians for Human Rights Asylum Network	Offers student-run clinic to document trauma
SANOFI	Provides free TDAP vaccine doses
South Carolina Free Clinic Association and South Carolina Foundation	Assists operational expenses and multiple health services
Tech Assisted Case Management (MUSC)	Provides glucose control management coupled with nurse care
Welvista	Provides access to over 180 medications to treat chronic illness

screen for depression, anxiety, and intimate partner violence at the beginning and later in gestation.

About two-thirds of the Clinic patients delivered previously at their country of origin (primarily Mexico, Central America, South America). The absence of prior pregnancy records limits the obstetricians' abilities to assess vaccinations, prior health conditions, and previous pregnancy outcomes. Extremes in maternal ages are uncommon, with 3% being less than 18-years-old and 14% being 35 years or older.

The Clinic has an excellent working relation and written contract with a nearby community hospital (Roper St. Francis). Although patients may deliver anywhere, they are urged to deliver at the contracted community hospital for cost considerations and improved communication. All patients are given updated hand-written prenatal record cards, and the hospital is provided the Clinic's prenatal electronic record to maximize transfer of information. Weekday appointments for the Clinic are made at the inpatient triage obstetric clinic adjacent to the hospital's Labor and Delivery Unit. This area is the site for consultation with a maternal-fetal medicine specialist, ultrasonographic imaging and fetal surveillance testing, and discussion with a hospitalist about any planned procedure (eg, external version of a breech, induction of labor, repeat cesarean delivery, trial of labor after cesarean). Final solutions to these discussions are at the discretion of the delivering physician and patient.

Approximately three-quarters of the Clinic's patients have accurate gestational dating by compatible menstrual and ultrasound dating. They tend to prefer waiting until their estimated date of delivery before a scheduled induction of labor with an accurately dated pregnancy. Those with only one prior cesarean are encouraged to undergo a trial of labor, although the prior uterine incision direction is unknown and the indication for prior surgery is often unclear. The decision is determined by obstetricians at the delivering hospital. The scheduling of a cesarean (usually repeat) occurs in 5% of the authors' entire population. The overall cesarean delivery rate is 20% to 25%.

All patients are encouraged to call the Clinic and return for at least one postpartum visit. Unfortunately, this occurs in only three-fourths of cases. To ensure that comprehensive needs are consistently met, postpartum visit checklists are used for either uncomplicated postpartum patients or those with medical or obstetric morbidities. The checklists ensure that essential elements of physical and mental well-being are routinely considered, any follow-up or specialty referrals are made, and future health risks are discussed.[11]

A repeat visit is often for long-acting reversible contraception placement, intrauterine device insertion, or quarterly medroxyprogesterone acetate (Depo-Provera) injections, which are provided at no cost and administered by the authors' providers. All infants receive Medicaid insurance coverage and are therefore not seen in the Clinic. Instead, an appointment at a nearby pediatrician's office is arranged at the hospital before discharge of the mother-infant pair.

Examples of Cost Savings

No reimbursement is taken from any patient. To be served at the clinic, all eligible patients must sign applications of proof of income below 250% federal poverty level and be uninsured. The companies, including laboratories, have programs that support populations such as those served at the Clinic.

Despite the at-risk nature of the patient's health backgrounds, additional costs are minimized by avoiding testing and consultation unless necessary and approved by the staff physician and clinic director. Nuanced counseling and referrals outside the Clinic will depend on a patient's demographics and comorbidities. Listed below are actions taken in the Clinic to provide outpatient care for the authors' pregnant patients at the lowest cost.

- The patients understand that they are responsible for transportation and for having a translator, either in person or through two-way cell phone calls.
- Telehealth communication has proven to be possible, although the authors' patients and providers prefer to meet in person.
- All ACOG-recommended prenatal laboratory testing is provided to every patient.
- All genetic testing is offered free of charge. Blood is drawn by the students.
- An ultrasound machine, bought by a donor, is used by volunteer obstetrician-gynecologists during the initial evaluation to confirm fetal viability, rule out twins, and estimate gestational age.
- A detailed fetal anatomic ultrasound is ordered to be performed between 18- and 24-weeks' gestation using the Clinic's ultrasound machine by the volunteer obstetricians and maternal-fetal medicine specialist. Scans are scheduled monthly and performed by an experienced sonographer at an hourly wage.
- An ultrasonogram is repeated for growth assessment in the third trimester only when necessary.[13]
- A donated nonstress test machine is used for biophysical assessments only if risk factors are identified by the Clinic's volunteer obstetrician-gynecologists.[13]
- Patients are encouraged, but not required, to deliver at the contracted hospital, which also provides a no-cost visit to the obstetric triage unit and access to the Clinic's EMR.
- The patient is well informed that any anticipated intrapartum interventions are decided upon by providers at each of the hospitals. The contracted hospital has no charges for patients to be evaluated after 36 weeks 0 days as arranged by the Clinic's staff.
- An induction of labor is offered in well-dated pregnancies at 39 weeks 0 days to 39 weeks 6 days gestation.
- Despite not knowing the direction of the prior uterine incision, a trial of labor is encouraged if there are no absolute maternal or fetal indications for cesarean delivery. Counseling includes a discussion of the risks of cesarean delivery, patient's comorbidities, and patient's preferences and goals if a prior cesarean had been performed.
- The Clinic food pantry provides food as often as monthly to their pregnant patients before and after delivery.

Measuring Effectiveness

Guidelines for spacing of prenatal clinic visits and ordering of prenatal tests comply with guidelines published by the ACOG.[2] Although the effects of prenatal care are difficult to measure, it is widely thought that early care fosters healthier pregnancies. Earlier care enables obstetric providers to identify and treat maternal conditions and behaviors that can adversely affect the initial stages of fetal development, provide medical advice, and assess the risk of a poor pregnancy outcome. Prenatal care may also provide an entry point to the health care system, especially for the Clinic's patients who do not have another source of care. Women who begin prenatal care at midgestation or later or who have no prenatal care receive less preventive care and education and have a higher risk of undetected complications.

Outpatient obstetric care confers some health benefits, although how it does so and the types and magnitude of benefits are complex and multifactorial. Accomplishments of care provided at the Clinic include the following.

- No eligible person has been turned away from initial or continued care.
- The few pregnant patients who leave the Clinic are for relocation reasons.
- There have been no known stillbirths.
- Most patients agree to prenatal genetic carrier and chromosome testing. There has been only one major chromosome aneuploidy uncovered. Positive genetic carrier test results have been performed on the presumed father.
- No patient has requested an induced abortion, although referrals to a nearby Planned Parenthood will be performed without prejudice.
- All patients who reach 36 weeks 0 days gestation are referred to the transition clinic at the contract hospital for orientation to the hospital system, tour of the facilities, and discussions about labor and delivery or any procedures.

SUMMARY

Undocumented immigrant women who are pregnant should receive prenatal care tailored to their specific needs, with an emphasis on basic needs (eg, housing, safety, food, transportation to appointment). Financial, cultural, and language barriers can impede undocumented immigrants from receiving adequate prenatal care. Adverse maternal and fetal outcomes may be more common but have not been well-quantified and cannot be compared with outcomes if care had been provided in their country of origin. Prenatal and postpartum planning frequently involves members of an interdisciplinary team to advocate for the basic needs of the mother and baby. An example of a community-funded clinic is described in minimizing cost and optimizing outcomes to undocumented immigrant pregnant patients. Partnering with health care organizations is described to support the free care to this otherwise underserved population.

CLINICS CARE POINTS

- Undocumented immigrant women who are pregnant should receive prenatal care that is tailored to their specific needs, with an emphasis on basic needs (eg, housing, safety, food, transportation to appointment).

- Financial, cultural, and language barriers can impede undocumented immigrants from receiving adequate prenatal care.

- Adverse maternal and fetal outcomes may be more common but have not been well-quantified and cannot be compared with outcomes if care had been provided in their country of origin.

- An example of a community-funded clinic is described to minimize cost and optimize outcomes of undocumented immigrant pregnant patients.

DISCLOSURE

The authors of this article have no relevant financial interests to disclose. Dr R. K is a paid director of the Shifa Clinic, while Dr Rayburn is a maternal-fetal medicine subspecialist who is a volunteer. This review was not funded.

REFERENCES

1. Rosen MG, Merkatz IR, Hill JG. Caring for our future: a report by the expert panel on the content of prenatal care. Obstet Gynecol 1991;77:782.

2. American Academy of Pediatrics Committee on Fetus and Newborn and American College of Obstetricians and Gynecologists Committee on Obstetric Practice. In: Kilpatrick SJ, Papile L, editors. Guidelines for perinatal care. 8th edition. Elk Grove, IL; Washington, DC: American Academy of Pediatrics; American College of Obstetricians and Gynecologists; 2017.

3. Fabi RE, Saloner B, Taylor H. State policymaking and stated reasons: prenatal care for undocumented immigrants in an era of abortion restriction. Milbank Q 2021;99:693–720.

4. Lockwood C.J. and Magriples U. Prenatal care: initial assessment, 2022, Wolters Kluwer, 1–71. Available at: https://www-uptodate-com.libproxy.unm.edu/contents/prenatal-care-initial-assessment?search=. Accessed August 29, 2022.

5. Walker PF, Barnett ED, Stauffer W. Medical screening of adult immigrants and refugees. Available at: www.uptodate.com=com.libproxy. Accessed September 3, 2022.

6. Workowski KA, Bachmann LH, Chan BA, et al. Sexually transmitted infections treatment guidelines, 2021. MMWR Recomm Rep (Morb Mortal Wkly Rep) 2021;70:1.

7. Lockwood CJ, Magriples U. Prenatal care: second and third trimesters. Wolters Kluwer; 2022. p. 1–31. Accessed October 29, 2022.

8. Cutts DB, Coleman S, Black MM, et al. Homelessness during pregnancy: a unique, time-dependent risk factor of birth outcomes. Matern Child Health J 2015;19:1276.

9. American College of Obstetricians and Gynecologists. Committee on Health Care for Underserved Women. Committee Opinion no. 454. Healthcare for homeless women. Obstet Gynecol 2010;115:396.

10. Brown HL. New Postpartum Visit: Beginning of Lifelong Learning. Obstet Gynecol Cl N Am 2020;47(3).

11. Society for Maternal-Fetal Medicine special statement. Postpartum visit checklists for normal pregnancy and complicated pregnancy. Am J Obstet Gynecol 2022;227:B2–8.

12. American College of Obstetricians and Gynecologists' Committee on Health Care for Underserved Women. Health care for immigrants. Obstet Gynecol 2023;141: 427–33.

13. American College of Obstetricians and Gynecologists' Committee on Obstetric practice, Society for Maternal-Fetal Medicine. Indications for outpatient antenatal fetal surveillance: ACOG Committee Opinion, Number 828. Obstet Gynecol 2021; 137:3177.

Moving?

Make sure your subscription moves with you!

To notify us of your new address, find your **Clinics Account Number** (located on your mailing label above your name), and contact customer service at:

Email: journalscustomerservice-usa@elsevier.com

800-654-2452 (subscribers in the U.S. & Canada)
314-447-8871 (subscribers outside of the U.S. & Canada)

Fax number: 314-447-8029

Elsevier Health Sciences Division
Subscription Customer Service
3251 Riverport Lane
Maryland Heights, MO 63043

*To ensure uninterrupted delivery of your subscription, please notify us at least 4 weeks in advance of move.

ELSEVIER

Printed and bound by CPI Group (UK) Ltd, Croydon, CR0 4YY

08/05/2025

01864724-0004